Leading & Managing Occupational Therapy Services

An Evidence-Based Approach

Leading & Managing Occupational Therapy Services

An Evidence-Based Approach

Brent Braveman, Ph.D., OTR/L, FAOTA
Clinical Associate Professor
Director of Professional Education
Department of Occupational Therapy
University of Illinois at Chicago
Chicago, Illinois

F.A. Davis Company • Philadelphia

F. A. Davis Company
1915 Arch Street
Philadelphia, PA 19103
www.fadavis.com

Copyright © 2006 by F. A. Davis Company

Printed in the United States of America

Last digit indicates print number: 10 9 8 7 6

Acquisitions Editor: Christa Fratantoro
Developmental Editor: Tom Robinson
Design Manager: Carolyn O'Brien

As new scientific information becomes available through basic and clinical research, recommended treatments and drug therapies undergo changes. The author and publisher have done everything possible to make this book accurate, up to date, and in accord with accepted standards at the time of publication. The author, editors, and publisher are not responsible for errors or omissions or for consequences from application of the book, and make no warranty, expressed or implied, in regard to the contents of the book. Any practice described in this book should be applied by the reader in accordance with the professional standards of care used in regard to the unique circumstances that may apply in each situation. The reader is advised always to check product information (package inserts) for changes and new information regarding dose and contraindications before administering any drug. Caution is especially urged when using new or infrequently ordered drugs.

Library of Congress Cataloging-in-Publication Data

Braveman, Brent.
  Leading and managing occupational therapy services an evidence-based approach/
Brent Braveman.
      p. ; cm.
  Includes bibliographical references and index.
  ISBN10: 0–8036–1192–7   ISBN13: 978-0-8036-1192-4
1. Occupational therapy services—Administration.
  [DNLM: 1. Occupational Therapy—organization & administration. 2. Evidence-Based
Medicine. 3. Leadership. WB 555 B826L 2005] I. Title.
RM735.4.B72 2005
615.8′515′068—dc22   2005006523

Dedication

To my mentors Susan Robertson and Gary Kielhofner for their guidance,
my parents Bill and Shirley, and
my friends Marty, Scott, Brent and Todd for
their support in this and all of life's projects.

Contributors

Regina F. Doherty, M.S., OTR/L
Massachusetts General Hospital
Boston, Massachusetts

Marcia Finlayson, Ph.D., OT(C), OTR/L
University of Illinois at Chicago
Chicago, Illinois

Gail Fisher, M.P.A., OTR/L
University of Illinois at Chicago
Chicago, Illinois

Gary Kielhofner, Dr.P.H., OTR/L, FAOTA
University of Illinois at Chicago
Chicago, Illinois

Debra Krause, M.A.
Chicago, Illinois

Elizabeth Peterson, M.P.H., OTR/L
University of Illinois at Chicago
Chicago, Illinois

Barbara Schell, Ph.D., OTR/L, FAOTA
Brenau University
Gainesville, Georgia

Preface

Purpose and Focus of the Book

The purpose of this book is to overview the primary roles, responsibilities, and functions of an occupational therapy manager. Additionally, in writing this text I sought to focus on strategies for using theory and evidence related to a wide range of occupational therapy knowledge as well as knowledge from related fields. This book presents a particular approach to leading and managing occupational therapy services—an *evidence-based* approach.

The term *evidence-based practice* has emerged over the past three decades in response to efforts in medicine and other disciplines to be more conscientious and explicit about the process of making clinical care decisions for individual clients. Evidence-based practice is a lifelong process of self-directed, problem-based learning that can inform decision making of all types by occupational therapy practitioners. Evidence-based practice involves identifying and defining a practice-related problem (remember that—in addition to clinicians—educators, researchers, and managers all *practice*), formulating a question consistent with this problem, and then going out to find and evaluate information that will help to answer the question.

Evidence-based practice requires that, as a practitioner, you constantly work to remain aware and up to date with literature in your field that is relevant to the type of work that you do. This does not imply that you will read everything in your field—that would be impossible. What it does mean is that you need to be aware of the journals, programs, researchers, and other resources that produce the information that can inform your work and the kinds of decisions you must make in your practice.

Topics

Part of the complexity of being a manager stems from the wide range of knowledge upon which a manager must draw in order to practice effectively. Given this dilemma, some management textbooks include a large number of topics and as a result have to either provide only general information that is hard to apply, or provide limited specific information that often becomes quickly outdated.

In choosing topics to include in this book, I focused on identifying the most critical and enduring topics related to management and sought to provide a balance of theory and practical information on each. Among others, topics chosen include leadership; the roles and functions of managers and supervisors; understanding organizations, health systems, and practice contexts; continuous quality improvement; program development; responsible participation in a profession; competency; managing change and solving problems; and effective communication.

Chapter Features

Several features of the book are intended to make the book "user friendly" and easy to read, and to highlight the relevance of the topics that are included to the management of occupational therapy services:

- Each chapter begins with a case example that reflects the *real-life management* experience of occupational therapy managers or other occupational therapy practitioners.
- Each chapter also returns to the case example and demonstrates how the information contained within the chapter can be applied to provide *real-life solutions*.
- Throughout the book, important concepts are highlighted in text *boxes* that summarize key points. Similarly, tables and figures are used frequently to provide summaries of evidence referenced in the text, or to illustrate concepts.
- Because data, information, and other forms of evidence are constantly evolving, each chapter concludes with a list of resources such as relevant journals, associations, or Web sites for more information.

Brent Braveman

Acknowledgments

I would like to acknowledge the following occupational therapy students for making contributions to this text by conducting literature searches.

Stefanie Conaway, OTS
Jenny Fox-Manaster, OTS
Andrea Gossett, OTR/L
Jessica Keller, MS, OTR/L
Danielle Lemon, OTS
Kavitha Padmanabhan
Elizabeth Stalzer, OTS
Rebecca Stein, OTS
Sarah Sullivan, OTS
Sun-Wook Lee
Roshawnda Wynn, OTS

A special acknowledgement to Navaraj Anandan, OTR/L, Angela Paynter, OTS and Sarah Reppenhagen, OTS who worked as Research Assistants and aided in preparation of this text.

For their careful review, the author would like to thank the following:

Diane Bailey, EdD, OTR, FAOTA
Tufts University
Medford, MA

Debra (Tiffany) Boggis, M.B.A., OTR/L
Pacific University
Forest Grove, Oregon

Georganna Miller, M.Ed., OTR/L
Xavier University
Cincinnati, Ohio

Kathryn Perrin, Ph.D., OTR/L, FAOTA
University of Mary
Bismarck, North Dakota

Ellen Rainville, M.S., OTR, FAOTA
Springfield College
Springfield, Massachusetts

Pat Sample, Ph.D.
Colorado State University
Fort Collins, Colorado

Deborah Yarett Slater, M.S., OTR/L, FAOTA
American Occupational Therapy Association
Bethesda, Maryland

Janie B. Scott, M.A., OTR/L, FAOTA
American Occupational Therapy Association
Bethesda, Maryland

Contents

CHAPTER 8

Managing Change and Solving Problems 197

Brent Braveman, Ph.D., OTR/L, FAOTA

CHAPTER 9

Developing Evidence-Based Occupational Therapy Programming 215

Brent Bravement, Ph.D., OTR/L, FAOTA, & Gary Kielhofner, Dr.P.H., OTR/L, FAOTA

CHAPTER 10

Turning Theory into Practice: Managerial Strategies 245

Barbara Schell, Ph.D., OTR/L, FAOTA, & Brent Braveman, Ph.D., OTR/L, FAOTA

CHAPTER 11

Evaluating and Improving Occupational Therapy Services 273

Brent Braveman, Ph.D., OTR/L, FAOTA, & Debra Krause, M.A.

CHAPTER 12

Communicating Effectively in Person and
in Writing   305

Brent Braveman, Ph.D., OTR/L, FAOTA

CHAPTER 13

Marketing Occupational Therapy
Services   333

Brent Braveman, Ph.D., OTR/L, FAOTA

CHAPTER 14

Responsible Participation in a Profession
347

*Regina F. Doherty, M.S., OTR/L,
Elizabeth Peterson, M.P.H., OTR/L, &
Brent Braveman, Ph.D., OTR/L, FAOTA*

CHAPTER 15

Introducing Others to Evidence-Based
Practice   371

*Brent Braveman, Ph.D., OTR/L, FAOTA, &
Marcia Finlayson, Ph.D., OT(C), OTR/L*

Marcia Finlayson, Ph.D., OT(C), OTR/L
Brent Braveman, Ph.D., OTR/L, FAOTA

Understanding and Applying the Concepts of Evidence-Based Practice to the Management of Occupational Therapy Services

Real-Life Management

Karen is an occupational therapy student who is completing her final fieldwork placement at a community facility serving older adults. When Karen started her placement, she expected to be treating clients seen through the outpatient rehabilitation and home care programs. She was surprised to find out that she was also going to be helping Beth, the Director of Occupational Therapy, prepare a proposal to expand the occupational therapy services in the facility's respite, community outreach, and educational wellness programs. The occupational therapy staff had previously not been involved in these aspects of the facility's services. As Karen works with Beth, she is struck by the range of information Beth draws on to argue her case for expansion—theory, clinical and marketing research, census data about the community, and data from third-party payers. The list seemed endless. Karen wonders how Beth is going to make sense of all of the information they have gathered. How is she going to decide if it was relevant? How is she going to put the information together to use it? Then there seem to be so many aspects of the proposal itself. Beth explains that it has to address a diversity of issues related to the management of occupational therapy services: staff supervision, communication, leadership, program development, continuous quality improvement, and funding, as well as decision-making processes about space, equipment, and other resources. Karen feels overwhelmed. Beth explains that, just as Karen is learning to use theory, models, and evidence to plan and implement intervention with patients, occupational therapy managers use theory, models, and evidence to plan and implement all facets of occupational therapy programming and services. Karen asks the simple question, "How do we get started?"

Key Issues

- Management of occupational therapy services involves a wide range of tasks and activities.
- Performing these tasks and activities involves finding and evaluating diverse data, information, and other forms of evidence to determine the best decision or course of action in a given situation.

- Finding, evaluating, and using data, information, and other forms of evidence means applying the process of evidence-based practice to management situations and problems.

Today's occupational therapy assistants, occupational therapists, and occupational therapy managers are constantly challenged to offer the best and most effective interventions possible within the constraints of available resources, including people, money, space, equipment, and time. The challenges we face today have come from a number of sources, one of which is the push in health care to ensure that activities and decisions are *evidence-based*.

When most occupational therapy personnel think about *evidence-based practice*, they think about using research to help them make decisions about what type of intervention has the greatest probability to work with a given client in a specific situation, considering their own clinical experience and knowledge, and the preferences of the client and his or her support networks. Rarely does evidence-based practice conjure up the image of an occupational therapy manager making decisions about program development, staffing patterns, equipment and space distribution, continuous quality improvement programs, or the style of leadership that he or she wishes to adopt. Yet, given the impact of each of these decisions on the operations and effectiveness of occupational therapy services overall, the manager would be wise to draw on the same evidence-based processes to make decisions for his or her practice that an individual therapist would use to select an intervention approach for a client. For example, a manager can draw on evidence to aid in decisions about staffing patterns in order to reduce turnover, or evidence about departmental layout to maximize patient safety.

The purpose of this book is to overview the primary functions of an occupational therapy manager and to provide strategies for using theory and evidence related to a wide range of occupational therapy knowledge and knowledge from related fields to guide performance as a manager. Therefore, the purpose of this chapter is to set the stage for this book by

1. Reviewing evidence-based practice principles and processes
2. Describing the relevance of evidence-based principles to the management of occupational therapy services

3. Identifying the types of evidence that can be used by occupational therapy managers as they perform various tasks and activities
4. Explaining a step-by-step process for finding, evaluating, and using evidence in occupational therapy management

Evidence-Based Practice: Reviewing the Basics

The term *evidence-based practice* has emerged over the past three decades in response to efforts in medicine and other disciplines to be more conscientious and explicit about the process of making clinical care decisions for individual clients. Much of the impetus for this movement can be traced back to the influential book by Archie Cochrane, *Effectiveness and Efficiency: Random Reflections on Health Services*, which was published in the United Kingdom in 1972. In his book, Cochrane highlighted the challenges of making informed decisions about health care because of the lack of access to careful, systematic, and up-to-date reviews of existing evidence, particularly randomized controlled trials (Cochrane Collaboration, n.d.).

Over the years, a number of individuals have responded to Cochrane's reflections by developing processes and practices that were initially named *evidence-based medicine*, and then later expanded to become *evidence-based practice*. Many of these early efforts grew from work at McMaster University in Ontario, Canada; the Cochrane Centre in Oxford, England; and the now well-known Cochrane Collaboration, an international organization (Cochrane Collaboration, n.d.; Sackett, Straus, Richardson, Rosenburg, & Haynes, 2000).

Although often misperceived as a "cookbook" approach that is focused on reducing the cost of health care, evidence-based practice is more accurately described as a lifelong process of self-directed, problem-based learning that can inform health care decision making (Dorsch, 2003; Law, 2002). It involves identifying and defining a practice-related problem (it must be remembered that—in addition to clinicians—educators, researchers, and managers all *practice*), formulating a question consistent with this problem, and then seeking out and evaluating information that will help to answer the question. Frequently, this information is from research literature, but, as you will see later in this chapter, there are different kinds of data and information that an occupational therapy manager may want to use. All of these types of information may be considered to be *evidence.*

Once a practitioner, regardless of his or her role, has gathered and evaluated the information found in a search, he or she will need to synthesize it together with what he or she knows from clinical experience and the values of an individual client. These three components—evidence, experience, and client values—are what are brought together to solve the problem and make a decision about what to do (Sackett et al., 2000). This does not seem particularly difficult, but engaging in evidence-based practice does carry with it some important responsibilities, which are discussed next and are summarized in Box 1–1.

Evidence-based practice requires that, as a practitioner, you constantly work to remain aware and up to date with literature in your field that is relevant to the type of work that you do. This does not imply that you will read everything in your field— that would be impossible. What it does mean is that you need to be aware of the journals, programs, researchers, and other resources that produce the information that can inform your work and the kinds of decisions you must make in your practice. For occupational therapy managers, this means

information from within the discipline of occupational therapy, but also from other disciplines and fields including health services research, business administration, organizational development, and psychology.

Evidence-based practice also requires that, as a practitioner, whether a therapist or a manager, you share what you have learned through synthesizing the literature with the person or people with whom you are working. Decision making about health care is not the sole responsibility of the health care provider—it is a joint responsibility with the client or consumer. Consequently, engaging in evidence-based practice means that you must be able to communicate well with your clients, whoever they may be—an individual patient, a family, the staff members you supervise as a manager, or the board of directors to whom you are accountable.

Law (2002) has described two other key aspects of evidence-based practice—judgment and creativity. *Judgment* refers to the responsibility to recognize that not all data, information, and evidence are created equal. Some sources of data, information, and other forms of evidence have questionable reliability and validity, cannot be confirmed by other sources, are not generalizable to the situation in which you work, or are based on studies that have not been conducted ethically (Christiansen & Lou, 2001; Law, 2002). Consequently, it is your responsibility to exercise good judgment in order to practice using an evidence-based approach. *Creativity* reflects the fact that translating what we find in the literature or other sources to the realities of our everyday work can be very challenging. It is not a simple or straightforward process. Therefore, as Law (2002) pointed out, practicing from an evidence-based approach means that you must be creative and think carefully about how to best apply what you are learning.

The ideas and concepts of evidence-based practice have been around for approximately 30 years, although they have really spread and been refined since the early 1990s. Initially, evidence-based practice was written off by many critics as a passing fad that would not take hold because of the time required, the discomfort most health care practitioners had with reading the research literature, and the belief that evidence-based practice was just another way to ration resources and cut costs. Nevertheless,

---

Box 1–1: Responsibilities Stemming from Evidence-Based Practice

- Staying up to date with the sources of information in your area of practice
- Communicating with others about what you have learned from synthesizing information
- Using good judgment about the information you have gathered by critically evaluating its quality
- Recognizing that translating evidence into everyday practice will not be easy and will require creativity

many factors have played a role in the rapid spread and continued refinement of the concepts and processes of evidence-based practice. These factors are listed in Box 1-2.

Although medicine was the first discipline to really discuss and publish articles and other forms of information about evidence-based practice, this type of practice is now a widespread phenomenon across the health care professions. Occupational therapy is no exception. A number of textbooks have been written about evidence-based practice in our field (Helewa & Walker, 2001; Law, 2002; Taylor, 2000); key professional journals, including the Canadian and British journals of occupational therapy, have produced special issues on the topic; and the *American Journal of Occupational Therapy* has been including an evidence-based practice forum in recent years (Tickle-Degnen, 2000a, 2000b).

The emphasis on using evidence to justify and support the decisions that you make is not going to go away. Your challenge now is to think about how to apply the concepts and processes of this way of conducting our practice throughout its continuum—from treating individuals to administering and managing entire occupational therapy departments.

Relevance of Evidence-Based Practice Principles to Management of Occupational Therapy Services

As you know, this book is about managing occupational therapy services. You have probably scanned through the table of contents by now, and have seen that the topics that will be covered are broad—leadership, communication, program development and evaluation, continuous quality improvement, budgeting, and many others. The tasks and activities that an occupational therapy manager performs are numerous, and yet many of the fundamentals of occupational therapy practice can be seen in the work of an occupational therapy manager. For example, a manager must evaluate the client and the client's situation; identify problems, concerns, and priorities; and develop an intervention plan, implement it, and then evaluate the outcomes. Table 1-1 provides a few examples of the types of clients an occupational therapy manager might have, and how the occupational therapy process might look when applied to these clients from the perspective of the manager.

Although the examples in Table 1-1 might make a lot of sense, the discerning reader should be asking, "How does the occupational therapy manager know that his or her approach is the best one? What is the evidence that choosing that particular intervention or way of proceeding is the most likely to lead to the desired outcomes?" The answer to these questions should be, "Because the manager applied evidence-based practice principles to his or her decision-making process and choice of interventions." As the example of Karen at the beginning of this chapter points out, occupational therapy managers perform a wide range of tasks and activities, and have to make many different types of decisions every day. Their choices and decisions can have a major impact on the overall functioning of occupational therapy services, and thereby on clients, families, therapists, support staff, other professionals, the organization, and potentially the broader community in which the occupational therapy services are offered. Because of these far-reaching impacts, the principles of evidence-based practice are relevant to management of occupational therapy services. Like the individual therapist, the occupational

Table 1-1 The Occupational Therapy Process Applied to the "Clients" of an Occupational Therapy Manager

	An Individual Therapist Having Difficulty Fulfilling the Demands of the Job	The Hospital Unit Staff Feels That The Occupational Therapy Services Are Not Meeting the Staff's Needs	A Board of Directors That Is Thinking About Cutting the Occupational Therapy Budget
Evaluate Client & Situation	New graduate is overwhelmed with job demands of working on a busy neurology service that has high-need clients.	Staff on an orthopedics unit has seen a 30% increase in clients with hip replacements, but there has been no increase in therapy services. Staff is being pushed to discharge earlier, but this can't be done without the aftercare input of occupational therapy staff.	The organization is experiencing drops in income, and has to cut budgets throughout the system. Members of the board of directors question the size of the occupational therapy budget.
Identify Problems, Concerns & Priorities	Therapist lacks confidence and has not connected with a mentor in the department. She came seeking help to improve performance.	There are only two occupational therapists assigned to this unit, and no Occupational Therapy Assistants (OTAs). The therapists work regular 8-to-4, Monday-to-Friday hours. The unit staff wants services more responsive to the unit's needs.	Members of the board are unfamiliar with occupational therapy services, and what is involved in providing them. They want to have a better understanding of the department's resource needs.
Select & Implement Appropriate Intervention	Manager decides to provide closer supervision and to connect therapist with another senior therapist for mentoring about managing workload demands.	Manager decides to reassign an OTA to assist on the unit half-time and to restructure occupational therapy work hours to provide part-time coverage on Saturdays.	Manager pulls together lay descriptions of occupational therapy, and brief case examples of the work in the facility that include information about the resources used during the cases. She also gathers stories from clients about the impact of occupational therapy services on their lives. This information is provided to the board members in a formal presentation, followed by a question-and-answer period.
Evaluate Outcomes	Therapist's confidence is increasing, and she feels more able to manage her job demands.	Unit staff's sense that occupational therapy services are better meeting the unit's needs, and the increased patient load and discharge schedule.	Extent of the cut to the occupational therapy budget.

5

therapy manager must carry out his or her job tasks and activities in an appropriate, responsible, ethical, and professional way in the ever-changing world of health care.

Types of Evidence Used by Occupational Therapy Managers

As Table 1–1 suggests, the types of interventions that an occupational therapy manager might employ are very diverse. Consequently, the types of evidence that might be necessary to guide his or her decisions are equally diverse. It is important to think broadly about the concept of evidence for management tasks and activities. But what are

those tasks and activities? Some of the most common ones are listed in Table 1–2, together with the chapters in which they are discussed in this book and the types of evidence that might be used by a manager during the process of performing them.

As Table 1–2 shows, research and theory are critical to the occupational therapy manager as he or she goes about making decisions and performing various tasks and activities. As in other areas of occupational therapy practice, it is important for the manager to draw on related knowledge to perform his or her job—theories on leadership, communication, and organizational development and behavior are critical. In addition, health services research that addresses issues such as the impact of different organizational structures and processes, staffing patterns, and service configurations on the health

Table 1-2   Sample Management Functions or Tasks

Common Tasks and Activities of Managers	Chapter	Types of Evidence That Might Be Used to Inform Manager as He or She Performs Tasks and Activities
• Strategic planning • Information gathering/staying informed about rules • Deciding on billing • Staffing patterns/plans	Chapter 2: Understanding Health Care Systems and Practice Contexts	• Organizational theory • Research on the impact and effectiveness of different staffing structures, patterns, and mix on patient outcomes • Statistics on billings outcomes
• Mentoring • Motivating others • Staff development	Chapter 4: Leadership: The Art, Science, and Evidence	• Research on effective leadership styles and strategies • Theory on leadership and mentoring • Performance reviews of manager • Performance of staff under manager's supervision • Statistics on staff retention
• Hiring • Firing • Mentoring • Motivating others • Staffing patterns/plans	Chapter 6: Roles and Functions of Supervisors	• Research on the impact and effectiveness of different staffing structures, patterns, and mix on patient outcomes • Theory on supervision styles • Workload statistics • Productivity statistics • Statistics on staff retention • Performance reviews of staff • Staff recognition within facility and outside of it

(continued)

Common Tasks and Activities of Managers	Chapter	Types of Evidence That Might Be Used to Inform Manager as He or She Performs Tasks and Activities
• Needs assessment • Program planning • Program implementation • Program evaluation	Chapter 9: Developing Evidence-Based Occupational Therapy Programming	• Research on existing programs and their effective components • Theory on program development • Census information on potential clients • Marketing research • Satisfaction surveys of clients attending program
• Designing processes (e.g., referrals, assessment, documentation) • Setting criteria for performance of staff and programs • Monitoring performance of processes, staff, and programs	Chapter 11: Evaluating and Improving Occupational Therapy Services	• Research on the impact of different processes on the efficiency of an organization • Data collected within the organization on a process • Benchmarking • Satisfaction surveys of clients
• Writing reports • Doing verbal presentations • Interacting with staff, upper management, public, and third-party payers	Chapter 12: Communicating Effectively in Writing and in Person	• Research on effective communication styles • Theory on communication • Feedback on reports and presentations • Extent of responsiveness from those with whom manager is communicating

outcomes of clients served are extremely important for the occupational therapy manager to read, evaluate, and apply to his or her work. This related knowledge will have to be used in conjunction with knowledge specific to occupational therapy in order for the manager to function in an evidence-based way. But what exactly does this mean? What are the specific steps involved in managing occupational therapy services from an evidence-based approach?

Process of Finding, Evaluating, and Using Evidence in Occupational Therapy Management

Using an evidence-based approach involves following six basic steps. These steps are outlined in Box 1–3. Over the next few pages, we will describe each

of these steps in detail. We have woven an example into these steps to illustrate the process more clearly.

Setting a Question

The first and most important step in evidence-based practice is identifying or *setting* a question. A good question is direct, clear, and focused. It should identify the population of interest, and the main concepts or ideas that you are interested in examining. The outcome that you are interested in also needs to be clearly specified. For more guidance about developing a good question, we suggest you visit one of the Internet resources on evidence-based practice provided in the Resources list at the end of this chapter. In addition to resources specific to evidence-based practice, reviewing information on conducting effective literature searches, which is commonly found on the library Web sites of many university libraries, will be helpful in the process of

---

Box 1–3: The Evidence-Based Practice Process

Step 1: Write a question related to a *practice problem.*

Step 2: *Locate resources* that may contain information relevant to the question.

Step 3: Conduct a *critical appraisal* on each resource.

Step 4: *Evaluate and summarize* overall findings.

Step 5: *Answer your practice question,* using your findings, your experience, and the input of your client or clients.

Step 6: *Implement the findings* within your practice.

---

developing an effective question to guide your search.

For our example, imagine being an occupational therapy manager who is about to complete annual staff performance appraisals. At a weekly staff meeting, you announce that appraisals will begin next month. Staff members at the meeting express the concern that, in the past, they felt that performance appraisals had been very subjective, and therefore unfair, particularly given their importance for annual merit increases in pay. As the manager, you decide to investigate this problem, and see if there is anything that you can do to improve staff perceptions about performance appraisal objectivity. You set the following question:

> *"What strategies have been presented in the literature to strengthen perceptions of employees that the performance appraisal process is fair and objective?"*

In this question, you have been clear, direct, and focused. The population of interest has clearly been defined as "employees." Although this is a broad population, it is often wise to start this way and then narrow the population as your search and evaluation of evidence proceeds. Your question has also clearly identified the main concepts of interest: performance appraisals and employee perceptions. The outcome of interest in this question is strengthening employees' perceptions of fairness and objectivity.

Locating Evidence

Once your question has been set, the next step in the evidence-based process is to find the evidence needed to answer your question. As Table 1–2 demonstrates, there is a wide spectrum of evidence that an occupational therapy manager might use in the course of his or her day-to-day work. Finding these potential sources of evidence can involve a number of different processes, for example, hand-searching journals or administrative reports, searching the Internet, or searching electronic bibliographic databases such as MEDLINE, CINAHL, or Wilson Business. "Hand-searching" literally means looking through the tables of contents or year-end indexes of targeted journals that are likely to have published articles on your question of interest. Hand-searching journals and administrative reports requires access to a library that has holdings that you are interested in reviewing, and can be time consuming.

It is important to distinguish between searching the Internet and searching electronic bibliographic databases. Electronic bibliographic databases are compilations of published research, scholarly articles, books, government reports, newspaper articles, and other recognized sources of information. There is a wide range of different databases, many having a disciplinary focus such as medicine, psychology, or education. For example, MEDLINE is a compilation of medically related publications, CINAHL focuses on publications from the allied health professions, and Wilson Business focuses on business and economics. OTSearch, an electronic bibliographic database provided by the American Occupational Therapy Association (AOTA), focuses on occupational therapy literature.

In comparison to an electronic bibliographic database, searching the Internet will not limit you to published articles and reports. Although you may find a journal article in the course of an Internet search, you will also find all sorts of other information that may have no direct relevance to the question or problem you are trying to address. Narrowing your search on the Internet can be very challenging, particularly because there are no set key terms or search words to use. In addition, much of what you will find will be of questionable credibility. Anyone can create a Web site or a Web page, as long as they have Internet access. Therefore, it is important to have strict criteria for selecting sites to review if you are going to use the Internet to find evidence. More information on appraising Web sites is provided later in this chapter. Generally speaking, it is a good idea to limit your Internet searches initially to government, university, and professional association Web sites. Ultimately, searching electronic bibliographic databases is probably going to be the most focused and productive option for finding information and evidence to support decision making in management of occupational therapy services.

Regardless of whether your search for evidence is done by hand-searching, using the Internet, or using electronic bibliographic databases, it is critical that your search is "a systematic, explicit, and reproducible method for identifying, evaluating, and interpreting the existing body of recorded work produced by researchers, scholars, and practitioners" (Fink, 1998). A good literature search will be systematic and methodical, clearly documented, and reproducible on subsequent days or by other people. To aid in achieving this goal of reproducibility, particularly when using electronic bibliographic databases, you should use the question you have already set to guide your search. Using your question means taking it apart to identify the key words and phrases that you will use during the search. The best way to start is by writing down the terms that correspond to the population specified in your question, as well as those that capture the main concepts and ideas. From the example we introduced earlier, we would write down "employee" and "performance appraisal" to start. During an actual search, these words and phrases are linked together using Boolean terms such as "AND," "OR," and "NOT" to focus the search and find the best and most relevant information. Using the "OR" term results in the largest number of citations by identifying any citation that includes any of the linked key words. Using the "AND" term limits citations to those including *all* key words. Using the "NOT" term eliminates citations including key words you do not wish to include in your search.

Next, you should select appropriate electronic bibliographic databases (e.g., MEDLINE, CINAHL, Wilson Business) for your search. Determining if a database is appropriate can be done by reviewing its focus (e.g., health) and content (e.g., names of

journals included). This information is typically available through the "Help" or general information section of a database. In the example we presented earlier, our question focuses on employee perceptions of performance appraisals. Given that performance appraisals are a task for managers, it is likely that databases addressing management and business-related topics will be the most relevant. When we looked for databases that had these foci, we found PsycINFO, Wilson Business, and Article First.

Once you have selected databases, it is a good idea to cross-reference the key words and phrases with the index terms in the database you decide to use, if possible. For our example, we started with the key words "performance appraisal." In the PsycINFO database, this term mapped to 15 different terms. We chose to narrow our search by focusing on the terms "job performance," "personnel evaluation," "rating," "employee attitudes," and "feedback." Finding the evidence that matches your questions is a process of initiating the search, making modifications to your search terms as necessary, and documenting your search and related decisions as you go. It is best to record the search words and phrases you use, and identify the combinations of terms that you use. The search can be limited or expanded as necessary. Ways of limiting your search include focusing on research articles only, or focusing on particular publication years. Expanding your search can be accomplished by using synonyms for your key words, and connecting these synonyms together with the Boolean search term "OR." Regardless of the way your search develops, it is critical to document it as you go, so that you can replicate it later if need be.

For our question, when we were using the PsycINFO database, the terms that we used ("job performance," "personnel evaluation," "rating," "employee attitudes," and "feedback") resulted in 22,166 citations. When we applied the English language limitation, this number was reduced to 21,117 citations. We then chose to limit the search to articles published between the years 1980 and 2004, and this reduced the number of citations to 15,082. We further limited our search by combining the results with the term "employee satisfaction" by using the Boolean term "AND." The final search resulted in 63 citations. Upon review of the citations and abstracts, we learned that seven of the citations were actually related to employee satisfaction with performance appraisal systems and that six of these were empirical. A similar search process in the Wilson Business database identified nine related citations, and in the Article First database, seven related citations. In some cases, you may have to go back and expand your search by using other key words or be willing to accept data, information, or other forms of evidence that are not as focused on your question as you might have hoped if directly related literature is not found.

Once you have identified a manageable number of sources from your search, you can review what you have found to determine if they are, in fact, relevant to your question. Although there is some variation in how different databases display the results of a search, some basic information is relatively standard. This information includes the title of the work that was located, the type of work that it is (e.g., journal article, book chapter, dissertation), author name(s), the specific source (e.g., journal volume, number, and pages or book publisher and location), the publication date, and usually an abstract or summary. You should review all of this information, particularly the abstracts or summaries, to determine if you want to obtain a copy of the specific source for further and more thorough review.

Because of the diversity of tasks and activities that the occupational therapy manager performs, searching the literature for evidence to assist in decision making will necessarily have to involve looking for all sorts of publications, such as books, journals, and, if it is appropriate, newspaper articles, government documents, and Web sites. It will be critically important to search the literature from disciplines other than occupational therapy. A good sign that your search is complete is that the articles that you are finding are citing other articles that you already have found.

Once you have completed your search, your next step is to evaluate what you have found. This step is known as critical appraisal.

Evaluating the Evidence

Critical appraisal is the process of judging the quality of a piece of information and determining its applicability to practice. It is a critical part of using an evidence-based approach to managing occupa-

tional therapy services. Critical appraisal has been identified as one of the steps of evidence-based practice that is the most difficult for occupational therapists, occupational therapy assistants, and other health care providers because they feel uncertain about reading research and making a determination about its quality and potential utility to inform and guide decision making (Dubouloz, Egan, Vallerand, & von Zweck, 1999).

Critical appraisal involves carefully reading and evaluating the reliability, validity, and overall quality of the source of data, information, and other forms of evidence that have been located. To assist with this evaluation process, one can draw on a large number of books, journal articles, and appraisal guidelines to learn about what to look for and evaluate across a wide variety of potential sources of evidence. For example, Greenhalgh (2000), Crombie (1996), and the occupational therapy evidence-based practice group at McMaster University have published guides for evaluating different types of research designs. In addition, in the mid-1990s, the American Medical Association published a series of articles by the Evidence-Based Medicine Working Group (see issues of *JAMA* published in 1994 and 1995). Other sources, such as the University of California at Berkeley Library (*http://www.lib.berkeley.edu/TeachingLib/*), have produced guides for evaluating information that is available through Web sites. Additional resources for evaluating information found on Web sites are provided at the end of the chapter.

Essentially what all of these different resources provide is a list of questions to ask yourself as you read an article or review a resource that has the potential to inform your decision-making process. Examples of some of the key questions that are asked in these guides are presented in Tables 1–3, 1–4, and 1–5.

Critical appraisal is a crucial step in the process of evidence-based practice. It is one thing to be able to locate data, information, and other forms of evidence, but, unless you can evaluate their quality and determine their utility for informing decisions, the evidence-based practice process will break down. Therefore, after reading the evidence you have found and answering the appraisal questions, it will be necessary to look across all of the material and decide what is worth using and trying to apply to practice. To aid in this process, it is a good idea

Table 1-3	Basic Appraisal Questions for Research Articles	
Area for Review	**Questions to Guide the Appraisal Process**	
Study significance	Is the reason for doing the study well developed? Do the authors convince you that doing this study was important?	
Purpose of research	Is the purpose of the study clear?	
Design	What is the design of the study? Does it match the purpose of the study?	
Sampling procedure	What is the sampling procedure? Does it correspond well to the question and the design? What are the strengths and limitations of the procedure with respect to being able to answer the question?	
Sample	What are the characteristics of the sample? Are there any potential biases inherent in the makeup of the sample that might interfere with the ability to answer the question?	
Data collection procedures and/ or measures	How were data collected for this study? What measures were used? What do you know about the methods/measures (consider reliability, validity, who developed it, for what purpose, pre- or pilot testing, etc.)?	
Intervention (if applicable)	What was the intervention? Is the intervention adequately described? Is the intervention conceptually congruent with the outcomes chosen?	
Results	What were the findings? Overall, do you feel that they are free of bias? If not, why not?	
Conclusions	Do you agree with the conclusions? What are the strengths and limitations of the study overall? Do you feel that the purpose of the study has been addressed (i.e., is the question answered)?	

Table 1-4	Basic Appraisal Questions for Review Articles and Non–Research-Related Reports and Documents	
Area for Review	**Questions to Guide the Appraisal Process**	
Purpose	Is the purpose of the material clear? What are the key points or messages?	
Main messages	How reliable do you feel the key points or messages are? Consider number, type, and age of citations; expertise of author(s); where material is published (e.g., peer-reviewed journal, professional magazine, etc.); consistency with other materials you have read.	
Population addressed	To what populations are the key points or messages relevant? How well do these populations correspond to the population(s) that you are interested in planning/making decisions for?	
Interventions, processes, and structures addressed	What types of interventions/processes/structures are addressed? To what extent might they apply in your setting?	
Outcomes addressed	What types of outcomes are addressed? Consider micro-, meso-, and macro-level outcomes. How relevant are these outcomes to your setting?	
Overall credibility	Overall, do you believe what is in this resource? Why or why not? What questions do you have remaining after reviewing this resource?	

Table 1-5	**Basic Appraisal Questions for Web Sites**
Area for Review	**Questions to Guide the Appraisal Process**
Reliability	To what extent can you count on the information provided at this site? Is the source trustworthy? How did the site's creators come up with the information listed here? Do they cite sources? Did they follow good research procedures? Do they have a bias? A reason to distort? Is this advertising?
Accuracy	Are these real numbers and facts? Do they match reality? How do you know they are real and on target?
Currency	How recent are the facts and figures? Does the site tell you? Does it matter? Might reported rates such as crime or employment have changed since the data were posted to the site?
Authority	Do the site's creators have any credentials to be providing this information? Any evidence of training or professional skill? Do they identify the author or provider by name? Who did this work?
Fairness	Have the site's creators presented the material selectively or in an unbalanced manner? Is there bias or slanting in the reporting? Did they leave some information out? Did they focus only on the positive? The negative?
Adequacy	Do the site's creators tell you enough? Do they provide sufficient data or evidence? Do they go into enough detail and depth?
Efficiency	Can you find what you need at this site relatively quickly, or is it loaded down with graphics and elements that prolong your visit and your searching unnecessarily?
Organization	Is the information laid out in a logical fashion so that you can easily locate what you need without wandering around and wasting time?

to give the material you are reviewing an overall quality rating. In other words, you should assign it a value to indicate the level of evidence the material offers.

There are many different typologies for applying a level of evidence to a resource that you are considering in your decision-making process. The majority of these typologies primarily address quantitative types of research such as randomized controlled trials, systematic reviews, meta-analyses, and quasi-experiments. Often, there is limited room within these typologies to consider the role or value of qualitative research, theoretical pieces, government or organizational reports, or administrative data (e.g., reports produced through aggregating discharge summary information). Some allow for the testimony of expert committees or the opinions of respected authorities, but these types of evidence are usually rated as the weakest form.

Although there are variations in the approaches used by different scholars and sources, most use similar approaches to assigning some sort of rating to indicate the rigor of the research and its overall quality. Table 1–6 includes three such typologies.

The first typology included in Table 1–6 is provided by the Cochrane Library, which is a resource for evidence-based reviews of clinical (primarily medical) interventions. The second typology is that used by the AOTA's Evidence-Based Literature Review Project. The third typology was presented by Dr. Margo Holm in her Eleanor Clarke-Slagle Lecture entitled, "Our Mandate for the New Millennium: Evidence-Based Practice" (Holm, 2000). As previously noted, you will find that there is more of an emphasis in these typologies on quantitative research using traditional experimental designs, but that some recognition of other forms of evidence is included.

Table
1-6

Strategies for Classifying Levels of Evidence

Level of Evidence	The Cochrane Library*	The American Occupational Therapy Association†	Moore, McQuay, and Gray (from Holm, 2000)
Strongest	A = Strong research-based evidence (multiple relevant, high-quality scientific studies with homogeneous results)	I = Randomized controlled trial	I = Some evidence from at least one systematic review of multiple well-designed randomized controlled studies
	B = Moderate research-based evidence (at least one relevant, high-quality study or multiple adequate studies)	II = Nonrandomized controlled trial, two groups	II = Strong evidence from at least one properly designed randomized controlled trial of appropriate size
	C = Limited research-based evidence (at least one adequate study)	III = Nonrandomized controlled trial, one group with pretest and post-test	III = Evidence from well-designed trials without randomization, or single-group pre-post, cohort, time series, or matched case-control studies
Weakest	D = No scientific evidence (expert panel evaluation or other information)	IV = Single-subject design NA = Narratives and case studies	IV = Evidence from well-designed non-experimental studies from more than one center or research group

*Available at *http://www.update-software.com/ebmg/*
†Note that some typologies, such as that used by the American Occupational Therapy Association's Evidence-Based Literature Review project, assign separate ratings for the study design, internal/external validity, and sample size.

By exploring any of the typologies in more depth, you will notice that a single article may be assigned multiple ratings, and that these ratings are indicative of different aspects of a resource. For example, the AOTA typology suggests assigning separate ratings for the study design, internal validity, external validity, and sample size, so the strongest evidence would receive a rating of I.A.1.a for a study with a randomized controlled trial, more than 20 subjects per condition, high internal validity, and high external validity (Tickle-Degnen, 2000b).

It is not as important which typology you use to rate the evidence you have found as it is that you have some systematic way of comparing the relative strengths and weaknesses of the evidence, and summarizing patterns and consistencies across articles. This need to compare and summarize across articles is particularly important when you are drawing from a large body of literature in which materials contradict each other.

Obviously, using a rating system such as that of the AOTA is most helpful when some of the evidence you are reviewing is of a quantitative type, so you can compare studies across a similar set of criteria. But what do you do if the managerial question you are exploring is not well researched or is not well suited to an experimental design? How do you evaluate evidence when the majority of it is not well suited to rating by the sort of typologies provided in Table 1–6? The answer has already been provided to some extent in Table 1–4. In this table, you were given a set of basic appraisal questions for non–research-related reports and documents. To expand on Table 1–4, we have developed a suggested typology for use in rating review articles, program descriptions, and non–research-related reports and documents. This typology is provided in Table 1–7.

It is important to keep in mind that few articles that you review will fit perfectly into a given rating typology. You must use your clinical expertise and judgment to determine whether or not a given resource fits more consistently with one of these ratings versus another. In addition, for some questions you might be trying to address, you may choose to be more conservative in your evaluation of the evidence. When decisions involve great expense or change, or if it will not be possible to easily reverse them, sometimes a more conservative approach is prudent.

Throughout this book, you will be presented from time to time with sample data, information, and other forms of evidence related to a variety of managerial topics. Because of the diversity of topics included in this book, choosing a single typology to

Table 1-7	A Suggested Typology for Rating Review Articles, Program Descriptions, and Non–Research-Related Reports and Documents
Level of Evidence	**Characteristics**
Strong	• Widely used and recognized. • Numerous other citations or examples of use are provided. • Discussions across the multiple citations or examples are consistent with each other. • Was developed specifically for use by occupational therapists or other practitioners in the setting in which you intend to use it. • Presented by an author, group, or resource with well-documented expertise in the relevant subject matter. • Presented by an author with clearly documented and relevant training and education. • Documented in a manner that clearly highlights the strengths, weaknesses, advantages, and disadvantages of the strategy, model, or approach. • Presented in a peer-reviewed publication or resource.

(continued)

Level of Evidence	Characteristics
Good	• Generally recognized by individuals familiar with the literature, but its use may be restricted to certain geographic regions or be associated with a particular setting or school. • Some other citations or examples of use are provided. Discussions across these citations or examples are generally consistent with each other, although some variability exists. • Was developed specifically for use by occupational therapists or other practitioners in a setting that is closely related to where you intend to use it. • Presented by an author, group, or resource with some documented expertise in the relevant subject matter, but length of expertise may be limited. • Presented by an author with related training and education. • Documented in a manner that allows the reader to extract the strengths, weaknesses, advantages, and disadvantages of the strategy, model, or approach. • Presented in a peer-reviewed publication or resource.
Weak	• Somewhat familiar, but not generally recognized even among individuals familiar with the literature. • Only one or two other citations or examples of use are provided. • Was developed for use by occupational therapists or other practitioners in a setting that has a few similarities to the one in which you intend to use it. • Presented by an author, group, or resource for which very limited information is available about expertise in the relevant subject matter. • Presented by an author with very limited training or education that is relevant. • Documented in a manner that makes it difficult for the reader to identify the strengths, weaknesses, advantages, and disadvantages of the strategy, model, or approach. • Presented in a trade or professional magazine that is reviewed by editors only.
Poor	• Being introduced for the first time and no other citation or example of use is provided. • Was developed specifically for use by another discipline or other practitioners in an unrelated setting. • Presented by an author, group, or resource for which no documentation of expertise in the relevant subject matter is provided. • Presented by an author whose training and education is not relevant or not documented. • Discussion is limited to application only, with no mention of the strengths, weaknesses, advantages, and disadvantages of the strategy, model, or approach. • The source or date of the publication cannot be determined. • No indication of any peer or editorial review.

evaluate the strength of the evidence proved difficult. In practice, we would recommend that you choose a typology that best fits the type of evidence that matches the question you are exploring. However, we were also concerned that continually shifting from one typology to another would be very confusing. For that reason, we have developed a simple typology that will be used throughout the book, regardless of the type of evidence being evaluated. This typology is presented in Box 1–4.

Once you have appraised the various sources of data, information, and other forms of evidence that you have uncovered, and assigned each of them a quality rating, the next step is to summarize and use this evidence.

Summarizing and Using the Evidence

In the example we have been using to illustrate the steps of the evidence-based process, we reviewed the abstracts of the articles from each database that appeared relevant to our question after narrowing the search results. We uncovered four articles that addressed our initial question regarding ways to strengthen employee perceptions of the fairness and objectivity of performance appraisals. One way of summarizing the evidence that you have found in order to consider if and how to use it is to construct what is called a *critical appraisal matrix*. A critical appraisal matrix for our example is provided in Table 1–8.

Critical appraisal matrices provide an opportunity to record the key characteristics, findings, strengths, and limitations of the materials that have been uncovered and appraised during a search in a

compact and manageable format. The organization of these matrices will depend on the topic of the search, how the information is going to be used, and what pieces of information we need to answer our question. In our example, we wanted to know about strategies for strengthening employee perceptions. Therefore, including a column on "strategies" in the matrix is prudent. In addition, we might want to include information on how the strategies were identified (i.e., methods), how many and what type of employees were being considered in the source of evidence, what the nature of the employment was (e.g., health or business), and what we thought of the overall quality of the material.

Once all of this information is extracted into the matrix, it is then possible to scan across the sources easily and quickly, looking for similarities and differences. From here, we can write a brief summary about what the answer to our question is (if there is one), and how or if the information is applicable to our situation.

Challenges of Using an Evidence-Based Approach

Most readers will have some familiarity with the steps of the evidence-based approach that we have just reviewed and described. Even if you have great skills in writing clear questions, searching the literature, and appraising and summarizing what you have found, challenges will still emerge. For the occupational therapy manager, the key challenges include getting access to facilities for searching, finding too much or not enough during a search, actually obtaining the materials that you have found, and just generally keeping up to date with relevant materials in the field. Let's explore each of these challenges a bit more.

The challenge for many occupational therapy managers is that they may not have easy access to electronic bibliographic databases if the facility they work in does not have a library that purchases subscriptions to these services, or alternatively, does not have access to a university-based library. A good alternative for many people is PubMed, which is freely available through the National Library of Medicine (*http://www.ncbi.nlm.nih.gov/pubmed/*).

Table
1-8

Sample Critical Appraisal Matrix

Author	Level of Evidence	Design	Strategies Investigated	N (Sample Size)	Results or Findings
Mani (2002)	Good	Survey using convenience sample	Correlations of satisfaction with the performance appraisal (PA) were done with demographic characteristics and a range of employee beliefs regarding their managers and the PA system	69 employees from four job classifications at a university	Overall satisfaction and trust of a supervisor correlated with increased satisfaction with the PA system.
Boswell & Boudreau (2000)	Good	Survey	Will use of a PA for evaluation versus employee development result in different perceptions of the appraisal?	128 employees at a production equipment facility	Employee perceptions that a PA was used for employee development positively correlated with employee satisfaction with the appraisal and the appraiser. Employee perceptions that a PA was used for evaluation were not related to employee satisfaction with either the appraisal or the appraiser.
Longenecker & Goff (1992)	Good	Questionnaire after in-depth interviews	Comparison of what managers evaluated as effective to what subordinates evaluated as effective.	60 managers and 401 division members at a Fortune 500 company	Appraisals were seen by both groups as *ineffective* when there were unclear performance standards, the manager lacked knowledge of subordinate performance, the manager was unprepared, the manager lacked skill in conducting appraisals, and the person doing the rating did not take the process seriously.
Goodson & McGee (1991)	Good	Survey	Relationship of goal development and PA activities to perceived objectivity	97 managers from one large department store	Employee participation in goal development, flexibility, and improvement discussions was found to be positively and significantly related to perceived objectivity of their PA, whereas participation in goal quantification related negatively.

For occupational therapists and occupational therapy assistants who are members of the AOTA, OTSearch is also freely available (*http://www.aota.org/*). For members of the Canadian Association of Occupational Therapists, OTDBASE is a free member service (*http://www.caot.ca/*). A fairly recent option for occupational therapy personnel is OTSeeker, freely available online at *http://otseeker.com/*.

Managers who begin to use an evidence-based approach to decision making will find that they face the same challenges that clinicians face when using evidence to guide their practice. At times, the amount and variety of evidence can seem overwhelming. For example, if you were to begin by searching the key words "leadership" and "research" in the PsycINFO electronic bibliographic database (limiting your search to leadership theories, styles, traits, and management), you would find more than 61,000 citations. This result can be narrowed to a more manageable number by applying simple strategies described earlier, such as limiting the citations to those in English, those published after a designated year or during a designated time frame, and those related to a particular leadership theory or practice.

At other times, very little information will be found or the evidence that is found may seem only generally related to your managerial question. For example, there is a fair amount of research on leadership styles, but little of it directly addresses leadership specifically within occupational therapy services. In such situations, an occupational therapy manager may need to read material from other fields and evaluate its applicability to his or her situation. For example, the U.S. Armed Services have conducted randomized trials comparing the outcomes of training using different leadership styles (Dvir, Eden, Avolio, & Shamir, 2002). Although this may not seem directly relevant to leading occupational therapy services, it is often important and necessary to read these related materials carefully. Depending on their focus and purpose, they can often hold some insights that the occupational therapy manager can reflect on and draw from in his or her daily work.

Nevertheless, in situations in which the evidence is thin or the relevance is not direct, it may be difficult to make decisions about how to use the information that has been uncovered. This reality means that a manager needs to be prepared for the possibility that there may be no clear answer to the question he or she was trying to address. An example is the task of finding a model to guide the steps of developing a new occupational therapy program. For managerial questions such as this, the only evidence that you may be able to find will be program descriptions or the opinions of subject matter experts. It is unlikely that you will find research equivalent to a "clinical trial" in which the effectiveness of the use of one model is compared to the effectiveness of the use of another. However, there are still strategies that can be used for evaluating the quality of evidence, such as a description of the application of a program development model, which we presented in Table 1–7.

Another common challenge that faces occupational therapy managers who are trying to use an evidence-based approach is actually obtaining the materials that you have found and want to appraise for further consideration and use. If this is a problem for you, check to see if the library at your facility has an interlibrary loan agreement with a university library in the area. You can also check the Web sites of local university libraries to determine whether or not they carry subscriptions to the journals or materials you are seeking. Fortunately, some journals are now making "full-text" articles available electronically, which means that you can download or print a copy of the entire article right at the time of your search. It is important to remember that, even though this service is provided, copyright laws still apply, and it is typically not legal to distribute multiple copies of the article without obtaining the publisher's permission. However, it is legal to download or print a single copy for your personal use.

Even for the manager who is regularly searching the literature for evidence to aid decision making, keeping up to date with new materials that are coming out can be challenging. Many new resources are now available to reduce this problem. For example, some journals now have *electronic table of contents (ETOC)* alerts in which the table of contents of the most recent issue of a journal is e-mailed to you free of charge. The Society for Academic Medical Education (*http://www.sacme.org/*) provides a list of journals that offer ETOC service. Another resource is medical news services that provide concise abstracts about recent publications, advances, and media coverage of medical subjects. Two examples of such services are CNN Health (*http://www.cnn.com/health/*) and IntelliHealth (*http://www.intellihealth.com/*). Finally, some federal agencies and nonprofit associations provide e-mail services through which information about current events, conferences or other learning opportunities, key research results, or updated demographic information is sent to you on a regular basis. For example, the Centers for Disease Control and Prevention (*http://www.cdc. gov/*) has a number of statistical reports on various health problems that are available through its Web site, and you can sign up to be notified by e-mail when updated reports are available.

Even in their best application, it is unlikely that the strategies suggested in this chapter or by other resources on evidence-based practice will eliminate all of your decision-making difficulties. However, it is likely that following the guidelines and suggestions that have been presented in this chapter will help to reduce some of your confusion and stress, and the product of your work will be of higher quality.

Chapter Summary

Today's occupational therapy assistants, occupational therapists, and occupational therapy managers are constantly challenged to offer the best and most effective interventions possible. Practicing from an evidence-based approach provides the foundation to act in a professional, responsible, and ethical manner. As explained in the introduction, the purpose of this book is to overview the primary functions of an occupational therapy manager and to provide strategies for using theory and evidence related to a wide range of occupational therapy knowledge and knowledge from related fields to guide performance as a manager. To set the foundation for the contents of this book, this chapter has reviewed evidence-based practice principles and processes; described the relevance of evidence-based principles to management of occupational therapy services; identified the types of evidence that can be used by an occupational therapy manager as he or she performs various tasks and activities; and explained a step-by-step process for finding, evaluating, and using evidence in occupational therapy management.

Useful Resources for Applying Evidence-Based Practice to Management of Occupational Therapy Services

As this chapter has explained, evidence-based practice is here to stay, and its principles and processes are relevant to management of occupational therapy services. Entire books have been dedicated to different aspects of evidence-based practice, or the applications of its processes by different disciplines or in different settings. It is not possible to cover all that is known about evidence-based practice in

Real-Life Solutions

After Beth explained to Karen the importance of using theory, models, and evidence to plan and implement the different facets of occupational therapy programming and services, Karen felt more comfortable. She especially appreciated how Beth was able to explain that a manager uses the same evidence-based process for answering a "practice-related" question as does a clinician. From her schoolwork, Karen knew about how to write answerable questions, search the literature, and evaluate what she had read. Although the materials that she would need to use to help Beth prepare the proposal to expand the occupational therapy services at the facility would come from many different sources and consist of a variety of types of evidence, Karen felt more prepared to engage in the process. Now she needed to turn her attention to learning about the specific issues related to administering and managing occupational therapy services: staff supervision, communication, leadership, program development, continuous quality improvement, and funding, as well as decision-making processes about space, equipment, and other resources.

this chapter, or to explain its steps in the level of detail that some readers might like. Therefore, in the final section, we have outlined some of the resources that we have found to be the most useful in the learning and application of evidence-based practice, particularly for management of occupational therapy services. You will notice that, at the end of each chapter, similar resources such as journals, organizations or associations, or other types of resources related to the chapter focus are provided.

Resources for Learning More About Evidence-Based Practice

Journals That Are Likely to Include Evidence Relevant to Management of Occupational Therapy Services

THE MILBANK QUARTERLY

The *Milbank Quarterly* has been published for over seven decades and features peer-reviewed original research and articles that review health care policy and provide analysis of current and evolving policy. Other content includes commentary from a range of professionals representing academicians, practitioners, researchers and policy makers. Articles and commentary found in this journal represent multidisciplinary perspectives on empirical research as well as the application of research and policy in a variety of settings. Social, legal, and ethical issues are addressed.

JOURNAL OF HEALTH SERVICES RESEARCH & POLICY

The *Journal of Health Services Research & Policy* includes articles presenting results of qualitative and quantitative multidisciplinary research from a wide variety of disciplines. In addition to the reporting of empirical results, articles also address current and evolving debates in the scientific, methodological, and empirical arenas.

HEALTH SERVICES RESEARCH

The journal, *Health Services Research,* provides researchers, policy makers and analysts, and health care administrators and managers with access to empirical findings as well as articles addressing policy and methodological issues. Readers interested in health care financing, the organization or delivery of health services, or in the evaluation of health delivery outcomes will find *Health Services Research* a useful resource. The journal provides a forum for the exchange of practices related individuals, health systems, and communities.

Professional Organizations Relevant to Management of Occupational Therapy Services

AMERICAN COLLEGE OF HEALTHCARE EXECUTIVES

http://www.ache.org

The American College of Healthcare Executives (ACHE) is an international professional society of health care executives working in a variety of settings including hospitals, health care systems, and other healthcare organizations. The ACHE is known for its credentialing and educational programs. The annual Congress on Healthcare Management is a nationally recognized and widely attended event. The ACHE publishes the *Journal of Healthcare Management,* and a magazine titled *Healthcare Executive.*

General Information on Finding and Evaluating the Literature

- Cochrane Collaboration and the Cochrane Library (*http://www.cochrane.org/index0.htm*)
- Health Information Research Unit at McMaster University (*http://hiru.mcmaster.ca/*)
- Database of Abstracts of Reviews of Effects (DARE) (*http://nhscrd.york.ac.uk/darehp.htm*)

Occupational Therapy–Specific Resources on Evidence-Based Practice

- OTSeeker (*http://www.otseeker.com/*)
- AOTA Evidence-Based Practice Project (*http://www.aota.org/*)
- Center for Evidence-Based Rehabilitation at McMaster University (*http://www.fhs.mcmaster.ca/rehab/centre.htm*)

Government-Related Web Sites and Documents

- Centers for Disease Control and Prevention (*http://www.cdc.gov/*)

- National Center for Health Statistics (*http://www.cdc.gov/nchs/*)
- Agency for Health Care Research and Quality (*http://www.ahcpr.gov/*)
- Centers for Medicare and Medicaid Services (*http://cms.hhs.gov/providers/edi/default.asp*)

Resources on Evaluating Information Found on Web Sites

- Beck, S. (1997). Evaluation criteria. In *The good, the bad & the ugly: Or, why it's a good idea to evaluate Web sources.* Available at *http://lib.nmsu.edu/instruction/evalcrit.html*
- The University of California Berkeley Library (*http://www.lib.berkeley.edu/TeachingLib/Guides/Internet/Evaluate.html*)

Reference List

Boswell, W. R., & Boudreau, J. W. (2000). Employee satisfaction with performance appraisers: The role of perceived appraisal use. *Human Resource Quarterly, 11,* 283–299.

Christiansen, C., & Lou, J. Q. (2001). Evidence-based practice forum: Ethical considerations related to evidence-based practice. *American Journal of Occupational Therapy, 55,* 345–349.

Cochrane, A. (1972). *Effectiveness and efficiency: Random reflections on health services.* London: Nuffield Provincial Hospitals Trust.

Cochrane Collaboration (n.d.). The Cochrane Collaboration brochure. The Cochrane Collaboration Web site. Retrieved November 5, 2003, from *http://www.cochrane.org/resources/brochure.htm*

Crombie, I. K. (1996). *The pocket guide to critical appraisal.* London: BMJ Publishing Group.

Dorsch, J. (2003). Evidence-based medicine: Finding the best clinical literature. University of Illinois at Chicago Library Website. Available at *http://www.uic.edu/depts/lib/lhsp/resources/ebm.shtml*

Dubouloz, C., Egan, M., Vallerand, J., & von Zweck, C. (1999). Occupational therapists' perceptions of evidence-based practice. *American Journal of Occupational Therapy, 53,* 445–453.

Dvir, T., Eden, D., Avolio, B. J., & Shamir, B. (2002). Impact of transformational leadership on follower development and performance: A field experiment. *Academy of Management Journal, 45,* 735–744.

Fink, A. (1998). *Conducting research literature reviews: From paper to the Internet.* Thousand Oaks, CA: Sage.

Goodson, J. R., & McGee, G. W. (1991). Enhancing individual perceptions of objectivity in performance appraisal. *Journal of Business Research, 22,* 293–303.

Greenhalgh, T. (2000). *How to read a paper: The basics of evidence-based medicine.* London: BMJ Publishing Group.

Helewa, A., & Walker, J. M. (2001). *Critical evaluation of research in physical rehabilitation.* Philadelphia: W.B. Saunders.

Holm, M. (2000). Our mandate for the new millennium: Evidence-based practice. *American Journal of Occupational Therapy, 64,* 575–585.

Law, M. (2002). *Evidence-based rehabilitation: A guide to practice.* Thorofare, NJ: Slack.

Longenecker, C. O., & Goff, S. J. (1992). Performance appraisal effectiveness: A matter of perspective. *SAM Advanced Management Journal, 52,* 17–23.

Mani, B. G. (2002). Performance appraisal systems, productivity and motivation: A case study. *Public Personnel Management, 31,* 141–159.

Sackett, D. L., Straus, S. E., Richardson, W. S., Rosenburg, W., & Haynes, R. B. (2000). *Evidence based medicine: How to practice and teach EBM* (2nd ed.). Edinburgh: Churchill Livingstone.

Taylor, M. C. (2000). *Evidence-based practice for occupational therapists.* Oxford: Blackwell Science.

Tickle-Degnen, L. (2000a). Gathering current research evidence to enhance clinical reasoning. *American Journal of Occupational Therapy, 54,* 102–105.

Tickle-Degnen, L. (2000b). What is the best evidence to use in practice? *American Journal of Occupational Therapy, 54,* 218–221.

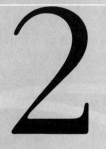

CHAPTER

2

Gail Fisher, M.P.A., OTR/L
Brent Braveman, Ph.D., OTR/L, FAOTA

Understanding Health Care Systems and Practice Contexts

Real-Life Management

Andrea is an occupational therapist who has been working in an outpatient clinic in a suburban area for 5 years. She has just accepted a position in a small-town hospital in a semirural area. The hospital has never employed an occupational therapist before, although some doctors have requested occupational therapy services for their patients.

The first week at her new job, Andrea, as both the Director of Occupational Therapy and the only occupational therapist, knew she had her work cut out for her. She needed to set charges, determine what occupational therapy services would be reimbursable by Medicare, and determine unmet needs that occupational therapy could address. She noticed that the hospital was not fully compliant with the Americans with Disabilities Act, and wanted to assist it in correcting these deficiencies. She also wanted to begin planning for hiring another practitioner within the next year to assist her, and needed to find out about the supply of occupational therapy personnel in her state and local area.

Andrea already had been contacted by the local school district, which was interested in contracting for occupational therapy services from the hospital. Rather than feeling overly challenged, Andrea knew that there were multiple resources to guide her as she analyzed the larger systems that impacted on her new role and her potential success. Andrea decided to start by networking with other managers who had faced similar challenges and to begin to collect data, information, and other forms of evidence to guide her decision making.

Key Issues

- Being knowledgeable about the contexts within which we practice is essential to succeed as an occupational therapy manager.
- Data, information, and other forms of evidence exist to assist managers to learn about reimbursement, legislation, trends, and other relevant subjects.
- Developing strategies for staying up to date regarding policies and other changes in the environment is essential because data, information, and forms of evidence are constantly being updated.
- Scanning the environment for indicators of future trends will keep you one step ahead in anticipating changes that will affect your practice and your organization.

An understanding of the larger systems within which you work is essential for managers. In Chapter 1, you were introduced to the different types of evidence and strategies for evaluating evidence. In particular, you learned to think more broadly about evidence and understand that, as an occupational therapy manager, you will rely on evidence beyond results of clinical research. Although other types of data and information (e.g., demographic trends or information about unmet needs of a population) might not fit perfectly with a researcher's conceptualization of evidence, the effective occupational therapy manager must be able to locate, evaluate, and integrate disparate types of information quickly. Learning to adapt the basic process of evidence-based practice introduced in Chapter 1 will aid you in making sound decisions based on the best available information.

In this chapter, evidence will be discussed in the context of management functions such as strategic planning, program development, budgeting, planning for staffing, and being up to date on the larger health care system and service delivery context as it evolves. Finding and using evidence about reimbursement, legislation, demographics, unmet needs, practice requirements, personnel, licensure, and future trends will allow you to make better informed decisions and plans in your role as a manager or even in your role as a therapist. This chapter will introduce you to a variety of sources and strategies for locating data, information, and other forms of evidence to help you make managerial decisions.

Health Care Systems and Occupational Therapy Service Delivery Settings

The health care "system" is a misnomer, but one that is commonly used to describe the larger service delivery context. What we have in the United States is a cobbled-together network of loosely connected pieces, including hospitals, long-term care facilities, outpatient centers, private offices of physicians and therapists, home care agencies, and community-based, not-for-profit agencies. Schools and early intervention (EI) centers are also part of the network, because they provide therapy and other health-re-

lated services. In Chapter 3, you will be introduced to various typologies for categorizing the organizations in which occupational therapy personnel most often work. One way of classifying organizations is by "setting" or naming organizations according to the function they serve in society. These settings may be placed along a continuum from those that are the most closely aligned with the medical model to those that are the least like the medical model (Box 2–1). Regardless of where it falls on this continuum, an organization may have other characteristics, such as being for-profit or not-for-profit, that influence how the organization interacts in the larger health care system.

The health care system in the United States is unique among nations. The United States is the only industrialized country that does not have health care funded by or provided by the government to all of its citizens, although it is clear that our government does play a large role in our health care system (the details follow later in this chapter). Our system is based on principles of the free market, with a large part of the system oriented toward making a profit. There are also some not-for-profit segments of the system, such as many community-based agencies and some hospitals, long-term care facilities, and home care agencies. Because the government is also involved in financing and regulating health care, there is built-in interaction between the government and the service providers (Sandstrom, Lohman, & Bramble, 2003).

Box 2–1: Continuum of Occupational Therapy Delivery Settings (Most to Least Medically Oriented)

Most Medically Oriented

- Hospital
- Long-term Care Facility
- Outpatient Therapy Center
- Home Health and Hospice
- Early Intervention
- Industrial/Work Rehabilitation
- School System
- Community/Social Service Agency

Least Medically Oriented

Dualism is a term that has been used to reflect the involvement of both government (at the national, state, and local levels) and private industry in the health care system (Sandstrom et al., 2003). Both advantages and disadvantages can be identified related to a dualistic system. Having the government involved in oversight of aspects of health care through accreditation, licensing, and certification systems may be seen as a safeguard to protect the public. Federal and state financing of some health care through systems such as Medicare and Medicaid provides access for a portion of our population that might not otherwise be able to afford care. However, governmental systems are often characterized as overly bureaucratic, slow to change, and relatively inflexible in administering policies and procedures in a way that allows for individual needs and situations.

The involvement of private industry and individuals in the system has contributed to innovation in care, as well as competition that typically is thought to act to keep costs lower, and provides for much greater choice and, in some cases, access among consumers. Yet great reliance on private providers makes oversight of quality and standardization of care very difficult, has allowed for tremendous fraud and abuse of reimbursement structures, and contributes to an abundance of some types of providers and shortages of providers in other, less lucrative specialties. For example, lucrative medical specialties such as plastic surgery have attracted larger number of medical residents, whereas primary care delivery has received less attention from medical students entering the field. Moreover, relying on private providers for a substantial portion of delivery of health care in our country results in potential conflict for the providers. These providers have a mandate to make a profit for the company's shareholders and must balance what is good for their financial "bottom line" with what is in their patients' best interest.

Health care economics is tremendously complex, but having an understanding of basic economic principles and their relationship to the health care system is useful for the occupational therapy manager if for no other reason than to help you understand the dynamic tensions faced by health care providers, payers, and consumers and why the health care system is so volatile. Further, it sometimes seems that a never-ending role for occu-

pational therapy managers is to interpret limitations and demands within organizational systems for those we supervise. Those who intend to move into roles in higher organizational administration or who desire to start and operate their own business would benefit from a more detailed investigation of health care economics. However, the scope of the discussion here will be limited to an overview of key concepts.

A basic economic principle to understand is that the goal of any economy is to *allocate limited resources* (Mansfield, 1980). Regardless of the type of economy within a given country or the health of an economy at a given time, there simply is a limited amount of human, financial, and capital resources that must be divided among competing needs. For example, Medicare is still the primary payment source for much of the occupational therapy intervention that is reimbursed by a third party in the United States. Yet we know that there is a limited Medicare budget that is under constant scrutiny as our federal government tries to manage growing budget deficits, and that there is competition for Medicare funds to pay for services ranging from prescription drugs to rehabilitation. Even in countries where "universal" health care provides health coverage for every citizen, limits are placed on who qualifies for various types of care and how long they must wait to receive it. For example, in Canada, although all citizens are insured and have access to health care, it takes nearly 25 weeks to get an appointment with an ophthalmologist, almost 21 weeks to receive orthopedic care, more than 18 weeks to get a heart bypass, more than 16 weeks to see a neurosurgeon, and nearly 12 weeks for a gynecologic exam (National Center for Policy Analysis, 2004).

Earlier it was mentioned that the U.S. health care system is based upon the *free-market system*. Drafke (2002) noted that the free-market system (which is based on capitalism) is one of the most prevalent economic systems in the world. Three key principles underlie free-market economies. The first key principle is that of *supply and demand*. Simply stated, as supply and demand diverge, the price of products should respond accordingly such that, when supply exceeds demand, costs to the consumer should go down, and when demand exceeds supply, costs to the consumer should go up. A second key principle of a free-market economy is that of *competition*. In many industries, competition helps to assure that consumers get higher quality products at lower prices. Consider, for example, electronics and the familiar phenomenon that occurs when new technology is introduced (e.g., DVD recorders). Initially, as availability of new technology is limited, quality expectations may be lower and prices are higher. However, as the number of companies producing a product increases and competition for buyers' attention grows, quality often improves while prices decrease. The third key principle of free-market economies is that of *free choice* based on information. However, a sometimes unrecognized assumption of a free-market economy is that consumers have access to information, the ability to gather information, and the ability to make informed choices when more than one provider is available. Further, it is typically assumed that economies work best when people are free to make what they want, buy what they want, and work where they want (Drafke, 2002; Mansfield, 1980).

When considering health care in the United States, however, application of principles from the free-market system is imperfect. Let's briefly examine the application of the principles of supply and demand, competition, and free choice to the health care market in the United States to identify how this market functions differently from markets for other goods or services. Supply and demand and competition are principles that interact in most markets. Often, as manufacturers, providers, or entrepreneurs note that there is growing demand for a product or service, they will move into that market. Production will increase eventually, increasing competition and supply, which in turn promotes quality and lowers prices. However, these principles do not function in the same manner in health care because of the complex interactions between availability and access to services (e.g., supply), need (e.g., demand), and the involvement of third parties in the payment for many services.

The involvement of third-party payers or insurers in the health care market limits the effects of supply and competition in a number of ways. For example, some forms of insurance limit access to providers and therefore limit competition to some extent (e.g., use of a preferred provider organization [PPO]). The intent of such a structure is to control costs by negotiating discounts with pro-

viders if those who are insured are forced to choose from a designated list of providers. However, we need to ask what can happen to quality when consumer choice is limited. For example, if persons are essentially forced into choosing a particular hospital system because of severe financial penalties if they go "outside of the PPO," how does the consumer know that all care delivered in that system is the best available? Although a given hospital might provide excellent cardiology services, it might not provide similarly effective orthopedic services. Yet the demand to improve these services that typically comes from a fully competitive free-market system is lessened by the restrictions on consumer choice. A second example of the limits on competition of health insurance is the use of "gatekeepers" in managed health care systems, whereby the decision to obtain specialty services such as a consultation with a dermatologist must first be approved by a general practitioner or nurse.

Competition in health care is limited in some ways as a result of both legal structures and to some extent societal values. Some aspects of competition are restricted by governmental regulation, such as the *certificate of need* process whereby a state typically requires health care providers to obtain permission for activities including construction of new health care facilities, acquisition of some types of major medical equipment (e.g., a new magnetic resonance imaging device), changes in ownership, or the addition of new services. Certificates of need are usually limited to major changes or additions, yet there is no doubt that to some extent they limit the ability of some providers to compete with others, and this means that the principle of supply and demand cannot be fully applied to health care.

Although advertising in health care has become more common, especially among hospitals and larger providers, it is still a relatively new phenomenon that is not universally well received. It is still seen by many as "distasteful" or "unprofessional" for health care providers such as physicians to widely advertise their services. Moreover, it is rare that prices for health care services are openly discussed in public formats so the costs of one provider might be compared to another, as is typical with most other products. Yet without access to all of this information, it is difficult for consumers to be fully informed, a prerequisite for making free choices. Additionally, when considering the relationship between cost and quality for most products, consumers will often choose to pay a lower price knowing that it also means accepting a lower level of quality. Yet, when making health care choices for oneself or one's family, who is willing to make a comparable decision? Consumers of health services typically expect and assume that they will get the best care possible regardless of the fee charged.

The assumption that information is readily accessible and understandable by all may be false. For example, in today's society access to information is clearly easier for those who also have Internet access and the skills and experiences to take advantage of it. To some degree, persons of lower socioeconomic status may have more difficulty obtaining information than those with more resources. Even if information is accessible, making health care choices can be incredibly complex. Terminology that health care professionals use routinely, such as PPOs, deductibles, co-payments, or out-of-pocket maximums, may be confusing to consumers, especially as our population becomes more diverse and a growing percentage of Americans have a language other than English as their first language. Finding objective information on providers in order to make informed choices about where to go for care can be daunting: Consider the task of moving to a new city and needing to choose a dentist, let alone a primary care physician, specialists, or a hospital. Finally, obtaining factual information about an illness or disease, the usual treatment, alternative treatments, and risks and benefits from busy physicians, nurses, or even occupational therapy practitioners is sometimes difficult, especially if you are not skilled in advocating for your needs. For all these reasons, being an informed consumer and making a "free choice" is much more difficult in the health care market than for most other products or services.

The complexity of our health care system and its inherent conflicts make enhancing cost, access, and quality across all elements of the system challenging. Raising costs to the consumers of the service may mean that fewer people can access the services they need. Service providers that cut costs to payers to appear more competitive may feel pressure to decrease the quantity or quality of services provided to the consumer. Reducing costs without reducing access to services or quality of services is a significant

challenge that our elected officials, providers, payers, and employers grapple with daily. Most changes to the system are incremental in nature, increasing access here, cutting costs there, and building in incentives for quality wherever possible. This is an evolving system that is continually changing. For that reason, the focus of this chapter is to point you to the relevant sources of data, information, and other forms of evidence. Rather than providing you with extensive details about specific reimbursement or legislation that may quickly be outdated, this chapter will focus on strategies for obtaining current data, information, and other forms of evidence on an ongoing basis. What is most important is for you to learn the skills to scan the environment for current information and future trends, and to stay abreast of developments relevant to your setting.

In addition to the health care system, occupational therapy practitioners practice in many other contexts, such as school systems, EI programs, and community agencies. Similar to the health care system, these practice settings are also influenced by changes in legislation, funding, and training requirements. The focus of relevant legislation may be different, but the need to be informed remains the same.

Evidence, Health Systems, and the Occupational Therapy Manager

A variety of data, information, and other forms of evidence is available to assist you in better understanding the segment of the health system in which you work, and for planning and implementing programs in health care, educational, or other types of settings. The type of evidence with which you are most likely familiar is evidence gained through empirical investigations. Common approaches to gathering empirical evidence are listed in Box 2–2. In addition to their use in research, these general approaches may be used to collect data (another form of evidence) to answer questions you will have as a manager. The type(s) of approach chosen will depend upon the question(s) you are trying to address.

However, at times it may be difficult to find formally published data, information, or evidence specific to your setting and your situation. At those times, you may rely more on informal evidence,

Box 2–2: Common Approaches for Gathering Data

- **Quantitative:** Numerical data
  - *Example of data obtained:* Mail survey, which includes a rating scale, sent to parents of children receiving special education to determine if they desire summer therapy programs at an outpatient clinic, followed by an analysis of the numerical data obtained
- **Qualitative:** In-depth interviewing and observing
  - *Example of data obtained:* Key informant interview with the director of the local senior citizens center to determine the need for a health promotion program delivered by occupational therapy students, followed by an analysis of interviews conducted with a number of key informants to determine common themes
- **Retrospective Observational Research:** Database approaches
  - *Example of data obtained:* Demographic statistics and trends in the incidence of stroke affecting people age 50 years and younger and the health care services that they utilized
- **Participatory Research:** Involving practitioners and consumers in the generation of knowledge, or in the generation of knowledge and taking action to improve services (the latter is Participatory Action Research)
  - *Example of data obtained:* Town hall meeting with consumers who have received occupational therapy to help plan for a new outpatient therapy center, followed by an analysis of the relevant comments

such as interviewing others in a similar position, Listserv communication, informal networking at conferences, and gathering information from colleagues or former classmates. In considering the value of this type of evidence, you should apply one of the appropriate typologies for evaluating evidence that were introduced in Chapter 1. In the next section of this chapter, we will briefly review common types of data, information, and other forms of evidence of use to the occupational therapy manager and how and where you might find it.

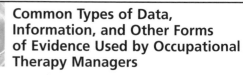

Common Types of Data, Information, and Other Forms of Evidence Used by Occupational Therapy Managers

Reimbursement

Who is paying for occupational therapy services and how much they are paying is core knowledge for managers. Several therapy-oriented texts provide a detailed analysis of payment sources and how they operate (Evanofski, 2003; McCormack, Jaffe, & Goodman-Lavey, 2003; Sandstrom et al., 2003). There are also Web sites that have up-to-date information for managers (see Resources section at the end of this chapter). Because the specifics of what various payers reimburse can change frequently, rather than discussing "who pays for what," it is more valuable to focus on understanding the long-standing facets of reimbursement in our health care system. If the reimbursement source is the government, there are official documents that detail the rules about what is covered and what is excluded (e.g., Medicare guidelines, eligibility for the State Children's Health Insurance Program [SCHIP]).

Deciding on rates for therapy services (i.e., what you will charge consumers for the services they receive) requires researching the relevant sources of reimbursement as well as market influences and the population served. Determining a specific fee for a service can be difficult at times. You may be able to obtain information from your peers or request information from other providers of service, and some service providers or payers may be willing to share their charge or reimbursement structures. You must be careful, however, because the process of agreeing with another service provider to set costs together at a determined level is known as *price fixing* and is illegal. Box 2–3 details information that managers need to know about sources of reimbursement as part of the process of setting rates for therapy services as well as determining potential sources of revenue.

For example, occupational therapy for Medicare patients will only be reimbursed if the payer determines that services are *"reasonable and necessary,"* and are expected to result in a *"significant and practical"* improvement in the individual's level of functioning within a reasonable period of time, and that a *"skilled"* service is required (i.e., not services that can be provided by an aide or family member) (Centers for Medicare and Medicaid Services [CMS], 2004). Reimbursement rates change and are influenced by legislative and presidential decision making, the gross national product, the state of the economy, and shifts in the number of Medicare beneficiaries and of people paying into the system through payroll taxes. Reimbursement for occupa-

tional therapy may also be influenced by payment changes for other professions. For example, because occupational therapy reimbursement for outpatient services is tied to physician reimbursement, their lobbying and advocacy work may have indirect benefits for therapists and vice versa (Cottrell, 2003). The American Occupational Therapy Association (AOTA) provides reimbursement updates to practitioners through its publications and electronic communications.

A few of the major reimbursement sources for health care are listed in Box 2–4, and a brief description of each is provided in the following sections of the chapter.

MEDICARE

Medicare is the largest payer of health care services in the United States, and also the largest payer of occupational therapy services (Sandstrom et al., 2003). Medicare is managed and funded by the federal government, and administered by the Centers for Medicare and Medicaid Services of the Department of Health and Human Services. There are specific guidelines for eligibility, covered services, and payment. Payments to hospitals primarily follow a model of prospective payment, identifying amounts that will be paid in advance based on patient characteristics, service needs, and facility characteristics. Outpatient services are reimbursed using a resource-based relative value scale (RVU), which takes into account the technical ability, knowledge, and skill of the provider; overhead and malpractice cost factors; and a local cost index (Sandstrom et al., 2003). Therapists in private practice must apply to be an approved Medicare provider before reimbursement is allowed.

Since the inception of Medicare, the CMS has contracted out vital program operational functions (i.e., claims processing, provider and beneficiary services, appeals, etc.) to a set of contractors known as Medicare Fiscal Intermediaries and Carriers. Intermediaries processed claims for inpatient services under Medicare Part A, and carriers processed claims for outpatient services under Medicare Part B. Most intermediaries and carriers covered one to six states. Under the Medicare Modernization Act of 2003, Medicare Part A and Part B contractors were integrated into a single authority referred to as Medicare Administrative Contractors (MACS). MACS are contracted for a period of 5 years to process Medicare claims (CMS, 2004).

These organizations develop coverage guidelines that may include descriptions of what they are looking for in documentation and exclusions of coverage. Medicare contractors and their Web sites are linked to the CMS Web site (*http://www.cms.hhs.gov/*). Contractors may post frequently asked questions, recommendations for documentation, and information on enrolling as a provider. The Office of the Inspector General of the federal government periodically evaluates service provision. In the past, it has evaluated whether occupational therapy delivered in skilled nursing facilities (SNFs) was medically necessary and met all the requirements of Medicare. In a 1998 study, it found that 25% of therapy services were medically unnecessary at five of the six SNFs surveyed. It also found that skilled services were frequently provided when nonskilled services would be more appropriate, the frequency of therapy was sometimes excessive, and time billed for therapy exceeded the actual time that services were provided (Office of Inspector General, 1998). The well-informed manager will be familiar with the facts that a reimbursement source has collected and how those facts are influencing its funding rules.

Because Medicare is administered by the federal government, passage of legislation can have a direct and dramatic impact on reimbursement for services. For example, in 1997, the U.S. Congress passed the Balanced Budget Act (BBA). This brought SNFs under prospective payment and dramatically changed the reimbursement to facilities. In addition, a $1500 annual limit per person, or cap, was placed on occupational therapy services provided in outpatient settings or SNFs (hospitals were exempted from the cap). The resulting downsizing of occupational therapy assistant jobs was significant (Fisher & Cooksey, 2002). It was critical for the occupational therapy managers who remained in the SNFs to understand the new rules for payment and to reconfigure the services delivered to fit the new payment model. These rules included the actual funding changes that based reimbursement on the intensity of therapy and nursing services needed, implementation dates, case mix and length-of-stay implications, reimbursement changes, personnel requirements, treatment implications (i.e., group vs. individual therapy), and the outpatient therapy cap. Moratoriums were temporarily placed on this cap for periods of several years at a time; however, at the time of this writing, the cap had not been permanently repealed. When changes of this nature occur, the best resources are AOTA federal affairs and reimbursement specialists, the AOTA Web site, and AOTA publications. There are also studies that have been conducted on the impact of the BBA on access to services that can provide justification for changing or maintaining current practices at an individual facility (Gage, 1999; McCall, Petersons, & Korb, 2003).

MEDICAID

Medicaid is jointly funded by the federal government and the states. Each state determines what Medicaid will pay for and who is eligible, providing at least the minimum required by federal law. Therefore, coverage for occupational therapy varies from state to state. You can often find details on Medicaid coverage on your state government Web site and on the Medicaid portion of the U.S. Government's CMS Web site (*http://www.cms.hhs.gov/medicaid/*). Some states require prior approval of occupational therapy treatment for all diagnoses, others waive the prior approval requirement for certain diagnoses, and still others do not require prior approval for treatment. Rates vary from state to state, and are prone to change depending on a state's fiscal situation.

In 1997, as part of the BBA, Congress created a new children's health insurance program called the State Children's Health Insurance Program. This program gave each state permission to offer health insurance for children who are not already insured to address the growing problem of children without health insurance. The SCHIP was designed as a federal-state partnership, similar to Medicaid, with the goal of expanding health insurance to children whose families earn too much money to be eligible for Medicaid, but not enough money to purchase private insurance. The SCHIP is the single largest expansion of health insurance coverage for children since the initiation of Medicaid in the mid-1960s (CMS, 2004).

The SCHIP provides coverage for children whose families' income is below 200% of the poverty level, but some states have expanded SCHIP eligibility beyond the 200% limit, and others are covering entire families and not just children. Benefits under the SCHIP often mirror Medicaid benefits for that state. More information about benefits and application processes specific to each state is available at *http://www.insurekidsnow.gov/* (CMS, 2004).

WORKERS' COMPENSATION

Workers' Compensation is mandated by the federal government and exists in all 50 states. In addition to paying wage replacement after a worker injured on the job has been off of work for 3 days, Workers' Compensation funds medical services, including therapy that is ordered by a physician. Each state has an industrial commission that determines payment and rules about what the employer or the employer's insurance company must cover. Because each state has its own industrial commission, the process of referral to and payment for therapy varies state by state. For example, some states are using a managed care model with tight case management practices. The rules about the employees' right to choose their own doctors also vary, and would influence to whom you would market your

work rehabilitation services. State industrial commissions may have data related to work injury rates, the most common work injuries, typical time off work, percentage of Workers' Compensation clients returning to work, and the percentage receiving rehabilitation or vocational services. These data will help you to ascertain the need for a new program or expansion of an existing program. When considering any type of insurance (e.g., Medicare, Medicaid, Workers' Compensation, or private insurance), it is critical that you consider what services are traditionally covered by the insured's "policy" and the extent to which you can negotiate payment for a service that is not covered. For example, it is very difficult to negotiate for services typically not covered by Medicare or Medicaid even if providing the services might result in an overall cost savings to the federal or state government. It is much more likely that you can negotiate payment for services on a case-by-case basis with a private insurer or with a Workers' Compensation insurer if you can demonstrate that covering the service will result in savings for the insurer.

REHABILITATION SERVICES ADMINISTRATION

What about local vocational and rehabilitation service agencies? This often-overlooked source of referrals and payments exists in every state. Through joint federal and state funding, the Rehabilitation Services Administration state-level agencies provide funding for vocational and independent living services for teens and adults with disabilities. A list of the state agencies and their Web sites can be found at *http://www.jan.wvu.edu/SBSES/vocrehab.htm*.

Relevant information that you need to know includes requirements for providers, criteria for payment for occupational therapy, referral mechanisms, and reimbursement rates. Because these are state-run agencies, each agency differs in how it operates. Gathering this information in person from the local vocational rehabilitation office may provide an opportunity to make personal contact with a referral source. Your state government Web site should have information on where these local offices are and how to make contact.

A related source of funding for vocationally relevant services is the Ticket to Work program funded by the Social Security Administration (SSA). This program offers persons with disabilities who receive SSA benefits funding and access to services to help them return to work and decrease their reliance on public benefits. The program was phased in to all 50 states during the period from 2002 to 2004. The "ticket" is a paper document that includes information about the person receiving services and is essentially a voucher that can be used to obtain funding for vocationally related services through state vocational rehabilitation agencies or employment networks. Employment Networks are private organizations or public agencies that agree to work with Social Security to provide services under the Ticket to Work program. More information on the Ticket to Work program is available at the program's Web site (*http://www.yourtickettowork.com/*), and information on other work incentives for persons with disabilities who are receiving Social Security benefits is available at the SSA Web site (*http://www.ssa.gov/*).

SELF-PAY

Another payment source to consider is out-of-pocket payment, which is sometimes referred to as "self-pay." More providers are making the decision to collect fees for services, and then the client or client's family can collect from their insurance company if able to do so. Trends in the use of alternative medicine, much of which has been paid for out of pocket, have demonstrated that people are willing to pay for something themselves if they think the benefits will be worth the cost (Wolsko, Eisenberg, Davis, Ettner, & Phillips, 2002). However, some clients would not be able to receive services if out-of-pocket payment was the only option. If you are considering moving to an out-of-pocket payment system, gathering data before making the decision would be crucial. How many of your current clients would continue if you switched to this method of payment? What would people be willing to pay for out of pocket? You must make sure you are able to articulate the value of your services and what people can expect when they foot the bill (Kimberg, 2004).

Legislation

AMERICANS WITH DISABILITIES ACT

In addition to legislation related to reimbursement, other laws are passed that directly affect our profession, our employers, and the people with whom we

work. The most relevant pieces of legislation are listed in Box 2–5. One example of civil rights legislation is the Americans with Disabilities Act (ADA) of 1990. This law built on the Rehabilitation Act of

---

Box 2–5: Key Legislation Affecting Occupational Therapy Practice and People with Disabilities

- **Americans with Disabilities Act (ADA):** Enacted in 1990. Provides for equal access for people with disabilities in employment, public transportation, private businesses, government services, and telecommunications.
- **Rehabilitation Act:** Enacted in 1973. Requires affirmative action hiring policies for federal agencies, nondiscrimination in hiring people with disabilities when the employer receives federal funding, and access to government buildings and services.
- **Individuals with Disabilities Education Act (IDEA):** Enacted in 1997; earlier version (Education for All Handicapped Children) passed in 1975. Provides for free and appropriate education for children with disabilities in the least restrictive environment. Includes requirements for the states to develop early intervention programs.
- **Health Insurance Portability and Accountability Act (HIPAA):** Enacted in 1996. Privacy rules require written consent before disclosing information and put restrictions on electronic data transmission.
- **Omnibus Budget Reconciliation Act (OBRA):** Enacted in 1987. Sets requirements to improve and monitor the quality of life of residents in long-term care centers. This requires that long-term care facilities assist residents in maintaining independence, living as full a life as possible, and being free from restraints whenever possible.

1973 and intended people with disabilities to have equal opportunity to participate fully in society. It has resulted in a number of changes in both physical and programmatic access for people with disabilities in the workplace, government buildings, community, and transportation arenas, although there is still much work to do. Managers should be familiar with this law because we are in a key position to provide education and resources to our clients, particularly people with newly acquired disabilities. Redick, McClain, and Brown (2000) found that, although 90% of the occupational therapists working in physical disabilities and home health who were surveyed thought it was important for therapists to know about the ADA and provide consumer education, the respondents had little knowledge of the provisions of the law. Only 44% had actually provided ADA education to clients, and less than half had referred clients to community resources or advocacy groups. Information on the ADA itself, accessible design standards, recent court cases, regional technical assistance centers, and the process for filing a complaint can be found on the Web site at *http://www.ada.gov/.*

The ADA may also affect how services are delivered at your setting. For example, the ADA specifies that all deaf patients have the right to interpreter services. New construction or renovation has requirements for bathroom accessibility, door width, height of drinking fountains, and availability of text telephones (TTYs). The ADA has guidelines regarding accommodations that employees or students can request (ADA&IT Technical Assistance Centers, 2002). An excellent resource for finding information on the ADA is the network of regional Disability and Business Technical Assistance Centers (DBTACs). These centers provide information, materials, technical assistance, and training on the ADA. In 2001, their responsibilities expanded to include providing those same services in the area of accessible information technology. This includes building accessible Web pages, assuring that distance learning programs are accessible, and assuring that technology purchases are those that are best able to work with assistive devices used by people with disabilities. Further information on DBTACs can be found at the ADA&IT Technical Assistance Web site (*http://www. adata.org/*).

How should a manager respond when a therapist with a hearing impairment requests a sign language interpreter for staff meetings? Is it reasonable for a therapist to request not to do transfers of patients over 120 pounds because of an old neck injury? Can you create a revenue source by screening job applicants for the hospital maintenance department to identify those who may be at risk for back injury? Consulting the ADA, accompanying resources, and technical assistance centers will provide the evidence you need to make legally sound decisions that also are consistent with your facility's policies. Published studies that report the outcomes and cost-benefit ratios of pre-employment screenings and environmental adaptation can be used to guide decision making in this area (Littleton, 2003).

Learning about the ADA or other new legislation may also be advantageous when considering consultation roles either as part of a practice or as a special area of practice. The 1999 Olmstead Decision, which requires that states provide community living options, has resulted in grants to aid states in moving people with disabilities from institutional care to community settings through the New Freedom Initiative (*http://www.cms.hhs.gov/ newfreedom/*). Occupational therapists and occupational therapy assistants have an important role to play in supporting this mandate (Cottrell, 2003). Other roles can include consulting with employers on reasonable accommodation requests and return-to-work issues, with architects on universal design and access guidelines, with planners on playground design and community access to public spaces, with attorneys on discrimination cases, and with local government regarding how to make programs accessible, particularly for persons with learning disabilities, intellectual disabilities, or other nonvisible impairments. The AOTA has a directory of specialists on their Web site (*http://www.aota.org/ featured/ area6/index.asp*), and members can be listed as specialists in ADA consultation and environmental modification, as well as a number of other areas, at no charge. Centers for Independent Living, which are run by people with disabilities, often provide ADA consultation and assist consumers with community access challenges. They exist in every state and can be located at *http://www.ilusa.com/ links/il-centers.htm.* Best practice in the area of ADA consultation is for therapists to partner with people with disabilities to provide a consumer as well as a professional perspective for clients.

INDIVIDUALS WITH DISABILITIES EDUCATION ACT

Another example of a piece of legislation that has had far-reaching effects is the Individuals with Disabilities Education Act (IDEA). Congress enacted the Education for All Handicapped Children Act (Public Law 94–142) in 1975 to support states and localities in protecting the rights of, meeting the individual needs of, and improving the results for infants, toddlers, children, and adolescents with disabilities and their families. This landmark law is currently enacted as the IDEA, as amended in 1997 (U.S. Department of Education, 2003). This law provides for a free and appropriate education for students with disabilities. If you work with children, you may get questions on the IDEA from patients/clients, family members, teachers, and other therapists. Understanding how occupational therapy fits within the larger educational system requires that you look beyond your immediate environment to understand the law that is responsible for the presence of occupational therapy in the schools. Checking the Web site (*http://www.ideapractices.org*) is the best way to get up-to-date information. Consulting AOTA official documents and networking with other managers can yield information on caseload, best practices, consultation roles, and billing practices. Publications also exist that provide evidence to support decision making regarding eligibility for occupational therapy, use of assessment data, and intervention models (Farley, Sarracino, & Howard, 1991; Muhlenhaupt, 2000). Conducting a literature search on billing practices in schools, for example, will provide information on the pros and cons of schools billing insurance or Medicaid for therapy services, as they are allowed to do.

The policy on billing at your local school district will influence expectations for documentation, goals, and the need for physician referral. Other evidence can be obtained from analyzing data on the number of children served under the IDEA in your district or region, the most common categories of disability classification used, the number of children receiving self-contained versus resource services, how many children have a one-on-one aide in the classroom, and so forth. As a manager, these data will help you to anticipate needs, have the appropriate number and type of personnel, and determine where and when your supervisory services will be most needed.

HEALTH INSURANCE PORTABILITY AND ACCOUNTABILITY ACT

Another example of legislation that is affecting practice is the Health Insurance Portability and Accountability Act (HIPAA) of 1996 (Jones, 2004). This legislation is regulatory in nature and is not tied to reimbursement or civil rights, although it does include statutes intended to protect the privacy rights of citizens in relation to "protected health information." *Protected health information* is defined under HIPAA regulations as

> "…*any information, whether oral or recorded in any form or medium that is created or received by a health care provider, health plan, public health authority, employer, life insurer, school or university, or health care clearinghouse and relates to the past, present, or future physical or mental health or condition of an individual; the provision of health care to an individual; or the past, present, or future payment for the provision of health care to an individual that could allow identification of an individual.*"

As a result of the HIPAA, managers have participated in facility-wide planning on implementing the patient privacy protections within their departments. This law has created some challenges because the electronic patient record has become the common mode of conveying information, and the protections are directly in reference to that. Private practices have had to develop their own privacy procedures that meet the intent of the law while keeping them simple enough for staff and patients to understand and interpret in a smaller setting (Jones, 2004).

IMPACT OF LEGISLATION ON PRACTICE

Determining the impact of legislation on access to services and practices may be helpful in guiding action in your own setting. The government conducts studies that provide oversight committees with information about the impact a law has had. For example, after the BBA was passed, the reduction of costs in home health agencies was much larger than expected, and a bill was passed to rescind some of the payment cuts. Often, papers are published about the impact of these statutes on our practice or the people we work with. The AOTA often sponsors position papers when a new law is enacted that affects our profession, such as the ADA. In addition, obtaining informal feedback from other places such as Listservs, directors groups, your state occupational therapy association, or associations in other states can be helpful.

Clinical Practice Requirements

When you are practicing in a particular setting, or contemplating practicing in that setting, learning the requirements for evaluation, documentation, treatment protocols, and discharge decision making is essential to survival. Each setting is unique, but there are common requirements that cross a number of settings. One good place to start your search for this information is with AOTA official documents such as position papers, standards for practice, or other documents that are written by AOTA representatives. Table 2–1 details the types of official documents available from the AOTA, and a full list of current official AOTA documents can be found at *http://www.aota.org/*.

Table 2-1	Types and Focus of AOTA Official Documents		
Type of Document	**Focus of Document**	**Example**	
Concept papers	Provide discussion of an issue or topic synthesizing different perspectives to assist reader in understanding in response to issues, concerns, or needs	"Service Delivery in Occupational Therapy" (1995)	
Guidelines	Present descriptions, examples, or recommendations of procedures related to the practice of occupational therapy	"Guidelines for Documentation of Occupational Therapy" (2003)	
Position papers	Present the official stance of the AOTA on substantive issues or subjects; for use within the profession or outside the profession	"Physical Agent Modalities: A Position Paper" (2003)	
Roles papers	Provide guides to major roles common in the profession of occupational therapy	"Roles and Responsibilities of the Occupational Therapist and the Occupational Therapy Assistant During the Delivery of Occupational Therapy Services" (2002)	
Specialized knowledge and skills papers	Provide detailed outline of specialized knowledge and skills needed for competent practice	"Specialized Knowledge and Skills for Feeding and Eating in Occupational Therapy Practice" (2000)	
Standards	Provide general descriptions of topics and define the minimum requirement for performance and quality	"Standards for Continuing Competence" (1999)	
Standards of practice	Define minimum requirements for performance and quality of care for services provided by occupational therapists and occupational therapy assistants	"Standards of Practice for Occupational Therapy" (1998)	
Statements	Describe and clarify an aspect or issue related to practice and are linked to the fundamental concepts of occupational therapy	"Applying Sensory Integration Framework in Educationally Related Occupational Therapy Practice" (2003)	

Adapted from the AOTA Web site (*http://www.aota.org*), 2004: Official Types of Documents.

The next place to look is guidelines from the payers in a particular setting. For example, in several settings, Medicare requires that data be collected and reported prior to reimbursement. In some settings, these data must also be collected on non-Medicare beneficiaries. These requirements minimally apply in SNFs and home health agencies. Table 2–2 provides a sample of settings in which Medicare reimbursement is prevalent, the system used by Medicare for reimbursement, required assessments used to gather data, and the implications for occupational therapy. Information on required assessments is also available in various manuals for different settings (e.g., SNF, inpatient rehabilitation facility) on the CMS Web site at *http://www.cms. hhs.gov/manuals/*.

Medicare and Medicaid typically have stringent requirements for initial, progress, and discharge documentation. This might include the initial jus-

tification for occupational therapy as a necessary skilled service, a monthly progress report, and a discharge summary. The CMS Web site is one useful source of information. Also, as mentioned earlier, contacting the Medicare contractor that pays the bills would be a good place to start. A list of these contractors by state can be found on the CMS Web site.

Managed care organizations may require that a clinical or critical pathway be followed as a quality assurance measure in medical settings. These pathways are typically established by the facility. For example, a clinical pathway may state that an occupational therapist should see a patient who will undergo hip replacement surgery the day before his or her surgery for patient education on precautions, and then evaluate his or her ability to apply these principles after surgery. A clinical pathway for an outpatient setting may involve a protocol for pa-

Table 2-2	**Medicare Payment Systems by Setting**			
	Hospital	Skilled Nursing Facility	Home Health Agency	Inpatient Rehabilitation
System Used to Determine Payment	Diagnosis-Related Groups (DRGs)	Resource Utilization Groups (RUGs)	Home Health Resource Group (HHRG)	Case Mix Groups (CMGs)
Criteria for Payment	Diagnosis and outliers (exceptions resulting from long or costly stay)	Level of intensity of nursing care and rehabilitation services needed	Mix of clinical and functional indicators and therapy need, paid for a 60-day period of service	CMG determined by Impairment Group Code and the Rehab Impairment Category, age, comorbidities, Functional Independence Measure motor and cognitive score
Evaluation Used	Medical diagnosis and secondary conditions	Minimum Data Set (MDS)	Outcomes and Assessment Information Set (OASIS)	Patient Assessment Instrument (Komives, 1991)
Implications for Occupational Therapy	Focus on early discharge, discharge planning, and prevention of readmission	Early assessment, deliver expected services, participate in MDS	Limited number of visits for all therapies combined, need to justify need for occupational therapy to other disciplines	Preadmission screening, work for maximal gain in the time provided, focus on functional gains, plan for discharge

Adapted from Centers for Medicare and Medicaid Services. (2004). Centers for Medicare and Medicaid Services Web site. Available at *http://www.cms.hhs.gov/*

tients who undergo carpal tunnel release and are covered under Workers' Compensation. This could include splinting, edema reduction, initiation of active movement, and follow-up ergonomic assessment of the workstation. It is essential that occupational therapy practitioners be at the table when these pathways are formulated, to ensure that our role is recognized and integrated within the care plan. Investigating the evidence to support occupational therapy involvement with patients with various diagnoses will prepare you for convincing others that occupational therapy intervention is a key component that should be included in the clinical pathway. Collecting ongoing outcome data for patients served will contribute to the body of knowledge and likelihood of occupational therapy being seen as an essential service.

In school system practice, there may be another set of expectations to follow regarding size of caseload, documentation, obtaining a physician prescription, and discharge guidelines. Some guidelines exist at the national and state levels, but many guidelines are formulated at the local district level (Carr, 1990). Each district, for example, may require different documentation of progress toward goals of the individualized education plan. One district may only require quarterly reports on goal attainment, whereas another may require therapists to complete a narrative note or a checklist after each occupational therapy session. Some districts bill insurance companies or Medicaid for therapy services (allowable by law after the 1997 amendments), and others do not. Another area of clinical practice that differs among school districts is their stance on how therapy services are to be delivered. Some districts support a consultation model, in which most of the occupational therapy services are delivered in the classroom or via consultation or training with teachers, assistants, and other staff. Other districts use a "pull-out" approach, in which the child receives therapy in a space outside of the classroom, and others may combine these approaches, depending on the needs of the child and the available space in the school. Some settings may use more group treatment, or work with the full class, and others use more individual treatment. Gathering evidence on the advantages, disadvantages, costs, and outcomes of these different models will assist you in implementing the approach that you determine meets the needs of the constituencies you serve.

Community agencies that are not medical in nature, such as day programs for seniors or mental health vocational centers, do not typically have the stringent requirements for assessment tools, documentation, and clinical practice as described previously. However, they might have internal protocols for progress measures and outcome evaluation, which are either mandated by the Commission on Accreditation of Rehabilitation Facilities or the prerogative of the agency. In these settings, you may wish to develop guidelines, protocols, and standards for intervention if they do not exist, and you are encouraged to use the strategies suggested throughout this book to make such guides based on the most current evidence.

Finally, you are encouraged to review studies and guidelines provided by other disciplines (e.g., knowledge related to occupational therapy practice but outside the occupational therapy domain) that may help you in developing services that meet commonly accepted expectations and that fit with other disciplines' services. For example, the fields of community psychology, physical therapy, special education, and nursing generate knowledge and documents of interest to and of use by occupational therapy practitioners.

Demographics

Planning new programs to address unmet needs, projecting revenue, and anticipating staffing requirements for the future require you to have knowledge about the population you serve. The processes of projecting revenue and staffing are described in Chapter 5, and the process of planning a new program is described in depth in Chapter 9. The type of data available to aid with these processes can range from national data sets to data collected in your own community or facility.

The U.S. Census, conducted every 10 years, provides a backdrop for other data more limited in scope. On the Web site of the U.S. Census Bureau (*http://www.census.gov/*), you can get access to all possible statistical data available from every subject for which the data were collected by the Census Bureau. The subject listings for which data are available are arranged in alphabetical order. The Web site provides links to national-level data on subjects such as disability, age groups, school enrollment, data on health care and social assistance, health insurance data, and occupation data. The figures presented within these data sets are mostly reported according to state or county.

Departments of public health of the state or city may also provide similar data, but on a state or local level. For example, the city of Chicago has 77 formally designated community areas and has developed Community Health Profiles on each area (Chicago Department of Public Health, 2004). These Community Health Profiles contain a mix of health status and health resource data. Each profile presents information for the specific community and, in some instances, comparable information for the city as a whole. In addition to a map that depicts the locations of health care facilities, each community profile includes

- Census statistics
- Estimated primary care capacity and utilization
- Health care resources
- Hospital capacity and utilization data
- Hospitalizations for ambulatory care–sensitive conditions
- Leading causes of death
- Leading causes of hospitalization
- Maternal and child health indicators
- Where residents obtain hospital care

These data allow you to compare your local population with the population in this area, and to look for trends over time. Other valuable data may include percentages of residents in your state who are covered by insurance, Medicare, and Medicaid. You can also find that information on the U.S. Census Bureau Web site.

Patterns of health care utilization by various subgroups have been analyzed in the literature, and such patterns are another example of demographic data you might find useful. For example, people without insurance tend to delay seeking primary care, and have more difficulty obtaining medical care than those who have insurance (Kasper, Giovannini, & Hoffman, 2000). This would also apply to uninsured individuals who delay in seeking a therapy evaluation or treatment out of concern that they will not be able to pay for it. Being knowledgeable about your potential market may indicate that outreach efforts to the uninsured population who might be eligible for government-funded health coverage are needed. Data on the number of

children served by EI programs or in the schools, their diagnoses, and length of treatment can also be helpful to compare local practices with state or federal patterns. This information may not routinely be published publicly, and you may have to be creative in obtaining it through methods such as developing personal contacts at organizations that might collect this information and be willing and able to share it with you. Another example of thinking creatively about finding and using statistical information to describe unmet needs might be using data on geographic distributions of providers to make an assertion that the absence or low percentage of providers in a geographic area indicates lower levels or absence of service. Table 2–3 lists examples of types of demographic data you might want to obtain, the geographic level to which the data refer, and places you might look to find the data.

Data, Information, and Other Forms of Evidence on Unmet Needs

Another type of evidence relevant to program planning is data about unmet needs. This information is obtained from a variety of sources, many informal and locally determined. You may need to gather much of this evidence yourself, in addition to accessing public information and relevant literature. (See Chapter 9 for a discussion of assessing needs in the process of developing evidence-based programs.) For example, when considering planning a new program or expanding an existing program, information must be gathered to ascertain need and also to identify other providers that are already involved in delivering services to meet that need. This information is needed to make a well-informed decision before proposing a new program or an expansion of an existing program, and assists in presenting the rationale for the new program. Box 2–6 summarizes different information-gathering strategies.

Comprehensive data gathering can provide the evidence you need to develop an effective and convincing business plan or program proposal to provide new services. During this process, you might ask potential clients to share their needs and desires

Table 2-3	Examples of Demographic Data and Where You Would Find It	
Information You Want	**Geographic Area**	**Where to Look**
Information about population by age, sex, race/ethnicity, socioeconomic status, disability status, education level, literacy level	• Nationwide • State • County • Local community	• U.S. Census Bureau Web site: has breakdowns for all levels, including a fact sheet on every local community, state, and county • Local departments of public health: vital statistics track demographic data
Causes of death, prevalence of illness or accidents	• Nationwide • State • County	• Centers for Disease Control and Prevention, National Center for Health Statistics • Vital and health statistics from the county or local government
Utilization of health services	• Nationwide • State • County • City	• National Center for Health Statistics • Vital statistics from state, county, or city health departments
Prevalence and description of a specific population, such as older adults or children in special education	• Local community • Nationwide	• Local department on aging • U.S. Department of Education, and national foundations or nonprofit organizations
Health trends	• National • State	• National Center for Health Statistics • Private foundations • Agency for Healthcare Research and Quality, U.S. Department of Health and Human Services

for services that are not available or not offered at convenient times or locations. They can also share their past or current experience with similar programs or services, and their frustrations and satisfaction with these services. You can ask about the likelihood that they would participate in the program you are trying to develop, explore the reasons why they would or would not participate, and iden-

---

Box 2–6: Strategies for Gathering Information About Unmet Needs

- **Key Informant Interview:** A one-on-one interview with individuals who have important information to share, such as decision makers, administrators, government officials, clients (current or potential service users), other providers, funding sources, or researchers.
- **Focus Group:** A 60- to 90-minute group interview of six to eight people to provide an in-depth exploration of needs, issues, and recommendations.
- **Written or Telephone Survey:** A survey of individuals, such as current clients, potential service users, referral services, and funding sources, about unmet needs and potential use of your services. Can include rating items on a scale and/or open-ended questions.

tify potential barriers such as transportation, financial limitations, family obligations, and language barriers.

Locating existing or planned programs in the area you are considering for expansion is another element in creating a comprehensive business plan. This includes identifying current programs that are provided by hospitals, social service agencies, outpatient centers, government agencies, health departments, and private agencies. This type of information can be found in local telephone directories or online listings, as well as the local newspaper. Another option may be to ask potential referral sources where they are currently referring clients for this service, and if they would refer clients to your facility if a program were available there. Once the relevant service providers are determined, you can visit them online or in person, gathering brochures and program information. There may be reluctance on the part of potential local competitors to provide information about the successes or challenges of their programs, but others with similar programs outside of your geographic area may be more willing to share information and collaborate.

Data about the community in which the proposed program will operate are helpful in determining needs and desired services. This could include information on well-respected institutions and organizations in the community, transportation systems, Internet and library access, social service agencies, and city and state government services. Data on local grants available to help with development of programs or delivery of services to your target population may also be available. This information can often be found by searching the Internet, reviewing Chamber of Commerce materials, or checking in local service directories.

Once the data-gathering phase is complete, the data, information, and evidence must be organized to form a convincing argument in the form of a business plan or program proposal (see Chapter 12). You can analyze the convergence of need, resources, and impetus for change with your desires, talents, and skills and those of key staff who would be involved. You can then identify factors you have uncovered that will be a positive influence on your planned intervention and plan how to maximize them, and identify potential barriers or negative influences and plan how to address them. This is the

foundation for developing a business plan and a marketing plan. The plan should build in methods of ongoing program evaluation and feedback loops for continuing to revise and improve your program, and you should include your key informants and service recipients in this process.

Gathering data, information, and other forms of evidence to support the need for program development and implementation is not always easy and sometimes requires creativity and perseverance. In some cases, information such as incidence, prevalence, and existing levels of service delivery may be found at national, state, and local levels relatively easily. For example, the Centers for Disease Control and Prevention (CDC) produces twice-yearly "AIDS Surveillance Reports" that provide incidence and prevalence data for human immunodeficiency virus/acquired immunodeficiency syndrome (HIV/AIDS) by age, gender, and race on a national and state level as well as for major metropolitan areas (http://www.cdc.gov/hiv/stats/hasrlink.htm). This can be combined with similar information that can be obtained from most city departments of public health. Further, by contacting local agencies such as community health centers or agencies that provide housing specifically for persons living with HIV/AIDS, you can obtain information about the needs of this population and services being provided. (See Chapter 9 for a full description of the process of gathering information for program development of an independent living and vocational preparation program for this population.) Additionally, information on funding for services for persons living with HIV/AIDS can be found on both government and nonprofit organization Web sites (e.g., that of the National AIDS Fund, available at http://www.aidsfund.org/). Although it is relatively accessible, you should not underestimate the time it takes to gather this sort of information. Gathering current and comprehensive data from multiple sites may take several hours or more of time.

In other instances it may be much more difficult to gather information related to the numbers of persons who have a condition, the nature of the condition, and the existing level of service delivery. Consider the following example. Let's assume you want to develop an EI program to serve children 3 years and under who are at high risk for developmental delay by providing developmental screenings, parent education, and group motor development classes. You know you need to conduct a critical review of empirical literature to justify the *effectiveness* of early intervention, but what other forms of data, information, and evidence do you need? You live in Seattle, Washington, and you assume you can use national, state, and local data to support your case. Where can you look to get information on the prevalence of premature infants, incidence of certain common diagnoses, and trends in service needs for this group, and how accessible is this information? The following case example demonstrates the initial steps of gathering data, information, and other forms of evidence to support the development of such a program.

Case Example: Gathering Data, Information, and Other Forms of Evidence to Justify Development of an Early Intervention Program

As a first step, you might conduct an Internet search using the terms "Seattle" and "early intervention" (a search for this example was conducted in April of 2004 using the MSN Web site). This search reveals a number of general Web sites on EI that provide statistics on the benefits of EI and on its cost-effectiveness.

In addition, your search reveals a number of sources, including the Infant Toddler Early Intervention Program (ITEIP) located within the Department of Social and Health Services for Washington State (*http://www1.dshs.wa.gov/iteip/sicc5a.html*). This program provides EI services, including family resources coordination, for eligible children from birth to age 3 years and their families. Although the Web site for the ITEIP provides information for consumers on accessing services, it provides only limited information on the extent of the need for these services. You do find an EI fact sheet that indicates that, during a 1-year period from October 2002 to September 2003, 6506 children were served, and the statistic that, during 2001–2002, there was a 14.4% increase in EI caseloads in Washington State (*http://www1.dshs.wa.gov/iteip/Publications.html*). Additionally, you find references (although somewhat old) to the cost-effectiveness of EI. This indicates that finding more current information on cost-effectiveness might strengthen your case for starting an EI program.

As you continue to review the results of your initial Internet search, you find a 2002 report from the Washington State Department of Public Health titled "The Health of Washington State" that includes a section on children with special health care needs (Washington State Department of Public Health,

2002). This report states that 17% of Washington's children have been identified as having a special health care need. Using this statistic and the birth rate in Seattle, you can estimate the number of children born in Seattle who will have a special health care need. As noted, not all information is easy to find. In this case you might find that, after several hours of searching, you are still not able to locate the number of live births in Seattle. After finally phoning the Seattle and King County Department of Public Health and leaving several messages, you receive a return call from a helpful Department of Public Health employee who informs you that, for the period of 2000–2003, there was an average of 6270 live births in Seattle (Ann Glusker, personal communication, April 23, 2004). You are now able to estimate that more than 1000 of the children born each year in Seattle will have a special health care need. Unfortunately, you note that, based on your initial search, it was very difficult to find specific information on the extent of the need for EI services, although several of the reports that you have reviewed cite intervention for children (especially those of lower socioeconomic status) as a priority for the coming decade.

If you expanded your search to target other data sources on state and national need for EI to further strengthen your argument, you might identify several sources. These would include

- The National Center on Birth Defects and Developmental Disabilities within the CDC (*http://www.cdc.gov/ncbddd/dd/default.htm*), which cites the national prevalence rates of developmental disabilities at an estimated 17% of U.S. children

(continued)

Case Example: Gathering Data, Information, and Other Forms of Evidence to Justify Development of an Early Intervention Program (Continued)

under the age of 18 years. You also get information that the state and federal education departments spend about $36 billion each year on special education programs for individuals with developmental disabilities who are 3 to 21 years old.

- The KIDS COUNT project Web site (*http://www.aecf.org/kidscount/kc1999/*), which reports that there has been an increase in low birth weight babies from 7% in 1990 to 7.5% in 1997. This resource also provides information that the prevalence of low birth weight babies in the state of Washington is 5.6%.
- The U.S. Census Bureau (*http://www.census.gov/main/www/subjects.html*), which reports that 6.1% of the total population in King County/Seattle is children below 5 years of age.
- The Childstats.gov Web site (*http://www.childstats.gov/*), which indicates that 8% of children ages 5 to 17 years have limitations in activity due to chronic conditions. Although you are interested in the birth to age 3 population, this suggests that adding information on the value of prevention will strengthen your argument.
- The CDC Web site, on which, in the A-to-Z index, you find a section called Child Health Statistics where you find the report "Summary Health Statistics for U.S. Children: National Health Interview Survey, 2002" (*http://www.cdc.gov/nchs/data/series/sr_10/sr10_221.pdf*). This report highlights that 5 million children nationwide ages 3 to 17 years have a learning disability.

After several hours of searching, you find that you still do not have a completely cogent argument for starting your program, because you are not yet able to make a comparison between the need for services and the level of existing services. However, you do find that you have made some progress and have several new ideas about information you are going to seek to strengthen your argument. Most importantly, as you have conducted your search, you have identified some valuable resources that may help you in the future. For example, you find that the University of California at San Francisco Disability Statistics Center has a very helpful Web site, Finding Disability Data on the Web (*http://dsc.ucsf.edu/main.php?name=finding_data*). This site explains various types of data sets that are available and how to find data that you need. A second resource that you find on the state of Washington ITEIP Website is an ITEIP Marketing and Outreach Kit. Although this resource does not help you justify the need for your EI program, it will be of great assistance in promoting your program if you are successful in starting it.

Your work is not over yet, but it is important not to become discouraged. Perhaps by thinking of your proposal as a puzzle, and the search as the process of finding the right pieces, you can even have fun gathering the remaining data you need! Other local resources, such as the Seattle school system, your state occupational therapy association (*http://www.wota.org/*), or your peers who provide similar services within Washington State or nationwide, may be of assistance in helping you find the specific information you need to complete your argument for starting an EI program.

 ## Data, Information, and Other Forms of Evidence on Personnel

In the personnel domain, there are several sources of data that will assist with well-informed decision making and more accurate forecasting of the need for and availability of new staff, as well as information about salaries. The U.S. Department of Labor, Bureau of Labor Statistics (BLS), compiles forecast information on a wide variety of fields every 2 years. It projects job demand and future trends, and also reports salary trends. For example, in its employment estimates for 2002 and projections to 2012, the BLS projected modest growth in occupational therapy positions, with employment projected to increase faster than average (21% to 35%

job growth). The BLS reported that demand should continue to rise because of increasing numbers of children and middle-aged and elderly persons needing services. It projected much faster than average growth (36% or more job growth) in occupational therapy assistant positions (U.S. Department of Labor, 2002).

Every few years, the AOTA completes a survey of occupational therapy practitioners. The results of the survey are available for purchase, and excerpts from the data are often available on the AOTA Web site or in AOTA publications such as *OT Practice*. Typical information includes annual salary, often broken down by state or region and number of years of practice in a given work setting, hours worked per week, and degree level. For example, the report indicates that 31% of respondents work part-time, and 20% of occupational therapists and occupational therapy assistants work for more than one employer (AOTA, 2000). This information could be valuable when planning staffing that utilizes part-time employees.

Data on the supply of new graduates may be important to the organizations that hire them. The National Board for Certification in Occupational Therapy (NBCOT) and the AOTA have recently sounded the alarm that there will be fewer new graduates entering the field in the next few years as enrollment drops result in fewer occupational therapist and occupational therapy assistant candidates taking the certification exam. The NBCOT reported in 2004 that there had been a 75% drop in the number of occupational therapy assistant candidates taking the examination over the period from 1998 to 2003, and a 39% decrease in occupational therapy candidates taking the examination during the period from 2000 to 2003 (NBCOT, 2004a, 2004b). Publications that examine workforce trends are available, and current data can be obtained from relevant sources (Fisher & Cooksey, 2002). Time trend data, which compare the number of new graduates who pass the exam over time, are available from the NBCOT Web site (*http://www.nbcot.org/*), and the total number of enrolled students is available to AOTA members in the Education Resources section of the AOTA Web site (*http://www.aota.org/members/area9/docs/ed03. pdf*). On reviewing the AOTA Web site, you will find that some areas and documents such as that just cited are limited to viewing by members only, a benefit of being a member of your professional association. Graduate data over time by state are also available from the American Medical Association's *Health Professions Education Databook* (American Medical Association, 2005).

Determining if there will be a shortage or surplus of desired personnel can assist you in determining appropriate starting salaries, salary increases, the appropriateness of the use of sign-on bonuses or other recruitment incentives, and the mix of occupational therapists and occupational therapy assistants that is most desirable and most feasible to attain. Student fieldwork programs often provide a supply of potential new graduate hires, and should be seen as a recruitment strategy during phases of increased job demand and/or decreased supply of practitioners. Obtaining data on graduates from local universities and colleges may also assist you in planning for personnel needs, and will guide you in how aggressive you need to be in mounting a recruitment campaign.

Monitoring the practice patterns of occupational therapy practitioners may also provide useful information for decision making. For example, the AOTA 2000 Salary Survey demonstrated a significant decrease in the percentage of occupational therapists and occupational therapy assistants employed by SNFs. At the same time, the percentage of occupational therapists and occupational therapy assistants employed in schools and EI programs was rising (AOTA, 2000). Table 2–4 shows the percentages of occupational therapists and occupational therapy assistants employed by setting and tracks changes in employment setting over time for the period 1982 to 2000.

Licensure and Certification

Understanding requirements for professional licensure and certification is critical when planning programs, especially if your programming will be provided in more than one state. Professional certification for both occupational therapists and occupational therapy assistants requires completion of an educational degree from an accredited program and passing the certification exam administered by the NBCOT. That examination provides initial certification for a period of 3 years. After that point, in

Table 2-4	National Employment Settings for Occupational Therapists and Occupational Therapy Assistants, 1982 to 2000							
	Occupational Therapists (%)				Occupational Therapy Assistants (%)			
Setting	1982	1990	1998	2000	1982	1990	1998	2000
General hospital	36	35	24	25	27	27	18	14
Skilled nursing facility, long-term care facility	10	9	23	13	23	20	46	38
Mental health facility	10	9	4	5	13	12	4	5
Home health agency	4	4	6	7	1	2	3	2
Private practice	4	8	6	5	1	3	1	5
Outpatient, physician's office	3	5	5	6	2	3	2	4
School system, early intervention program	18	19	22	29	11	17	17	26
Community-based	2	1	2	1	13	12	2	2
Academic	5	4	6	6	2	1	2	3
Other	9	6	2	3	8	3	2	1

Data from American Occupational Therapy Association. (2000). *Member compensation survey.* Bethesda, MD: American Occupational Therapy Association.

order to maintain the right to use the Occupational Therapist, Registered (OTR) and Certified Occupational Therapy Assistant (COTA) designations, practitioners must complete requirements for continuing competence. Recertification must be completed every 3 years if one desires to maintain the OTR and COTA designations. A variety of activities can meet this requirement, including formal continuing education, mentorship, fieldwork student supervision, and research (NBCOT, 2004c).

As of 2002, all states regulated the practice of occupational therapy. As of 2004, for occupational therapists, 46 states had licensure laws, 2 had registration laws, 1 had a certification law, and 1 had a trademark law. For occupational therapy assistants, 46 states had some type of regulation, including 43 states with licensure laws, 1 with a registration law, and 2 with certification laws; 4 states did not regulate occupational therapy assistants. Box 2–7 defines each of these types of regulation.

The laws that govern occupational therapy practice vary considerably from state to state, so it is important for you to be familiar with the regulation in your state and neighboring states. Box 2–8 shows the different components that may be addressed by a licensure or practice act. If you or one of your supervisees does not follow the requirements for

physician referral, supervision, documentation, signature, provisional license, or continuing competence, penalties may be invoked that range from verbal or written warning to loss of license. Not being familiar with the licensure requirements in your area is not an adequate excuse, because this is a law all occupational therapy professionals are expected to know and follow.

Imagine that you have just accepted a management position in another state. How do you find out whether the state has a practice act/licensure law, and what you need to do to apply? Once you begin your new position, can you hire a new graduate before he or she passes the NBCOT exam? Do you need a physician referral in order to initiate intervention? What is the minimum supervision time that occupational therapy assistants are required to have? The AOTA Web site's licensure section has all of the answers in database format and downloadable reports (AOTA, 2004). Table 2–5 presents a comparison of the answers to these questions from the AOTA database for two neighboring states, Mississippi and Alabama (as of April 2004; this information is subject to change). You should note how variable these components are, and recognize that they may change over time because they are determined by legislation passed by each state.

Box 2–7: **Types of Practice Regulations**

- **Licensure:** Provides highest level of public protection by prohibiting unlicensed individuals from practicing occupational therapy or referring to themselves as occupational therapists/occupational therapy assistants. Licensure laws reserve a certain scope of practice for those who are issued a license.
- **Mandatory Certification:** Protects the public by prohibiting uncertified persons from referring to themselves as occupational therapists/occupational therapy assistants. Unlike licensure, individuals under certain circumstances can practice if they do not refer to their services as occupational therapy. Certification laws may provide for a definition of occupational therapy.
- **Mandatory Registration:** Protects the public by prohibiting unregistered persons from referring to themselves as occupational therapists/occupational therapy assistants, although they can practice if they do not refer to their services as occupational therapy. Registration laws may provide for a definition of occupational therapy.
- **Trademark or Title Control Legislation:** Prohibits individuals who have not met specific education and entry-level examination requirements from referring to themselves as occupational therapists/occupational therapy assistants, although they can practice under certain circumstances if they do not refer to their services as occupational therapy.

Box 2–8: **Common Components of Practice Acts**

- **Scope of Practice:** Defines the domain of occupational therapy, such as defining the roles of occupational therapists and occupational therapy assistants. May include specifics such as orthotics, physical agent modalities, activities of daily living intervention, and environmental modification, or may be more general in nature.
- **Referral Requirements:** Specify if a physician referral is necessary for evaluation and/or treatment.
- **Temporary License/Work Permit:** Defines the process for unlicensed personnel to obtain permission to work while waiting for their licenses.
- **Continuing Competence:** Specifies the requirements for continuing education and other means to demonstrate continuing competence.
- **Occupational Therapy Assistant Supervision Requirements:** Define what type of supervision is required for occupational therapy assistants, including amount of time, frequency, and documentation requirements.

Trend Data and Future Forecasts

In addition to uncovering evidence from all of the previously described areas, it is important to anticipate upcoming trends and changes to be prepared for the future. In fact, a keen awareness of these trends allows you to *shape* the future, because you are able to position your department in front of the pack in addressing emerging needs. It is your responsibility as a manager to constantly scan the environment for information on emerging trends and ways of thinking about practice and health systems. There are numerous places to look for this information, both within and outside the field. For example, the "Presidential Address" delivered by the president of the AOTA at the association's annual conference often addresses future directions of the profession (Kornblau, 2004). Other fields and disciplines often have similar forums, and because such addresses are typically published in the professional literature, they are easily accessible. Keeping abreast of AOTA Executive Board and Representative Assembly decisions via the AOTA Web site is also a key strategy. A good tool for keeping up with the

Table 2-5	Comparison of Two States' Practice Act Regulations		
Component of Act	Mississippi	Alabama
Referral requirement	Physician referral not necessary	Physician, chiropractor, dentist, or optometrist referral necessary with annual confirmation of the diagnosis. Referral not required to provide services to people with educationally related needs.
Temporary license/permit	Limited permit provided until the exam scores are received, allowed to renew one time if exam is not passed	Temporary permit until the exam scores are received; if the exam is not passed, the permit is revoked.
Continuing education requirement	20 contact hours every 2 years	30 contact hours every 2 years.
Supervision of occupational therapy assistants	Occupational therapist must be available by phone; joint supervisory patient visit every 7 treatment days or 21 calendar days	5% of occupational therapy assistant work hours per month must be spent in one-to-one supervision with an occupational therapist

Adapted from the AOTA Web site (http://www.aota.org); licensure information adapted from state occupational therapy statutes and regulations, as of 2004.

latest developments in health care, financing, and legislation is using Internet services that screen news headlines for the topics you are most interested in, and then send you the relevant headlines and links to full text. The *New York Times* offers such a service at *http://www.nytimes.com/*. Another option is to scan an Internet site that lists headlines from health care–related articles that appear in newspapers around the country, such as the Yahoo.com full-coverage news on health-related topics, including health care, available at *http://www.yahoo.com/health/*. Some private resources, including health-related foundations, track changes in health care trends over time. An example of such a foundation is the Robert Wood Johnson Foundation (*http://www.rwjf.org/*). Other relevant literature includes Healthy People 2010 and subsequent versions, a compendium of desired health outcomes to be achieved by the target year (U.S. Department of Health and Human Services, 2004). Also, literature on emerging disabilities will be relevant. This includes studies of disability prevalence and changes over time, future projections on demographic changes and how they will impact the need for

health services, and new areas on the horizon that are "hot." Reading occupational therapy literature about new program models and innovative service delivery is also recommended (Starnes, 2000).

Chapter Summary

This chapter described the complex "system" of health care and other service delivery systems in which occupational therapy practitioners work. The dualistic health care system was described, and you were introduced to basic free-market economic principles and learned how they can only be applied to the health care market in limited ways. These concepts included supply and demand, competition, and free choice.

In Chapter 1, you were introduced to a range of types of evidence, and in this chapter you were further encouraged to consider a broad range of data, information, and other forms of evidence beyond the results of empirical investigations. You learned that strategies commonly used in research can also be used to gather these other types of evidence that are useful in planning and justifying occupational therapy programming. Evidence may be gathered on reimbursement and the payment practices of specific sources of reimbursement (Medicare, Medicaid, Workers' Compensation, out-of-pocket, and SSA), legislation, clinical practice requirements, demographics, personnel, and licensure/certification requirements. Perhaps most importantly, this chapter demonstrated a range of strategies for finding data, information, and other forms of evidence, some of which is readily accessible and some of which must be found through creativity and perseverance.

At the beginning of the chapter you were introduced to Andrea, who had accepted a new job as the sole occupational therapist in a rural health facility. Andrea used the information presented in this chapter to develop occupational therapy services at her facility.

Resources For Learning More About Health Care Systems and Practice Contexts

Journals That Often Publish Articles Related to Health care Systems and Practice Contexts

HEALTH AFFAIRS: THE POLICY JOURNAL OF THE HEALTH SPHERE

Health Affairs is a bimonthly, peer-reviewed journal that explores health policy issues of current concern in both domestic and international spheres.

HEALTHCARE FINANCING REVIEW

The *Healthcare Financing Review* is available through subscription from the Centers for Medicare and Medicaid Services (CMS). Readers who wish to

Real-Life Solutions

Andrea decided to begin by learning about the larger system issues by researching reimbursement sources, determining which of the patient populations at her facility were covered, what sort of occupational therapy interventions were covered, the reimbursement rates, and the requirements for referral and documentation. She consulted with the AOTA and obtained resources on determining charges and reimbursement, and obtained copies of key documents produced by the association to help guide her practice and to give credence to services as she presented them to other managers in the facility.

Despite the fact that she was initially intimidated, Andrea made contact with her Medicare contractor and obtained copies of relevant guidelines for outpatient occupational therapy under Medicare. She also began to network with her peers in her city and state, and across the country through Listservs and Internet discussion boards, to learn more about Medicare reimbursement. Further, Andrea began to plan for a needs assessment, which would include an analysis of local demographics and illness/injury patterns, socioeconomic status, risk factors, and services currently available. She sought

reference materials on developing surveys and other tools to collect information from payers and consumers.

The ADA Web site furnished specifics on providing accessible parking, elevators, and signage, as well as funding available for adapting the workplace for employees with disabilities. At first it seemed overwhelming that so much information was available, but soon Andrea began to feel more proficient at searching the Internet to take advantage of the many resources available, including the Web sites of government agencies at the national, state, county, and local levels, as well as those for private foundations.

Andrea also contacted the state regulatory agency and investigated the requirements for supervision of occupational therapy assistants and recently graduated occupational therapists. She knew she would be hiring another therapy practitioner in the near future, because the evidence pointed to significant unmet needs and the potential to build a successful occupational therapy practice in a rural context. Andrea was sure that the skills she was acquiring in finding and evaluating data, information, and other forms of evidence would support her efforts.

gain an improved understanding of the Medicare and Medicaid programs and the U.S. health care system will find this a helpful resource. In addition to policy-relevant research, published articles present varied perspectives on issues including health care policy, and the planning and delivery of health care services. Articles include analyses on a broad range of health care financing and delivery issues and promote discussion and debate from a diverse audience that includes policymakers, planners, administrators, insurers, researchers, and health care providers. The *Review* appears quarterly, with an additional statistical supplement issue every year.

JOURNAL OF PUBLIC HEALTH POLICY

The *Journal of Public Health Policy* publishes scholarly articles on the epidemiologic and social foundations of public health policy. Results of empirical research related to the development of public health policy as well as the implementation of such policy are included.

HEALTH SERVICES RESEARCH

Health Services Research provides researchers, policy makers and analysts, and health care administrators and managers with access to empirical findings as well as articles addressing policy and methodological issues. Readers interested in health care financing, the organization or delivery of health services, or in the evaluation of health delivery outcomes will find *Health Services Research* a useful resource. The journal provides a forum for the exchange of practices related individuals, health systems, and communities.

Professional Associations Concerned With Health Care Systems and Practice Contexts

AMERICAN HEALTHCARE ASSOCIATION

http://www.ahca.org/index.html
    The American Healthcare Association (AHCA) is a nonprofit association of state health organizations. Member organizations include both nonprofit and for-profit organizations representing the areas of assisted living, nursing facility, developmentally disabled, and subacute care providers. The AHCA represents the long-term care community to the general public as well as the federal and state governments and business leaders. In addition to other functions, the AHCA serves a role as an ad-

vocate for change within the long-term care field. The association provides members and the public with information, educational resources and tools to improve the delivery of quality care.

AMERICAN PUBLIC HEALTH ASSOCIATION

http://www.apha.org/
    The American Public Health Association (APHA) provides a forum for health researchers, health service providers, administrators, teachers, and other health workers to interact and to exchange ideas and varied perspectives. In addition, the APHA is concerned with a variety of societal and health care system issues. Among others the APHA identifies issues of interest such as federal and state funding for health programs, pollution control programs, and policies related to chronic and infectious diseases, a smoke-free society, and professional education in public health.

Web Site Resource List

VOCATIONAL REHABILITATION STATE OFFICES

http://www.jan.wvu.edu/sbses/vocrehab.htm
    This Web page contains information about and links to vocational rehabilitation state offices.

U.S. CENSUS BUREAU

http://www.census.gov/main/www/subjects.html
    This Web page is a comprehensive index to data available from the U.S. Census Bureau Web site. It provides access to all possible statistical data available from every subject for which the data were collected by the U.S. Census Bureau. The subjects about which the data are available are arranged in alphabetical order. The page provides links to national-level data on subjects such as disability, age groups, economic census data on health care and social assistance, health insurance data, and occupation data. The data presented are mostly organized at state levels.

CENTERS FOR DISEASE CONTROL AND PREVENTION

- National Center for Health Statistics (*http://www. cdc.gov/nchs/about.htm*)
- Diseases and Conditions Section (*http://www. cdc.gov/node.do/id/0900f3ec8000e035*)
- Publications (*http://www.cdc.gov/nchs/hus.htm*)

    The CDC home page has a section on diseases and conditions with an A-to-Z listing. Although the list omits some common diagnoses, such as Alzheimer's disease, each listed condition has a Web page that may include a fact sheet, relevant Web site links, publications, and/or information about prevalence of certain conditions across the United States.

The National Center for Health Statistics (NCHS) of the CDC is the United States' principal health statistics agency. The agency compiles statistical information on health-related issues. The Web site contains data from various national surveys on various health concerns that range from disability, nutrition, and hospice care to statistics on vital life events (births, deaths, marriages, infant mortality, etc.). The Web site also has links to many other government agencies, including state and local health departments and Web resources and publications, as well as software and products you can download or order.

The NCHS has several publications that provide background information about trends in health care needs and service utilization. For example, *Health, United States* is an annual report on national trends in health statistics. The 2003 report includes a highlights section, a chartbook, and 151 trend tables. This report and those of previous years are downloadable in .pdf format, and include summaries of key points as well as detailed breakdowns for population subgroups in a number of categories, such as income level, race/ethnicity, and age.

National Center on Birth Defects and Developmental Disabilities

http://www.cdc.gov/ncbddd/dd/default.htm

This agency is an important resource within the CDC that provides information and statistical data on the prevalence rates of developmental disabilities. The Web site also provides links to other resources such as the National Institute of Child Health and Human Development and the Administration for Children and Families, Administration on Developmental Disabilities.

Office of Disability Employment Policy, U.S. Department of Labor

http://www.dol.gov/odep/

The Office of Disability Employment Policy (ODEP) provides statistics on employed disabled persons, as well as the Workforce Investment Act of 1998 WIA 188 Disability Checklist. The Web site provides information on a wide range of issues related to disability and the workforce, including guidelines for implementation of the ADA and for return-to-work programs for workers who are injured, that is arranged in alphabetical order.

The National Organization on Disability

http://www.nod.org/

In cooperation with the Harris Poll, the National Organization on Disability (N.O.D.) provides timely survey research data on the participation of people with disabilities in American life. Recent information includes the 2000 N.O.D./Harris Survey of Americans with Disabilities, which covers the participation gaps between Americans with and without disabilities in 10 major life activities, and the 2000 N.O.D./Harris Survey of Community Participation, which focuses on people with disabilities and their involvement in community life. The Web site also provides links to other disability-related surveys and studies.

Centers for Medicare and Medicaid Services

http://cms.hhs.gov/researchers/

This Web page provides statistical data on Medicaid and Medicare, ranging from estimates of future Medicare and Medicaid spending to enrollment, spending, and claims data.

State Children's Health Insurance Program

http://www.cms.hhs.gov/schip/default.asp

This Web page, which can be accessed by linking from the CMS Web site, overviews the SCHIP program.

Insure Kids Now

http://www.insurekidsnow.gov/

This Web site is a U.S. Department of Health and Human Services site for consumers that provides links to the states' Web pages that describe the details about the SCHIP, including eligibility, services provided, and application procedures.

National Institutes of Health

http://www.nih.gov/

The National Institutes of Health Web site has health information for consumers, health news and events, media contacts (radio/video), grants and funding opportunities, and scientific resources (special interest groups, library catalogs, journals, research training and labs, statistical computing).

The Annie E. Casey Foundation

http://www.aecf.org/kidscount/kc1999/

KIDS COUNT, a project of the Annie E. Casey Foundation (AECF), provides national and state-by-state statistical data on the status of children in the United States. The Web site offers several interactive online databases that allow visitors to create free, customized data reports. It includes the ability to generate custom profiles, line graphs, maps, and rankings, and to download raw data. The following files from the KIDS COUNT 1999 Databook (in .pdf format) can also be downloaded from the site:

Profiles: Gives detailed information about a single state or the nation as a whole

Graphs: Presents state indicators graphed over time

Maps: Provides color-coded maps of the United States based on KIDS COUNT data

Rankings: Provides access to views of all 50 states, ranked according to an indicator

Raw Data: Provides the opportunity to download all of the KIDS COUNT data as Microsoft Excel files or comma-delimited files

Administration for Children and Families, U.S. Department of Health and Human Services

http://www.acf.hhs.gov/news/stats/index.html

This Web page provides statistical data highlights on child care, child support, child welfare, the Head Start program, refugees, and welfare.

Administration on Aging

http://www.aoa.dhhs.gov/prof/Statistics/statistics.asp

This web page provides statistical data on older adults along different dimensions, including indicators of well-being, disabilities data, and 2000 census data on aging.

Bureau of Labor Statistics, U.S. Department of Labor, and Occupational Safety and Health Administration

http://www.osha.gov/oshstats/work.html

This Web page contains Occupational Safety and Health Administration (OSHA) workplace injury and illness statistics, including data on in-jury/illness incidence rates; state occupational injuries, illnesses, and fatalities; and injury and illness characteristics.

American Hospital Directory

http://www.ahd.com/

The American Hospital Directory Web site provides online data for more than 6000 hospitals. Its database of information is built from Medicare claims data, cost reports, and other public use files obtained from the CMS. The data also include annual survey data from the American Hospital Association. Detailed information is available for subscribers.

General Accounting Office

http://www.gao.gov/

This Web site contains reports of health care disparities among ethnic groups and by gender, SSA disability decision-making data, and the like.

Centers for Independent Living

http://www.ilusa.com/links/ilcenters.htm

This Web page contains a listing of Centers for Independent Living, organized by state. These centers are run by people with disabilities and typically provide advocacy, peer counseling, information and referral, and community education.

Healthy People 2010

http://www.health.gov/healthypeople/

The Healthy People 2010 home page has new objectives from the January 2000 "Partnerships for Health in the New Millennium" Conference. Visitors can view broadcast sessions or the full text of the conference online.

Office of Minority Health Resource Center

http://www.omhrc.gov

The Office of Minority Health Resource Center Web site has health information and statistics on various ethnic populations (Asian-American, African-American, Hispanic, Native-American, etc.), health brochures and videos in various languages (covering topics such as diabetes, teen pregnancy, and hypertension), publications (*Closing the Gap*), funding resources, and a network of resource people to contact.

USA Counties 1998 (U.S. Census Bureau)

http://www.census.gov/statab/www/county.html

This reference Web page from the U.S. Census Bureau contains data (e.g., vital statistics, health) covering all 3142 counties in the United States. Many items provide several years of data. Sources include the Census Bureau, other government agencies, and private organizations. The Web page also provides links to other statistical references available from the U.S. Census Bureau.

Geospatial and Statistical Data Center, University of Virginia Library

http://fisher.lib.virginia.edu/collections/stats/ccdb/

This resource provides Internet access to the electronic versions of the 1988, 1994, and 2000 County and City Data Books. Some items that are covered include health, vital statistics, and demographics. This service provides the opportunity to create custom printouts and/or customized data subsets.

Reference List

ADA&IT Technical Assistance Centers. (2002). Structure of the ADA. ADA & IT Technical Assistance Centers Website. Available at *http://www.adata.org/whatsada-structure. html*

American Medical Association. (2005). *Health professions career and education directory.* Chicago: American Medical Association Press.

American Occupational Therapy Association. (2000). *Member Compensation Survey.* Bethesda, MD: American Occupational Therapy Association.

American Occupational Therapy Association. (2004). State occupational therapy statutes and regulations. American Occupational Therapy Association Web site. Available at *http://www.aota.org/members/area4/links/link12.asp?PLACE =/members/area4/links/LINK12.asp*

Carr, S. H. (1990). State guidelines for school-based occupational therapy: 1989 survey. *American Journal of Occupational Therapy, 44,* 755–757.

Centers for Medicare and Medicaid Services. (2004). Centers for Medicare and Medicaid Services Web site. Available at *http://www.cms.hhs.gov/*

Chicago Department of Public Health. (2004). Community health profiles. City of Chicago Department of Public Health Web site. Available at *http://www.cchsd.org/cahealth-profiles.html*

Cottrell, R. P. F. (2003, March 10). The Olmstead decision: Fulfilling the promise of the ADA? Implications for occupational therapy. *OT Practice,* pp. 17–21.

Drafke, M. W. (2002). *Working in health care: What you need to know to succeed.* Philadelphia: F. A. Davis.

Evanofski, M. (2003). Occupational therapy reimbursement, regulation, and the evolving scope of practice. In E. B. Crepeau, E. S. Cohn, & B. A. B. Schell (Eds.), *Willard & Spackman's occupational therapy* (10th ed., pp. 887–896). Philadelphia: Lippincott, Williams & Wilkins.

Farley, S. K., Sarracino, T., & Howard, P. M. (1991). Development of a treatment rating in school systems: Service determination through objective measurement. *American Journal of Occupational Therapy, 45,* 898–906.

Fisher, G., & Cooksey, J. A. (2002). The occupational therapy workforce: Part one—context and trends. *Administrative and Management Special Interest Section Quarterly, 18,* 1–4.

Gage, B. (1999). Impact of the BBA on post-acute utilization. *Health Care Financing Review, 20,* 103–125.

Jones, J. (2004). Implementing HIPAA's privacy rule. *Advance for Occupational Therapy Practitioners, 20*(6), 51.

Kasper, J. D., Giovannini, T. A., & Hoffman, C. (2000). Gaining and losing health insurance: Strengthening the evidence for effects on access to care and health outcomes. *Medical Care Research and Review, 57,* 298–318.

Kimberg, I. (2004). The shape of things to come. *Advance for Occupational Therapy Practitioners, 20*(6), 7.

Komives, S. R. (1991). The relationship of same and cross gender work pairs to staff performance and supervisor leadership in residence hall units. *Sex Roles, 24,* 355–363.

Kornblau, B. L. (2004). A vision for our future. *American Journal of Occupational Therapy, 58,* 9–14.

Littleton, M. (2003). Cost effectiveness of a pre-work screening program for the University of Illinois at Chicago physical plant. *Work, 21,* 243–250.

Mansfield, E. (1980). *Principles of microeconomics* (3rd ed.). New York: W. W. Norton.

McCall, N., Petersons, A., & Korb, J. (2003). Utilization of home health services before and after the Balanced Budget Act of 1997: What were the initial effects? *Health Services Research, 38,* 107–112.

McCormack, G. L., Jaffe, E. G., & Goodman-Lavey, M. (2003). *The occupational therapy manager* (4th ed.). Bethesda, MD: AOTA Press.

Muhlenhaupt, M. (2000, December 4). OT services under IDEA 97: Decision-making challenges. *OT Practice,* pp. 10–13.

National Board for Certification in Occupational Therapy. (2004a). Declining trend in COTA applicants. National Board for Certification in Occupational Therapy Web site. No longer available.

National Board for Certification in Occupational Therapy. (2004b). Declining trend in OTR exam candidates. National Board for Certification in Occupational Therapy Web site. No longer available.

National Board for Certification in Occupational Therapy. (2004c). Professional development requirements. National Board for Certification in Occupational Therapy Web site. Available at *http://www.nbcot.org/WebArticles/anmviewer.asp? a=55&z=13*

National Center for Policy Analysis. (2004). Canada's health care system a disaster. National Center for Policy Analysis Web site. Available at *http://www.ncpa.org/ea/eajf93r.html*

Office of Inspector General. (1998). *Medical necessity of physical and occupational therapy in skilled nursing facilities* (Report No. OEI-09-97-00120). Washington, DC: U.S. Department of Health and Human Services.

Redick, A. G., McClain, L., & Brown, C. (2000). Consumer empowerment through occupational therapy: The Americans with Disabilities Act Title III. *American Journal of Occupational Therapy, 54,* 207–213.

Sandstrom, R. W., Lohman, H., & Bramble, J. D. (2003). *Health services: Policy and systems for therapists.* Upper Saddle River, NJ: Prentice Hall.

Starnes, W. (2000, January 31). Expanding to the community: Preparing yourself for new opportunities. *OT Practice,* pp. 14–17.

U.S. Department of Education. (2003). History of the IDEA. U.S. Department of Education Web site. Available at *http://www.ed.gov/policy/speced/leg/idea/history.html*

U.S. Department of Health and Human Services. (2004). Healthy People 2010. Healthy People 2010 Web site. Available at *http://www.healthypeople.gov/*

U.S. Department of Labor. (2002). Occupational outlook handbook 2002–2003. Bureau of Labor Statistics Web site. Available at *http://www.bls.gov/oco/home.htm*

Washington State Department of Public Health. (2002). The Health of Washington State. Washington State Department of Public Health Web site. Available at *http://www.doh.wa.gov/HWS/MCH.shtm*

Wolsko, P. M., Eisenberg, D. M., Davis, R. B., Ettner, S. L., & Phillips, R. S. (2002). Insurance coverage, medical conditions, and visits to alternative medicine providers: Results of a national survey. *Archives of Internal Medicine, 112,* 281–287.

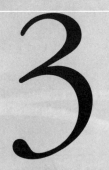

Brent Braveman, Ph.D., OTR/L, FAOTA

Understanding and Working Within Organizations

Real-Life Management

Kate has been working in a large hospital system for 2 years since graduating from an occupational therapy program. The system comprises different types of facilities, including a general hospital, a free-standing rehabilitation hospital, a skilled nursing facility, and several outpatient centers. She has followed with interest what seems to be a constant state of change in the organization. It seems that staff and services are continually changing not only within the facilities in which she has worked but also in the larger system.

Kate often hears expressions of frustration from her peers that seem to indicate that they don't understand why many of the changes are being made. Kate is interested in pursuing additional education but knows that she is not interested in a research career. She is considering enrolling in a Master of Business Administration or a Master of Health Care Administration program because she has always had an interest in how successful organizations operate and she is interested in learning more about the business side of health care. Because the curriculum in her occupational therapy program had a strong emphasis on theory, she wonders if there are theories related to how organizations are structured and managed that she'll learn about as she furthers her education. Additionally, she wonders how these theories might be helpful to her first as a clinician and later as she pursues her long-term goal of becoming an occupational therapy manager.

Key Issues

- Rational systems, natural systems, and open systems are three perspectives on organizations, and each provides helpful ways of understanding the operation of an organization.
- Factors from both the organization's external and internal environments affect organizational performance, and recognizing such factors and their influence can make you a more effective manager.

- Learning to observe how an organization's culture and values are demonstrated in the daily life of an organization can help you be more effective as a manager.
- There are numerous methods to classify organizations by *type*, and each method can aid in better understanding the organization's interactions with its environment.

Occupational therapy personnel work in a wide spectrum of organizations, including hospitals, schools, community-based organizations, and private businesses. There has been considerable theory development related to organizations, and a considerable body of research exists on various aspects of organizational development and function. Notable scholars have devoted entire careers to the study of organizations and organizational behavior. Chapter 2 provided an introduction to the health care system and other systems in which occupational therapy managers are employed. This chapter will provide an introduction to some key concepts useful in understanding the organizations that employ occupational therapy managers.

Occupational therapists and occupational therapy assistants are well familiar with improving function by examining the fit between an individual and his or her environment. As an occupational therapy manager, you can more effectively direct and coordinate services and be a more effective advocate for the profession, the staff that you supervise, and consumers of occupational therapy if you improve your fit and the fit of your department with the environment of your organization. A first step is to develop an understanding of how your organization functions. To do this, you must come to recognize and understand the factors that have influenced your organization's development, its current operations, and its future. In Chapter 1, it was noted that managers *practice* just as clinicians do, and that becoming familiar with the data, information, and other forms of evidence available on organizations is necessary to practice effectively as a manager.

An observation made throughout this book is that, all too often, occupational therapy managers "fall" into their roles without adequate preparation and training rather than consciously choosing to pursue a career in management. Whether their roles are planned or occur by circumstance, it is also true that often occupational therapy managers remain insular, with too heavy a focus on the knowledge base of the profession, and fail to avail themselves of the considerable body of theory and evidence developed by other fields such as organizational development and behavior. You are encouraged to explore and use the full range of theory and evidence available to guide your practice as an occupational therapy manager.

In this chapter, we will explore theoretical views and frameworks of the types of organizations, the relationship between organizational structure and function, the culture of organizations, and the fit between personal values and worldviews and "fit" within various types of organizations. Recent trends in theories related to organizational function and research will also be presented.

A Brief History of Organizations

Organizations have played a critical role in the evolution of modern culture. The great social transformations in history have essentially been organizationally based. The expansion of the Roman Empire, the spread of Christianity, and the growth and development of capitalism and socialism have been accomplished through organizations (R. H. Hall, 1996). Organizations have been present throughout history, including in early Chinese and Greek civilizations. For example, early tax collectors were "organized." Organizations assumed increased importance in regard to organized labor and developing economies in the late 1600s and the 1700s, especially as technological improvements contributed to the industrial revolution. In addition to technology, expanding trade markets and a growth in population created increased demand for goods and paved the way for new factories that brought with them the need to improve work methods and productivity. Specialization in work skills flourished during the 1800s as the concept of "division of labor" began to get a foothold and the advantages of specialization related to skill development, saved time and efficiency, and the development and utilization of specialized tools were recognized.

Frederick Winslow Taylor introduced one of the first theories of organizations, and he found an eager audience in the managers and foremen of the factories of the second part of the 19th century. Taylor used "scientific management" to analyze work tasks and to make changes in production methods that resulted in increased productivity and a lessened need for labor. Taylor's early work on a theory of organizations has taken root in common thinking about organizational functioning. Today, theorists recognize that organizations play an even more central role in modern-day Western civilization. Organizations have come to serve as the structure through which most critical societal needs are met. These needs include, among others, education (schools and universities), production and distribution of goods (factories and wholesale firms), health care (hospitals and community medical centers), travel (airlines, train companies, bus companies, and taxicab companies), preservation of culture (museums, art galleries, and libraries), communication (phone companies and Internet service providers), and entertainment (restaurants, movie theaters, and television and radio studios) (Scott, 1992).

R. H. Hall (1996) noted that organizing is a requisite for social change. Without organization, change cannot occur. A social cause alone, however strongly felt by its supporters, in itself is not adequate for change. However, by organizing, supporters of a cause can foster social change that may be lasting and of great importance. Changes in civil liberties, including the civil rights movement, equal opportunities for women, gay and lesbian rights, and the rights of disabled persons, have all been moved forward by groups forming organizations to garner political power and influence.

Today the vast majority of persons are employed by and look to different types of organizations to provide their source of income and productivity and to meet most of their basic needs. It has been estimated that, in economically developed nations, anywhere from 75% to 90% of those individuals working for a living do so for a wage or salary in a formal organization, or what Elliott Jaques referred to as a "managerial hierarchy" (Jaques, 1998).

The study of organizations has emerged only during the last century and has been promoted by various fields of study, including sociology and anthropology, and more recently within academic departments such as schools of business administration. March (1965) traced the origins of the study of organizations as an academic discipline back to the period of 1937 to 1947 in Europe. The study of organizations was further supported with the translation into English of the works of Max Weber, a German sociologist who is cited as publishing one of the first discussions of formal organizations or *bureaucracies* within modern society early in the 20th century (Weber, 1946). A much larger proliferation of literature began to be published in the 1940s and 1950s as organizations became even more central to economic and industrial development and production in the post–World War II United States.

Organizations as Systems

Scholars of organizational development have used three distinct perspectives to describe organizations as systems (Scott, 1992). These three perspectives view organizations as *rational, natural,* or *open systems.* Although the most common way of introducing how health care organizations function is to discuss them as "open systems," each perspective adds to the overall understanding of the function of health care organizations, and each perspective continues to be used to guide research, theory development, and the application of theory to everyday managerial action.

Descriptions of organizations as *rational systems* use language that one might expect as indicated by the term *rational.* Rationalists view organizations as having characteristics that differentiate them from other types of social groups, such as families. This view of organizations focuses on the following characteristics:

- Organizations benefit from having specific goals for their existence, and the more specific the goals, the higher functioning the organization is likely to be.
- Organizations are systems that are highly formalized, with tight lines of authority and accountability that serve to support the organization in meeting its goals.
- Organizations function through the implementation of rules and the tight coordination of organizational units.

Rationalists place high importance on the specificity of goals because goals can provide a set of criteria to guide decision making, and believe that more successful organizations have more specifically defined goals. Likewise, it is believed that the more formal the structure of an organization, the more predictable its behavior may become, leading to decreased resources being required to guide an organization. Rationalists such as Weber (1968) proposed that strictly defined structures and clearly delineated lines of authority and accountability for performance would improve organizational efficiency. Hence, an organizational leader who adopts a rationalist perspective may place high value on activities such as strategic planning and tend to favor organizational structures that are stable and formal, with clearly delineated lines of authority and accountability.

Whereas rationalists view organizations as systems constructed purposefully to pursue specific goals, *natural system* theorists view organizations primarily as collectives with characteristics similar to those of other social groups that are more important than the characteristics identified by rationalists (e.g., specificity of goals, authority, etc.). Natural system analysts focus on the "human element" that employees bring to an organization, including their personal values and convictions as well as the fact that individual agendas of employees can impact organizational functioning. A primary theory within the natural systems perspective is that of *human relations theory* (Scott, 1992). Human relations theory is constructed on the assumptions that

- Most individuals find work and the expenditure of physical and mental effort to be as natural as play or rest.
- External control and threat of punishment are neither the only nor the most effective means for bringing about effort toward organizational objectives.
- The most significant rewards are those associated with the satisfaction of the ego and self-actualization needs.

Organizational leaders who adopt a naturalist perspective may stress activities related to the personal and professional development of personnel and favor organizational structures that are relatively more fluid and that promote individual growth.

An *open systems* perspective of organizations arises from *general systems theory*, which proposes that a change in any one part of a system causes inherent change in the total system and that living organisms maintain structure through continuous change (von Bertalanffy, 1968). An open system is a system that is capable of self-maintenance within a larger context or environment. Open systems theory has been used widely in the studies of organi-

zations and of human behavior and is the systems perspective most commonly used to describe health care organizations in management texts (Liebler, Levine, & Rothman, 1992; McCormack, Jaffe, & Frey, 2003).

Open systems theory points to three fundamental contradictions of organizational life (Mumford & Peterson, 1999):

- There is a constant need to balance the tendency toward stability with the need for change.
- Although they need to work together to produce a product or service, members may not agree on goals or strategies for coping with change.
- Managers must cope with meeting performance objectives and the bottom line while recognizing the unique needs of people who comprise work units.

Organizational leaders who adopt an open systems perspective may tend to focus on activities that include monitoring and assessment of internal and external organizational environments and favor a balance of formal planning and human resource development activities.

Basic to the premise of organizations as open systems are the concepts of (1) input, (2) throughput, and (3) output. Input can be thought of as the resources and influences that flow into the organization (e.g., physical resources such as money and materials or psychological and human resources in the form of energy and knowledge) that allow the organization to complete its basic functions. Throughput can be thought of as the processes that occur within an organization or the processing of input to achieve the organization's end goals. Output is simply what the organization sends back into the larger environment in terms of goods or services. Feedback is provided from the environment in which the organization functions and in return becomes an additional source of input. The key features of an open system are presented in Box 3–1, and a simple visual depiction of an open system is presented in Figure 3–1.

Although an open systems perspective provides a simple way to think about the influences on and the functions of organizations, more complex frameworks are needed to help managers within an organization perform their jobs effectively. This is true because even very large and complexly structured organizations may be conceptualized as

Box 3–1: Key Features of Open Systems as Applied to Organizations

- **Input:** Entry of resources, energy, and information into the system.
- **Throughput:** Processing of input to achieve organizational goals.
- **Output:** Goods or services produced by an organization and returned to the external environment.
- **Feedback:** Knowledge or information returned to the organization from external sources or from internal sources interpreting the result of output.
- **Environment:** Organizations exist within environments that provide input to the system and received output from the organization.

open systems. Viewing an organization as a hierarchical system adds the perspective that organizations may be structured differently in order to manage input into the system and produce the goods or services related to their mission or the reason they exist.

Organizations have characteristics that may be examined as a first step toward understanding the day-to-day functioning of the organization. The following is a partial list of characteristics to consider:

- Organizations have boundaries that serve to define membership and to include some members of the population and exclude others.
- Organizations involve social relationships in which individuals within the organization interact with each other, and with persons outside of the organization.
- Organizations involve a hierarchy of authority in which power to make decisions and commit resources is unequally distributed.
- Organizations involve a division of labor in which tasks are typically divided among employees based on skill, capacity, and the types of rewards associated with completion of tasks.
- Organizations exist outside the lives of their members and therefore have goals, missions, and a reason to exist on their own.

Any complex system or organization is composed of multiple subsystems. For example, a hospital may both comprise smaller subsystems such as divisions, departments, or product lines and itself operate within a larger system or "network" of health care providers. Similarly, a school is composed of individual classrooms that function to some degree as subsystems but is located in a school district comprised of individual schools that each function as distinct organizations. Within each system or subsystem, a hierarchy, or some form of levels, may be found. How these levels interact in terms of status, power, authority, and accountability may vary a great deal, but the main point to consider is that most systems in which occupational therapy personnel work both are made up of smaller subsystems and are themselves typically components of larger systems. Occupational therapy managers may benefit by becoming adept at analyzing and understanding systems both within and outside of their organization. Managers who can do so, and who can recognize, respond to, and even predict the influence of environmental changes, will increase their value to the organization and the profession. In addition, a manager who develops an understanding of how organizations work can be more effective at setting questions related to managerial functions and finding relevant data, information, and other forms of evidence needed to answer these questions.

Although many veteran managers may appreciate the value of educating their staff about the influences of the greater system in which the occupational therapy department or organization functions, they are likely to also express that it can be difficult at times to convince line staff of this importance. Entry-level practitioners are often con-

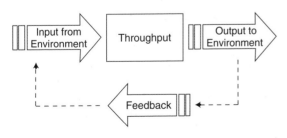

Figure 3–1 An open system.

sumed by the stressors of learning a myriad of new skills, coming to terms with their professional style, understanding the dynamics of the levels of the organization in which they interact directly, and sometimes learning to integrate basic habits of daily work into their lives. Given these demands, it is reasonable to understand that placing energy into comprehending the larger political, economic, and legislative contexts in which an organization functions might not appear as a priority for the typical occupational therapy staff member. One need only consider the basic organization of a typical medical-model setting in which occupational therapy service providers work to recognize just how far removed the staff members are from the "outside world" in terms of daily work (Figure 3–2). By coming to understand more about how organizations function, the occupational therapy manager can help to filter information for the oc-

cupational therapy staff members and call their attention to the environmental influences that will have the most impact on employees.

Organizational Environments

Occupational therapy personnel are well aware of the importance of the interaction and fit between an individual and his or her environment as it relates to the capacity of the individual for satisfactory occupational performance. Likewise, organizations operate within environments, and the capacity of the organization to meet environmental demands and anticipate and prepare for future demands impacts the performance capacity of the organization. In today's world, the organizations in which occupational therapy service providers work may interact not only in local environments, but sometimes on a state, national, or even global basis. It is useful as an occupational therapy manager for you to understand the environments in which your organization operates and the forces and pressures to which the organization must respond.

Managers can have great influence on those whom they supervise. Managers can be mentors, inspiring others to work beyond their own expectations for performance and helping those they supervise to make a positive contribution to the organization and their community. However, managers can also add to a subordinate's sense of dissatisfaction, frustration, and lowered productivity. Working to actively monitor and understand the internal environment of the organization can help to have a positive influence on the job satisfaction and performance of subordinates.

External Environments

R. H. Hall (1996) made the interesting and important observation that, with regard to the influence of external environmental factors on health care organizations, environmental factors have both *theoretical* and *practical* outcomes for these types of organizations. In other words, we cannot rely on theory or evidence alone to help us understand the decisions that a health care organization may make. For example, although hospitals may increase services or invest monies in updated facilities based

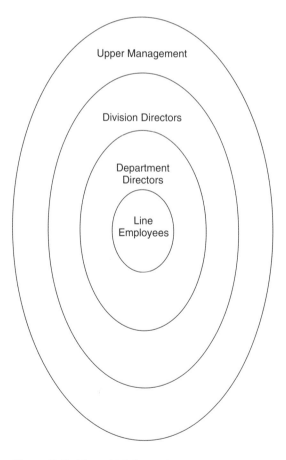

Figure 3–2   The multiple layers of a typical organization.

upon patient needs, this may not be the only or even the primary environmental influence to which they are responding. Hospitals and other health care or public service organizations also need to compete in a competitive, market-driven environment. As noted by Fennell (1980), "Hospitals also expand their services not because of the needs of their patient populations but rather because they believe that they will not be judged as fit themselves if they cannot offer everything that other hospitals in the area provide." In Chapter 2 you were introduced to the concept of supply and demand. Based upon this economic theory alone, we might expect that an organization would make the rational decision to not invest monies in inpatient hospital beds if the market in which it operates were already saturated. However, in the year 2000, Cook County in Illinois began construction on a new 464-bed hospital in Chicago despite the fact that, during that same year, the average occupancy rate for Illinois hospitals was only 58.5% and it was estimated that, in the city of Chicago and its suburbs, there might be as many as 10,000 more inpatient hospital beds than required (Illinois Hospital Association, 2003). The practical outcome of remaining competitive in the market by improving the physical facilities outweighed the theoretical outcome of contributing to an already saturated marketplace.

There are a number of specific arenas within the external environment that should be of concern to occupational therapy managers. These include

- The *legislative arena* at a state and national level, because new laws influence access to services, reimbursement, and the scope of care that can legally be provided.
- The *economic arena*, because the availability of resources and the local, state, and national economy influence organizational plans for the future.
- The *technology arena*, because finding and managing information becomes more sophisticated and complex and new products and services are constantly introduced.
- The *demographic arena*, because the age, socioeconomic status, racial mix, and other characteristics of local and national populations change.
- The *sociocultural arena*, because societal values and beliefs about what is acceptable and expected are constantly shifting.

Organizations survive and sometimes thrive in turbulent environments by responding to change at multiple levels. The issues or problems of external adaptation and survival specify the coping cycle that any system must be able to maintain in relation to its changing environment (Schein, 1992). Edgar Schein, a noted organizational psychologist and a Professor of Management at the Massachusetts Institute of Technology Sloan School of Management, described five stages of a cycle of adaptation for an organization. The stages of the cycle are outlined in Box 3–2. When reviewing the stages suggested by Schein, it is of interest to note that the most commonly identified functions of management (i.e., planning, organizing and staffing, directing, and controlling) are easily recognizable within them.

Typically an organization's mission (a statement of why the organization exists) remains fairly stable and can be thought of as a rudder that guides the organization in the direction envisioned by its founders. Highly successful organizations maintain a sense of focus but are flexible in serving multiple functions and meeting the needs of numerous constituent groups. For example, the major initiatives pursued, products produced, and services provided by a community or health care agency typically

---

Box 3–2: The Stages of Organizational Adaptation to External Change

1. *Mission clarification:* obtaining and maintaining a shared and functional understanding of the organization's core mission, functions, and products.
2. *Goal setting:* developing consensus on goals that match the stated organizational mission.
3. *Means to goal obtainment:* developing consensus on the means and methods to reaching stated goals.
4. *Measurement:* establishing clear criteria to use to measure how well the organization is doing to meet stated goals.
5. *Correction:* developing consensus on appropriate remediation or strategies to take if goals are not being met.

reflect the organization's core mission, but the interests and desires of key personnel or customer groups may also be reflected in programming and service offerings that come and go over time. The extent to which large amounts of the organization's financial and human resources are diverted from the core mission to these "side projects" is one measure of the success of organizational leadership in making the organization's mission "real." Organizational missions are not impervious to challenge, however, especially when the survival of the organization itself comes into question. Few organizations ever willingly state, "Our mission has been achieved, so we are disbanding," or "It is clear in the marketplace that our competitors are better equipped to serve the public than we are, so we are closing up shop in the best interests of the public." In today's society, one commonly recognized function of an organization is to provide a living wage for those it employs, and reaching this goal can at times seem to take precedence over goals related to the very reason an organization was created in the first place.

It might seem that, if an organization's mission is kept front and center in the minds of personnel through the actions of leadership, then establishing goals to match the mission would be an easy task. However, doing so is more complicated than you might imagine. Establishing a common understanding of mission does not automatically translate to having a shared understanding of how that mission is best served or the strategies that should be pursued. It is through the management functions of strategic and operational planning (discussed in Chapter 5) that a concrete and articulated set of specific goals with specific time frames are developed. Planning is an ongoing process that must include consistent monitoring of the external environment to cue the organization to when it must adapt strategies and pursue contingent actions.

Organizations cannot reach their goals unless there is a clear and articulated consensus on the specific means and methods by which they intend to do so. Moving from long-range planning focused on the goals of the year or next few years to day-to-day planning for tomorrow and next week requires vigilant attention on the part of all levels of leadership and management. Managers must decide how to best *organize* resources to accomplish work tasks

and must assure that the right combination of skills and talents are assembled for the work to be done. Schein (1992) made the interesting observation that deciding how things will be done often also inadvertently assigns ownership of who will do what in many ways. He noted that various amounts of status, access to rewards, and certain privileges inevitably accompany the assigned roles, and the means by which things get done in the external environment become "property" in the internal environment. Such a sense of ownership can both facilitate the work of an organization if personnel are appropriately involved in making decisions, and inhibit work if changes to processes are perceived as threats or as a means of lowering one's status in the workplace.

Pre-established criteria or indicators of performance allow an organization to monitor whether it is meeting its goals and to identify when contingent action must be taken to get it back on course. Such *operational definitions*, if properly applied, remove any doubt regarding expectations for middle managers, who are often responsible for direct supervision of those who do the primary work of the organization. These operational definitions also allow managers to take swift action when it becomes apparent that a unit is not on target. Applying such criteria is often described as the *control* function of management. Again, such steps may seem as if they would be relatively simple, but often agreeing on performance "targets" as well as the process for measuring performance against a target can be difficult. Common criteria for performance that are encountered by occupational therapy personnel and managers include volume or productivity targets. Agreeing on performance criteria, such as the number of billable hours per day per therapist to be provided, may be difficult enough, but coming to consensus on how to factor the many situations therapists encounter into such criteria becomes very difficult indeed. Information, including some of the most basic financial information, can be analyzed and interpreted in a variety of ways. Assuring not only that operational definitions are in place but also that there is discussion about the underlying rationale for criteria can help maintain consensus.

Finally, when things are not going according to plan and it appears that goals are not being met, organizations must make decisions about what strategies are to be assumed. Alternatively, sometimes organizations exceed expectations for performance, and managing unexpected success and taking full advantage of such situations are also forms of contingent actions.

Internal Environments: Organizational Culture

The term *culture* is widely accepted to mean a learned, shared set of basic assumptions or shared way of doing things that is based upon the underlying values and beliefs of the members of a particular society or of a group. Shared values serve to impact the actions of the members of an organization in several ways. Shared values

- Help turn commonplace, routine work into valued activities
- Create a connection between the mission of the organization and society's values
- Provide a source of competitive advantage to the organization

Individual values are developed through interactions between a person and the environment and culture in which he or she resides. As we might expect, because the experiences of individuals vary even within the same cultural context, different persons develop different values. Values are typically thought to be resistant to simple influences and to persist over time because they develop over periods of many years as we interact with the world. A commonly recognized method of classifying values was developed by psychologist Milton Rokeach, who identified two classes of values: *instrumental values* and *terminal values* (Rokeach, 1973). Instrumental values relate to the *means* for achieving ends, such as self-sufficiency or honesty. Terminal values relate to the *ends* that a person wishes to achieve, such as financial independence or a high level of self-esteem. It has been hypothesized that, as workers age, a shift occurs so that terminal values are less influential and instrumental values exert more influence on worker actions. If this is true, understanding the difference in how these values can be supported in the workplace can be useful for the occupational therapy manager.

The relationship between organizational values and individual values has important implications for the workplace. As one might expect, it is generally believed that having a high level of *congruence* between the values of an organization and those of individual employees facilitates improved organizational performance. When values do not match, or are *incongruent*, it is typically expected that level of conflict may be higher and that organizational performance may be lower. The connection between value congruence and organizational performance has an implication for managers. If it is true that individual values are resilient to simple influences and not easily changed, it may be easier for managers to select employees who have values that match and support those of the organization than to try to instill a set of values within employees after they are hired. Although fully assessing the values of potential employees may be beyond the scope of time and resources available to most managers while recruiting employees, a manager can effectively communicate recognized organizational and department values by

- Sharing copies of mission and vision statements for the organization and department during the recruitment process
- Including current staff in the interview process and encouraging candidates to ask questions of staff regarding shared values and common practices and what it "feels like" to work for the organization, as well as providing examples of group norms that represent shared values
- Sharing explicit statements of personal values as a manager and making expectations clear by giving examples of how he or she hopes that values are translated into action and behavior by staff

One aspect of the concept of organizational culture that is useful is that it implies structural stability in a group. This stability means that there are elements of an organization or group that can be *observed*. Moreover, these elements are often just below the level of consciousness of most organizational members. An astute manager can use these observations to his or her advantage when joining an organization or attempting to create change. As noted by Schein (1992), "If the concept of culture is to have any utility, it should draw our attention to those things that are the product of our human need for stability, consistency, and meaning." Schein identified 10 phenomena associated with

Box 3–3: Observable Phenomena Related to Organizational Culture

1. *Behavioral regularities*, including the language used and the customs, traditions, and rituals that evolve, such as expectations to attend department functions, including holiday parties or company picnics.
2. *Group norms*, or implicit standards and values, such as a norm of offering to cover each other's patients during vacations.
3. *Espoused values*, or publicly announced principles and values, such as customer service.
4. *Formal philosophy*, or the broad policies and ideological principles that guide a group's actions toward employees, customers, and other key stakeholders, such as rewarding seniority among employees or providing special privileges to loyal customers.
5. *Rules of the game*, or the unspoken rules for getting along that are often described as "the way we do things around here," such as staying late in the office to finish paperwork and submit it on time.
6. *Organizational climate*, or the feeling that is conveyed in a group by the way members interact with each other, customers, and other outsiders, such as staff routinely asking "May I help you?" when they see someone who appears to be lost in the building.
7. *Embedded skills*, or the special competencies that group members display in accomplishing certain tasks such as communicating with parents who do not speak English about their children's therapies.
8. *Habits of thinking, mental models, and/or linguistic paradigms*, or the cognitive frameworks that guide the perceptions, thought, and language used by the members of a group, such as commonly used conceptual practice models.
9. *Shared meanings*, or the emergent understandings that are created by group members as they interact with each other, such as meanings associated with eating lunch together, or in regard to common events, such as having all referrals assigned to an evaluating therapist in a timely manner.
10. *Root metaphors*, or the ideas, feelings, and images groups develop to characterize themselves that become embedded in the physical spaces and material artifacts of the group, such as group photos, awards given to the department, or souvenirs on display from group outings.

Adapted from Schein, E. H. (1992). *Organizational culture and leadership.* New York: Jossey-Bass.

organizational culture that may be overtly observed. These phenomena and common examples of each are listed in Box 3–3.

We must understand that we are not born into a culture, but rather are born into a society that teaches us its culture (Schermerhorn, Hunt, & Osborn, 1982). Similarly, as we enter a new organization, we may come to understand the underlying or shared values and beliefs as we become exposed to the way things are done within the organization. The notion of organizational or "corporate" culture is pervasive in the management literature and has been widely investigated. In their influential book, *In Search of Excellence*, Peters and Waterman (1982) stressed the contribution that the development of specific organizational cultures made to what they defined as "best-run" organizations. They noted that

> "The dominance and coherence of culture proved to be an essential quality of the excellent companies. Moreover, the stronger the culture and the more it was directed toward the marketplace, the less need there was for policy manuals, organization charts, or detailed procedures and rules. In these companies people way down the line know what they are supposed to do in situations because the handful of guiding values is crystal clear."

Schemerhorn et al. (1982) identified three levels

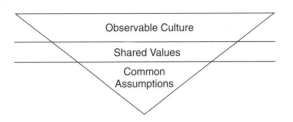

Figure 3–3 Three levels of analysis in studying organizational culture. (Adapted from Schermerhorn, J. R., Hunt, J. G., & Osborn, R. N. [1982]. *Managing organizational behavior* [5th ed.]. New York: John Wiley & Sons.)

of analysis for organizational culture, as shown in Figure 3–3. Briefly, these levels include

First level: Observable culture, or "the way we do things around here," including the unique stories, ceremonies, and corporate rituals that make up the history of the organization

Second level: Shared values that link organizational members together and provide a motivation for organizational behavior

Third level: Common assumptions or taken-for-granted truths that collections of corporate members share as a result of their joint experience

These levels of analysis can be used by a new or veteran manager who wishes to understand more about the values, beliefs, and shared assumptions of the members of the organization. Listening to the stories told about the organization, sharing observations about common practices with other managers and listening to their interpretations, and carefully noting the feedback and reaction you receive both in times that you are succeeding and when you are struggling are strategies that you can use to gain insights into your organization's culture.

Organizational cultures will present both opportunities and challenges to you as a new manager as you enter an organization and must interpret the explicit and implicit messages that you receive about the way that things are to be done. Through shared experiences, veteran organizational members will likely have developed ways of accomplishing day-to-day work that tacitly incorporate strategies to meet challenges previously encountered and overcome. It is likely that members will have also developed strategies that tacitly manage the expectations, demands, and work styles of other

units within the organization. Unconscious ways of working such as those just described may not only provide key insights into the underlying values and assumptions of an organization's members, they may also serve to improve the effectiveness and efficiency of work groups. Unfortunately, systems, processes, and procedures sometimes outlive their usefulness, and you may find that it seems that members of an organization complete tasks in an almost ritualistic fashion without being quite sure why. The tendency to challenge such behavior as ineffective, wasteful, or unneeded is understandable, but you must remember that, in doing so, you may be perceived as challenging not just the way things are done but also the underlying values that drove members to assume the action in the first place.

All organizations have some things in common, most notably that each organization exists for a particular reason (e.g., the organizational mission) and that each makes particular contributions to society by its output or products. Recognizing the commonalities among organizations is helpful in understanding how they function; however, it is also useful to recognize the differences between organizations. The next section of the chapter will overview some typologies for making distinctions between organizations.

Types of Organizations

Relatively large numbers of systems for classifying organizations, or *typologies*, have been presented in the organizational development literature. However, R. H. Hall (1996) made the point that any single typology may or may not be useful depending on the needs of the reader. Taking a cue from Hall, the following is not intended as a specific system of classification but is actually a mix of typologies that focuses on making the distinctions that are most helpful for the occupational therapy manager to understand the types of organizations in which occupational therapy personnel most often work.

Bureaucracies and Associations

Jaques (1998) made a distinction between a bureaucracy, or a typical managerial authority structure, and an association. This distinction is helpful in understanding the relationship between the types of organizations in which most occupational therapy personnel are employed and the voluntary organization that represents occupational therapists and occupational therapy assistants, the American Occupational Therapy Association (AOTA), or similar associations that represent other health disciplines or professionals. Although the term *bureaucratic* has generally come to hold a negative connotation, indicating an organization that is inefficient and overly structured, in organizational development literature it simply indicates the type of authority structure found in most businesses where employees are paid for the work they produce and is not meant to hold either a negative or a positive connotation. *Associations* are formally named organizations comprised primarily of participants who do not derive their livelihoods from the organization's activities. When speaking of the AOTA, it is important to distinguish whether you mean the occupational therapists and occupational therapy assistants who pay to be members of the association in order to have their professional interests represented, or you mean the paid staff members who work for the bureaucracy (the authority structure), or both. The distinction between bureaucracies and associations has become less clear in modern times as associations have assumed more responsibility for activities such as continuing education, marketing, and product development, yet it is still helpful at times to recognize the unique combination of paid and volunteer leadership in professional associations and how it influences decision making.

For example, in the AOTA, the executive director is a paid employee (often *not* educated in occupational therapy) who is hired by the board of directors. The board of directors is composed of mostly occupational therapists or occupational therapy assistants elected to the board by members of the association in voluntary elections. The executive director leads a group of paid employees composed of occupational therapy personnel and non–occupational therapy personnel hired for their expertise in marketing, sales, program development, information management, or other skill sets required to carry out the work of the association and meet the varied needs of the membership. There is also a

very large volunteer leadership structure comprising members who are elected or appointed, or who volunteer to assume various roles, led by the president of the AOTA, who is elected for a 3-year term. One important part of most associations is a policymaking group that is typically composed of elected members who represent various segments of the association. For example, the AOTA's Representative Assembly (RA) is composed of representatives elected from the 50 states and persons who fill other key volunteer leadership positions. The RA sets policy for the association, such as strategic directions, the cost of membership dues, and the membership structure, and charges association bodies with projects to meet the needs of the membership and to promote occupational therapy. Other professional associations have similar policymaking and decision-making groups.

For-Profit and Nonprofit Organizations

A simple but sometimes important way of distinguishing between organizations is whether they are *for-profit* or *nonprofit* organizations. To the outsider, at first glance it might be difficult to distinguish between for-profit and nonprofit organizations that have similar missions and produce similar products and services. For example, there are both for-profit and nonprofit hospitals and skilled nursing facilities that provide similar services to similar populations and that are structured in almost identical ways. Simply by examining their organizational charts, or even the mission statements, you might not be able to distinguish the for-profit from the nonprofit organization. Further, if you were to speak to managers from each type of organization, you might hear very similar descriptions of what their responsibilities and concerns entail. Both are likely to report being responsible for the traditional management functions (e.g., planning, organizing and staffing, directing, and controlling) and facing the same pressures of operating with limited resources to produce a quality product with high levels of productivity. Moreover, managers in nonprofit organizations may be as concerned as if not more concerned than managers in for-profit organizations with helping to create a positive "bottom line," or assuring that the organization makes money in any given year. In fact, nonprofit organizations must make a profit in order to be able to maintain and improve physical facilities, buy new equipment, and pay for the same expenses faced by for-profit organizations, such as advertising and marketing. So, if for-profit and nonprofit organizations can have so much in common, you are likely asking, "How are they different?"

There are many financial and legal differences, such as whether the organizations are taxed on their profits or must pay taxes on goods that they purchase, how the organizations are legally structured, and who is legally responsible for debt and contractual obligations entered into by the organization. In addition, a primary difference is that the for-profit organization exists to make money for a group of investors and the nonprofit exists solely to meet its mission and reinvests all profits into the organization. Another difference may be represented in the decisions the organizations make about the nature of the programming they provide and how flexible they are willing to be in accepting various forms of payment for services. Managers in for-profit organizations are likely to feel more pressure to examine the impact that service design and delivery will have on reimbursement and to maximize services that are highly reimbursed while avoiding, when possible, services that are not reimbursed. It must be noted, however, that even many for-profit organizations provide some level of "indigent" or uncompensated care.

The for-profit sector of the profession not only includes large health care organizations but also includes the private practitioner and business entrepreneurs who may provide traditional occupational therapy services or other services such as the manufacture and sale of assistive and adaptive equipment. Owning and operating your own business can be rewarding both financially and professionally but is also very challenging, and requires the development of business and marketing skills in addition to a devotion to hard work and to making the business successful. Resources for the private practitioner or business entrepreneur can be found through the AOTA, the Small Business Association, and other associations, including associations dedicated to helping women or people of color to succeed as small business owners. The next section of this chapter will provide a brief description of the most common types of private businesses and the advantages and disadvantages of each type.

Common Types of Private Businesses

SOLE PROPRIETORSHIPS

The majority of small businesses start out as sole proprietorships (Small Business Administration, 2003). Sole proprietorships merge together the business and its affairs and the owner's personal affairs, and therefore, from the standpoint of nearly all legal rights and responsibilities, the business and the owner are considered to be one and the same. In sole proprietorships, the owner directs business activities and may hire employees; however, this does not alter the legal nature of the business. The owner of a sole proprietorship has legal ownership of all assets of a business but also assume responsibility for all debt. If credit is used in the operation of the business, it is important to maintain separate financial records for business and personal finances. Interest payments on personal debt are not a deductible expense for federal and state income tax purposes; however, interest payments on business borrowing are fully deductible.

Advantages of sole proprietorships are

- They are the easiest and least expensive form of business ownership to organize.
- They can be established, bought, sold, or terminated very quickly.
- They do not require public notification to start, terminate, or be modified beyond routine permits and licenses.
- The size and structure can change, and others (family, etc.) can be involved according to the proprietor's wishes.
- Complex business planning or organizational arrangements (bylaws, organizational charter, etc.) are not required by law.

Disadvantages of sole proprietorships are

- Both personal and business assets are at risk unless they are protected in a trust or some other protective mechanism.
- Mixing business and personal finances can make it more difficult to measure the financial success of the business.

- The business ends with the death of the proprietor, and a new business must be formed if others wish to continue the business.
- In family sole proprietorships, each generation must purchase or inherit the business assets, paying any applicable taxes and costs, upon death of the sole proprietor.
- The availability of credit and ability to respond to opportunities may be restricted because of limited resources.
- Conflicts or disagreements within the family can stagnate the business and delay needed decision making.

PARTNERSHIPS

A partnership is an association of two or more persons formed to carry on a business for profit. All partnerships should be based on a written partnership agreement that lays out in advance how decisions are to be made in the case of disagreement and how funds and property are to be handled upon dissolution of the partnership. With few exceptions, a partnership is not an income tax–paying entity because profits from the partnership flow directly to the partners' personal tax returns. Unless arrangements are made to continue the partnership beyond death or withdrawal of a partner in the partnership agreement, the partnership is dissolved in such situations.

Advantages of partnerships are

- They are relatively easy to establish because the partners may combine resources.
- The partners may capitalize on their skills and interests by specializing in certain aspects of management or operations.
- There may be a greater capacity for obtaining credit by partners than what either partner might obtain on his or her own.
- The necessary record-keeping and income tax filing requirements are only slightly more complicated than for individuals.
- They provide opportunities for family members or friends to work together in starting or operating a business.

Disadvantages of partnerships are

- The personal assets of all partners are put at risk.
- Business is disrupted upon the death or withdrawal of a single partner.

- Alienation of a partner with minority interests can occur if partners with majority interests vote together and block the interests of the minority.
- They must be carefully planned to allow succession to a new generation or the next generation, and tax laws related to inheritance apply.
- They can lead to fragmented leadership if the division of management responsibility among the partners results in no one having an overall understanding of the financial standing of the partnership.
- They may be difficult to end without undue financial loss and/or interpersonal conflict with the other partners.
- They can lose productivity and profitability if conflicts or disagreements among the partners immobilize business decision making.

LIMITED LIABILITY CORPORATION

The limited liability corporation (LLC) is a form of business that, unlike a sole proprietorship, is separate and distinct from the personal and business affairs of its owners. The LLC is a newer form of *hybrid* business that is now permissible in most states (Small Business Administration, 2003). It is designed to provide the limited liability features of a corporation and the tax efficiencies and operational flexibility of a partnership. One or more persons may organize an LLC by preparing and filing copies of articles of organization with the designated state agency. The name, the purpose for which the LLC is organized, its principal place of business, the resources to be invested in it, and the identity and addresses of managers must be stated in the articles. Upon issuance of a certificate of organization by the designated state agency, the LLC can begin business activities.

An LLC may be dissolved when (1) the identified life span specified in the articles of organization expires, (2) the members unanimously agree in writing that it should be dissolved, (3) any other dissolution cause specified in the articles of organization occurs, or (4) it is dissolved by a court. Operating procedures are also articulated in the articles of organization. With the exception of liabilities for unpaid taxes, members and managers of an LLC are not liable for LLC debt or liabilities.

Advantages of LLCs are

- They provide the owners with a flexible and

adaptable form of business organization that provides liability protection comparable to the protection provided by incorporation.

- They can be established at moderate cost in a relatively short time.
- All members, one or more members, or a nonmember individual or business entity may manage an LLC.
- The interests of the owners can be transferred to others upon approval of the members of the LLC as articulated in the articles of organization.

Disadvantages of LLCs are

- They can be more difficult to establish than sole proprietorships or partnerships and require legal assistance and public notification.
- Conflict can arise among members because it may be more difficult to correctly anticipate ownership and management issues.
- Corporations are monitored by federal, state, and some local agencies and so may require more paperwork to comply with regulations.
- Incorporation may result in higher overall taxes.

S CORPORATIONS

An "S Corporation" is a corporation that is taxed under Subchapter S of the Internal Revenue Code and receives Internal Revenue Service (IRS) approval of its request for Subchapter S status. Eligibility for S corporation tax status is based on compliance with IRS regulations regarding the number and characteristics of stockholders, type of stock issued, and other characteristics specified in the regulations. Because it is a separate legal entity, the corporation finances and records are established and maintained completely separate and distinct from the finances and records of the stockholders. One or more officers of the corporation are authorized to conduct business on behalf of the corporation. If the corporation is new and has a limited credit record, personal guarantees by one or more officers or stockholders may be required to obtain the necessary credit to conduct business, which then may create personal liability for those individuals.

Advantages of S Corporations are

- The liability of stockholders is limited to their investment in the corporation and their personal assets are protected.

- These corporations can raise additional funds through the sale of stock.
- They can continue operating despite the death of one or more stockholders.
- They accommodate multiple owners but provide for decision-making mechanisms that base influence on percentage of ownership.
- They allow for change of ownership through sale or gift without disturbing business operations.
- They may benefit from communication between stockholders, legal counsel, and other groups to maximize management knowledge.

Disadvantages of S Corporations are

- Personal guarantees from officers or stockholders may be required if the corporation has limited credit.
- Conflict can erupt if a small but powerful group of stockholders join together and limit decision making.
- Minority stockholders may be limited from being able to recover the value of their investment in the corporation.
- Stock ownership can become fragmented among many persons who are not active in or knowledgeable about the business through gift or sale to others.
- The corporate shield of limited liability may be lost in some instances when corporate formalities are not followed, and shareholders can become personally liable in rare instances.

C CORPORATIONS

A "C corporation" is a corporation that is taxed under Subchapter C of the Internal Revenue Code and receives IRS approval of its request for Subchapter C status. As a legal entity, the C corporation is separate and distinct from the owners of the corporation (stockholders). The C corporation must pay taxes on its taxable income prior to making dividend distributions to stockholders. It is allowed to issue more than one type of stock and can have any number of stockholders. One or more officers or employees of the corporation are authorized to conduct business on behalf of the corporation. As with an S corporation, if the corporation is new or has a limited credit record, a lender may require personal guarantees by one or more officers or stockholders before approving a credit application from the corporation. If personal guarantees are given, the signer(s) usually have unlimited liability for the debts of the corporation. Some legal costs are incurred in setting up a C corporation, and the formation and continued operation of a corporation is required and is accomplished through filings with the designated state office.

Advantages of C corporations are

- The perpetual life of the corporation makes possible its continuation, and the relatively undisturbed continued operation of the business, despite the incapacity or death of one or more stockholders.
- Fractional ownership interests are easily accommodated in the initial offering of stock.
- The purchase, sale, and gifting of stock make possible changes in ownership without disturbing the corporation's ability to conduct business.
- The required separation of finances and records for the corporation reduces the risk of unrecognized equity liquidations.
- To the extent the corporate shield is maintained and other investments and savings of the stockholders are not at risk, the personal life of stockholders is simplified.
- The annual meetings of stockholders and consultations with legal counsel can provide stimulus for improved communication with the stockholder group (usually a family group) and can provide more comprehensive guidance for management.
- Life insurance up to $50,000 per person, health insurance, housing costs, and other benefits for employees (including stockholder-employees) can be tax-deductible expenses for the corporation.

Disadvantages of C corporations are

- They must pay income tax on their net income before distribution of dividends to stockholders, and the dividends are taxable to the stockholders, resulting in double taxation of corporation income distributed to stockholders.
- Personal guarantees from corporate officers may be required if credit is limited, resulting in loss of the corporate shield to limit liability.
- Conflict among a small group of stockholders may stagnate decision making.

- Stock ownership can become fragmented among many persons who are not active in or knowledgeable about the business through gift or sale to others.
- Corporation paid benefits for stockholder-employees may become costly and exceed the ability of the business to pay.

For more in-depth information on starting a business and on the advantages and disadvantages of various forms of structuring private practices or entrepreneurial ventures, you are encouraged to review the resources at the end of the chapter, particularly those provided by the U.S. Small Business Administration (*http://www.sba.gov/*). Your local Chamber of Commerce may also provide a network of peers and learning opportunities for persons interested in starting and managing their own business.

Organizations by Societal Sector

A common-sense way that organizations have been classified is according to their societal "sector," such as medical, educational, or community-based. Although R. H. Hall (1996) pointed out that this manner of classifying organizations is limited because there are dimensions of organizations that can overlap in unpredictable ways (e.g., many universities operate hospitals), this classification is functional and commonly used to describe the settings in which occupational therapists and occupational therapy assistants work. For example, it is common to refer to occupational therapy service providers who work in the "school system," and much has been written about the increased number of occupational therapy personnel who have returned to practice in the "community." Classifying organizations in this manner is useful because, for the occupational therapy manager and practitioner, it typically has significant implications for the type of services provided.

Hospitals and other medical-model settings are still a popular area of practice for occupational therapy across the full age span of patients and the entire continuum of care from acute trauma to skilled nursing facilities. These settings are often referred to as "medical-model" settings because the focus of much of the intervention is on remediation of an underlying physical impairment in order to restore health and function. It should not be assumed, however, that practicing in a medical setting prevents the delivery of holistic care, the provision of occupation-based practice, or the use of strategies to lessen disability by adapting the environment. Effective managers in medical-model settings must develop a working knowledge of a wide range of reimbursement policies because these can have dramatic effects on the services provided, patterns of staffing, and organizational structure. For example, the 1997 Balanced Budget Act drastically decreased the amount of covered services in skilled nursing facilities and imposed caps on Medicare reimbursement for outpatients.

A large percentage of occupational therapists and occupational therapy assistants work in school systems and provide services under the Individuals with Disabilities Education Act (IDEA), which was discussed in Chapter 2. As with hospitals, choosing to practice in a type of organization such as a school system typically has implications for the nature of practice. Often, services in a school are provided through consultative models by collaborating with a student's teacher and adapting the environment to promote learning while providing limited individual service. Occupational therapy managers who work in the school system often supervise therapists over a large geographic area, therapists in a number of different schools, or therapists from other disciplines, including physical therapy and speech-language pathology.

Occupational therapists and occupational therapy assistants work in a wide range of community-based organizations, including those providing early intervention, work rehabilitation, mental health, and adult day programs (Scaffa, 2001). Although it is common to refer to "community-based organizations" as a single type of organization, the diversity within these organizations must be recognized. Community-based organizations can be small organizations focused on the delivery of a single type of service to a very specific population, or they can be large and serve a range of needs experienced by the community they serve. The range of roles assumed by occupational therapy managers in community-based organizations must be recognized. Whereas it is common for the role of the occupational therapist or occupational therapy assistant in a medical-model setting such as a hospital to be more narrowly defined because of the presence of numerous other disciplines, occupational therapy service providers in community-based organizations often assume a wider variety of duties. In addition to managing and providing traditional occupational therapy services, they may assume responsibility for supervision of volunteers, case management of clients, or organizing and running special events.

Regardless of type, organizations can be structured in various ways. Understanding the relationship between organizational structure and performance is important and can help the occupational therapy manager more effectively navigate the flow of daily challenges. The next section of this chapter will provide a brief overview of concepts related to organizational structure.

Organizational Structure

Organizations can be structured in a wide variety of manners from simple to extraordinarily complex. Depending on the size and age of an organization, it may have undergone a number of restructurings intended to improve efficiency and effectiveness, and often to reduce costs. These restructurings may have been planned and executed in a logical manner, or they may have happened organically as the organization grew, added new services, or had to respond to environmental influences. A good place to start to understand the structure of an organization is the organizational chart. An *organizational chart* is a management tool that visually depicts the following aspects of an organization (Liebler et al., 1992):

- Major functions, usually by department
- Relationships of functions or departments
- Channels of supervision
- Lines of authority and of communication
- Positions by job title within departments or units

It is important to remember a number of things when considering an organizational chart. First, the organizational chart typically is a static picture of an organization. It may be out of date, may not reflect current vacancies or temporary employees such as consultants, and may not accurately reflect staffing that changes based on volume or work demand. Second, organizational charts usually represent only formal chains of command and authority and do not indicate informal communication systems between departments or units, or power and informal authority that may evolve as members remain in an organization for extended periods of time.

Examining the organizational charts of many large organizations may provide evidence to support that systems are not only "open" but often quite organic in how they grow and structure themselves over time. The architect Louis Sullivan noted that "form follows function." Of course, Sullivan was referring to the physical structures of organizations, but his idea has often been used to explain how the organization of personnel and resources follow the function completed by an organization. Unfortunately, it sometimes happens that organizational forms remain as artifacts that no longer serve the purpose for which they were developed and may even contribute to dysfunction in the organization.

According to R. H. Hall (1996), organizational structures serve three basic functions (Box 3–4). First, structures are intended to produce organizational outputs and to achieve organizational goals. Second, structures are designed to minimize or at least regulate the influence of individual variations on the organization. Structures are imposed to ensure that individuals conform to the requirements of the organization and not vice versa. Third, structures are the settings in which power is exercised, in which decisions are made, and in which the organization's activities are carried out. These three purposes are important to remember because changes in structure may also change how the organization achieves its goals and may unintentionally increase or decrease the formal power and authority of individuals.

Although few large organizations perfectly fit the profile of any "named" organizational form or structure, there are a few basic structures commonly found in health care organizations that are useful for a new manager or practitioner to understand. These structures include the *dual pyramid* form of organizing, *product line* or *service line management* organizations, and *hybrid* or *matrix* organizations. The term *dual pyramid* has been used to

> **Box 3–4: The Three Purposes of Organizational Structure**
>
> 1. Structures produce outputs to achieve organizational goals.
> 2. Structures minimize or regulate the influence of individuals on the organization.
> 3. Structures are the settings in which power is exercised, decisions are made, and activities are carried out.
>
> Adapted from Hall, R. H. (1996). *Organizations: structures, processes and outcomes* (6th ed.). Englewood Cliffs, NJ: Prentice Hall.

describe the common structure found in many medical-model settings, such as acute and general hospitals. The symbol of a pyramid has been used to represent a typical organization of personnel, with upper management at the top of the pyramid and line staff at the bottom (Figure 3–4).

In the *dual pyramid* form of organizing, the traditional relationship between medical staff and administration results in the pyramid structure shown in Figure 3–4 being duplicated. One pyramid represents the structure of professional staff organized in departments, including top management (with the chief executive officer at the top of the pyramid); allied health professionals such as occupational therapy, physical therapy, and social work in the middle; and all support services, such as engineering, housekeeping, and human resources personnel, as line employees. A second pyramid mimics that structure but represents the organization of the medical staff, with the chief medical officer at the top of the pyramid, department heads as middle management, and staff physicians as line employees. The major role of the medical staff organization is to recommend to the hospital board of directors the appointment of physicians to the medical staff (Sultz & Young, 1997). Medical staff also provides oversight and peer review of the quality of medical care in the hospital.

Both pyramids report to the ultimate authority, which is typically a board of trustees or board of di-

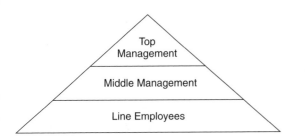

Figure 3–4   The pyramid form of organizing.

rectors. However, there are two distinct chains of command, which results in authority and accountability systems being separated depending on function within the organization. The "bricks" of the pyramid are based upon the function that individuals complete or upon education and training. An example of a typical dual pyramid structure is provided in Figure 3–5.

An alternative form of organizing to the dual pyramid is the *product line* or *service line management* form of organizing. In a product line management organization, personnel are organized according to the service or product that they provide rather than according to the specific function that they complete or according to departments based upon education or training. A board of directors maintains ultimate authority, and the chief executive officer and chief medical officer often still maintain parallel but distinct responsibilities and authority. An example of the organizational chart for an organization with a product line management form of organizing is provided in Figure 3–6.

A *matrix* or *hybrid* organization is one that combines elements of organizing by department, as found in a dual pyramid form of organizing, with the functional approach found in the product line management form of organizing. Combining the key elements of the dual pyramid and product line management forms provides increased flexibility. In matrix organizations there is typically a more fluid organizational chart, including the use of project management teams and strategies in which subject matter and technical experts are borrowed from departments or functional units to lead key projects on a temporary basis. Project teams may form for periods of weeks to months to guide the implementation of a new organizational system and disband when their work is done. This results in a constant shifting of the organizational chart.

Each of the methods of organizing has advantages and disadvantages, and understanding how they influence the function of your organization can help you capitalize on the benefits and compensate for the limitations within your system. Health care organizations formed in a dual pyramid structure rely on departmentation according to discipline or professional education and training to provide for strong supervision of staff and oversight of clinical performance. As such, communication within a professional discipline is facilitated and the daily work of a unit may be completed more efficiently. For example, planning staffing levels or coverage for staff members who might be absent becomes easier in this type of organization. Continuous quality improvement (CQI) of processes and outcome measurement of single types of interventions are also easier to measure in a dual pyramid organization. This is due to the typical presence of a department manager or supervisor from each discipline who has direct access to

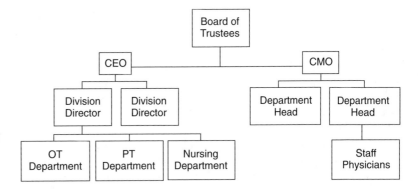

Figure 3–5   A sample dual pyramid form of organizing. (CEO, chief executive officer; CMO, chief medical officer; OT, occupational therapy; PT, physical therapy.)

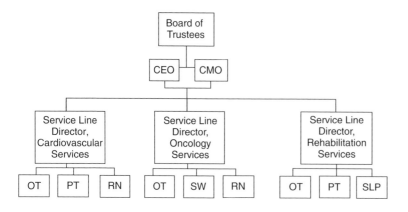

Figure 3–6   A sample product line management form of organizing. (CEO, chief executive officer; CMO, chief medical officer; OT, occupational therapy; PT, physical therapy; RN, nursing; SLP, speech-language pathology; SW, social work.)

staff and data related to routine processes and interventions. For the same reason, it may be easier for discipline-specific managers to work with staff from their own discipline to plan for professional development and continuing education. There are also disadvantages to the dual pyramid form of organizing. Communication across disciplines may be more complicated and pose potential hazards for developing and managing new programs. Problem solving and process improvement in existing programming may be cumbersome because staff members may feel it necessary to communicate up through the chains of command. The advantages and disadvantages of both the dual pyramid and the product line management form of organizing are summarized in Table 3–1.

Regardless of the form that an organization takes, another important concept to recognize related to organization form and function is the difference between what have been termed *line functions* and what have been termed *staff functions*. Line units or employees conduct the major business that is directly related to the primary outputs of the organization. For example, in a typical hospital, physicians, nurses, and therapists complete line functions. Staff functions or employees assist the line units by providing specialized services and bring specialized supportive knowledge such as human resource management, accounting, or information technology. Staff functions are critical to the operations of an organization, and a new occupational therapy manager would benefit from establishing and maintaining relationships with contacts in other departments, including areas such as human resources, planning and marketing, information technology, engineering, and accounting.

Trends in Organizational Development, Behavior, and Function

In recent decades, many organizations that employ occupational therapy service providers have faced considerable change as a result of new legislation, turbulent economic times, increased competition in the marketplace, and myriad other factors. An example would include responding to decreased reimbursement under the Balanced Budget Act of 1997 that resulted in large numbers of providers of rehabilitation to skilled nursing facilities "downsizing" by laying off occupational therapy and physical therapy personnel. Other examples include the impact of decreased levels of reimbursement under managed care and the effects of the September 11th terrorist attack on the economy and charitable giving to nonprofit organizations, including those that employ occupational therapy service providers. At the same time, occupational therapists and occupational therapy assistants have had an increasing influence in community-based practice and in the area of work disability in industry, and new opportunities have presented themselves in these types of organizations. As organizations struggle to keep pace with their changing environments, a number of trends have emerged. Three of these trends will be briefly reviewed in this section.

Table 3-1	Advantages and Disadvantages of Common Forms of Organizing	
	Dual Pyramid	Product Line Management
Communication	Communication within a discipline is facilitated.	Communication between disciplines becomes harder.
Planning	Planning for activities such as professional development and clinical supervision is facilitated but program planning becomes harder.	Program planning and planning for interdisciplinary activities such as program evaluation is facilitated but functions within disciplines become harder.
Budgeting	Tracking and planning for finances related to single-discipline costs is facilitated but that for interdisciplinary activities (e.g., cost per unit of care) is harder.	Tracking and planning for finances related to programmatic costs is facilitated (e.g., cost per unit of care) but that for discipline-specific activities is harder.
Staffing	Some needs, such as providing coverage for leaves or vacancies, may be easier, but the need to communicate with other managers increases. Recruitment activities are facilitated.	Staffing activities influenced by other disciplines, such as scheduling programmatic elements, may be facilitated, but coverage for leaves or vacancies becomes more difficult. Recruitment of staff may be more difficult or you may need to rely upon managers from other disciplines for assistance.
CQI, Program Evaluation, and Outcomes	Improving discipline-specific processes is easier, as is measuring single-disciplines outcomes and indicators of program evaluation, but interdisciplinary programs require extra effort.	Improving interdisciplinary or program processes is easier, as is measuring program outcomes and indicators of program evaluation, but discipline-specific elements require extra effort.
Professional Development	Development of discipline-specific skills related to assessment and intervention may be facilitated by the ease of access to disciplinary specialists.	Development of interdisciplinary skills related to the needs of a population or program development or implementation may be facilitated.

Continuous Quality Improvement

Most health care organizations, such as hospitals, have had formal systems to evaluate and improve quality for many years. In the last two decades, however, there has been a shift from what was referred to as *quality assurance* to *continuous quality improvement*. Chapter 11 explores CQI in depth, including the history of CQI and the common concepts, strategies, tools, and techniques used for "process improvement," so only a brief explanation will be provided here. The primary change that has resulted in moving from quality assurance to CQI has been a shift from focusing on gathering data on stable processes to *control* or *assure* quality to a focus on customer satisfaction by improving the efficiency and effectiveness of the common or *critical processes* completed in the course of everyday work. This shift has included both a change in management philosophy, including increased involvement of employees in decision making about how to best meet the needs of customers, and a change in the strategies for examining the flow of work. The principles behind CQI (commonly known as *total quality management* in industry) find their origins in the 1940s and 1950s in efforts to rebuild the post–World War II economy in Japan. Since that time, these principles have been effectively implemented in a wide range of industries in the United States, including the automobile, hotel, and manufacturing industries, and most recently have been widely implemented in health care settings.

Operations Improvement/ Process Re-engineering

A second trend in organizations, particularly in medical-model health care settings such as hospitals, has been a focus on cost savings through *operations improvement* and *process re-engineering*. Operations improvement should not be confused with CQI. They are not the same thing, but neither are they mutually exclusive. Many hospitals have undertaken both CQI and operations improvement efforts at the same time. In CQI, the relationship between costs and customer satisfaction is such that it is believed that, by focusing on customers needs, you also improve efficiency and effectiveness and hence reduce costs. In operations improvement approaches, you are likely to re-examine work processes and change or "re-engineer" how things are done, but the primary focus is on reducing costs. In addition to an examination of work processes, operations improvement includes an examination of staffing and ways of doing business, such as purchasing practices focused on eliminating unnecessary costs.

A key difference between CQI and an operation's improvement initiative is *who* is involved and *how* they are involved. In CQI, an outside consultant or consulting firm may very often be involved in initial orientation and training of staff. After training of organizational leadership is complete, the consultants turn over all responsibility for CQI effort to the organization, and it becomes the responsibility of the organizational leadership to plan for ongoing training of staff. A focus of CQI is involving staff at all levels (e.g., all key stakeholders in the process) in process improvement. As a result, staff members may feel positively about their involvement in making decisions and creating change within the organization.

Consultants are also a typical part of operations improvement initiatives, as is training of organization leadership and department managers. However, in operations improvement initiatives the focus is definitely on cutting costs from the budget, and less attention may be paid to involving all levels of staff in the process. Still, these initiatives may often include a brainstorming or idea generation phase in which employees are invited to submit ideas. Naturally, both CQI and operations improvement efforts will be heavily influenced by the values of organizational leadership, and may be experienced as positive or negative processes by managers and staff depending on how the initiatives are rolled out. It is important to understand, however, that operations improvement initiatives do not target the management philosophy of organizational leadership, as does CQI. Rather, the central target is cost cutting. The fees of operations improvement consulting firms and their reputations may be heavily dependent upon their success in cutting costs from a budget in a relatively short period of time. Some of the most common strategies used in operations improvement efforts include

- Combining departments to eliminate duplications of effort in both management and support positions, such as receptionists and secretarial support
- Leveraging tasks to the most appropriately trained but lowest paid staff members, resulting in decreased use of professional staff and increased use of assistants and support staff
- Purchasing strategies such as buying all office supplies from the same supplier so that larger volumes are purchased at one time and discounts can be negotiated
- Process re-engineering and automation of processes to eliminate rework and delays and to eliminate or decrease the number of work hours devoted to routine processes

Organizational Learning and Learning Organizations

Organizational learning and *learning organizations* are concepts that have appeared in the organizational development and organizational behavior literature over the last three decades and have been met with mixed reaction. Whereas some organizational development theorists have had high praise for the concepts, others have dismissed these ideas as fads.

Argyris (1977) defined organizational learning as the process of "detection and correction of errors." Organizations detect and correct errors, or "learn," through individual employees who function as agents of change and learning for the organization. Argyris stated, "The individuals' learning activities, in turn, are facilitated or inhibited by an ecological system of factors that may be called an organizational learning system." When a person or an organization learns by processing information and experiences, the range of potential behaviors of the employee or organization is changed. Although the process of learning can be extremely complicated, the types of learning that occur with organizations have been described simply as learning related to (Haines, 2002)

- New knowledge, or the understanding of concepts, facts, and opinions
- New attitudes, or the willingness and motivation to act
- New skills, or the ability to demonstrate or perform an action or function

WHAT IS A LEARNING ORGANIZATION?

Senge (1990) defined the learning organization as the organization in which "you cannot *not* learn because learning is so insinuated into the fabric of life." He described a learning organization as an organization in which "a group of people [are] continually enhancing their capacity to create what they want to create." McGill, Slocum, and Lei (1992) defined the learning organization as "a company that can respond to new information by altering the very 'programming' by which information is processed and evaluated." Simply stated, a learning organization is one in which the organization strives to have everyone working at their best, and to recognize how this happens and to consciously facilitate that state. A key concept related to the learning organization is that of *generative* or *double-loop* learning.

ADAPTIVE LEARNING VERSUS GENERATIVE LEARNING

Much of the traditional view of organizations is based on *adaptive learning*, or what some refer to as "single-loop learning." Adaptive learning or single-loop learning focuses on solving problems in the present without examining the appropriateness of current learning behaviors. Adaptive organizations focus on incremental improvements, often based upon the past track record of success. Essentially, they don't question the fundamental assumptions underlying the existing ways of doing work. Senge (1990) noted that increasing adaptiveness is only the first stage; companies need to focus on generative learning or "double-loop learning" (Argyris 1977). *Generative learning* emphasizes continuous experimentation and feedback in an ongoing examination of the very way organizations go about defining and solving problems. In Senge's (1990) view, generative learning is about creating—it requires "systemic thinking, shared vision, personal mastery, team learning, and creative tension [between the vision and the current reality]." Generative learning, unlike adaptive learning, requires new ways of looking at the world.

To become most adaptable through the use of generative or double-loop learning and to survive in fast-changing and unpredictable environments, organizations need to learn to incorporate experimentation as a way of daily life. Learning organizations must become comfortable with frequent change in structures, processes, domains, goals, and the like, even in the face of apparently optimal adaptation (Hedberg, Nystrom, & Starbuck, 1976; Starbuck, 1983). The consequences of an ongoing state of experimentation are that organizations learn about a variety of design features and remain flexible.

WHAT IS THE MANAGERS' ROLE IN THE LEARNING ORGANIZATION?

Senge (1990) suggested that the leaders of learning organizations must adopt the role of designer and teacher. He argued that leaders can build a shared vision and challenge the status quo by suggesting alternative mental models to those that have traditionally driven managerial action. In other words, leaders are responsible for learning.

The key ingredient of the learning organization is in *how* organizations process their managerial experiences. In learning organizations, managers *learn* from their experiences rather than being *bound* by their past experiences. In generative learning organizations, the ability of an organization or manager is not measured by *what* it knows (that is the product of learning), but rather by *how* it learns—the process of learning. Management practices encourage, recognize, and reward openness, systemic thinking, creativity, a sense of efficacy, and empathy.

EVIDENCE ON LEARNING ORGANIZATIONS

Although there is a growing body of literature on the concept of learning organizations, the attributes thought to foster their development, and descriptions of the implementation of discrete strategies, there is relatively little empirical evidence. An increasing number of models have been proposed to describe how learning organizations might develop, but few have been empirically validated (Lahteenmaki, Toivonen, & Mattila, 2001).

The research that has been conducted has to date been qualitative, descriptive studies typically in a case-study format (Gardiner, 1999; B. P. Hall, 2001; Kasl, Marsick, & Dechant, 1997). These studies have described the characteristics of managers thought to empower employees to learn as well as the limitations of existing perspectives. Although the evidence to support the concept of learning organizations is not yet sufficient to provide strong evidence for managerial action, the general findings are not inconsistent with better developed perspectives on learning, employee development, and mentoring and so may warrant a review by an occupational therapy manager interested in employee learning. A sample of evidence on learning organizations is summarized in Table 3–2.

Table 3-2 Summary of Selected Evidence on Learning Organizations

Author	Study Type	N	Level of Evidence	Results
Mojab & Gorman (2003)	Literature review using Marxist-feminist analysis	Not stated	Poor	Authors suggest based on their review that learning organizations have limited capabilities to support democratic, grassroots, and gender-conscious organizations and do little to promote the economic interests of women.
Lahteenmaki et al. (2001)	Literature review	Not stated	Poor	Identifies proposed gaps in organizational learning research, including a lack of empirical validation of concepts, continued focus on individual learning rather than social structure, and the continued proliferation of new models rather than efforts to validate currently proposed models.
B. P. Hall (2001)	Case study	1 shipping company	Poor	Values exploration and values mentoring of organizational leaders increases leadership decision-making capability and the consciousness of the system as a whole, which are critical factors in developing the organization as a learning environment.

(continued)

Author	Study Type	N	Level of Evidence	Results
Ellinger & Bostrom (1999)	Semistructured interviews using critical incident analysis	12 managers from 4 organizations	Weak	13 behavior sets were identified that were associated with coaching from an empowerment paradigm. 11 behaviors have previously been associated with managerial taxonomies, but 2 new behaviors were identified that were closely associated with learning organizations.
Gardiner (1999)	Case study	2 engineering organizations	Weak	Developing a true learning organization is very difficult, and it may be more realistic to describe a learning orientation. Key attributes were vision, empowerment, appropriate rewards, effective communication, and trust.
Kasl et al. (1997)	Case study	1 petrochemical company and 1 data-processing company	Poor	Team learning is a dynamic process in which both learning processes and the conditions that support them change qualitatively as the team learns. The passage of time becomes a dimension of learning such that shared experiences of a team contribute to a team's capacity for deep understanding.

As was asserted in Chapter 1, many of the topics overviewed in this introduction to organizations would lend themselves to the development of questions to be answered through the identification and evaluation of evidence. The literature presented in Table 3–2 is just one example of such evidence.

Chapter Summary

Organizations play a critical role in the functioning of modern life in industrialized nations. Most occupational therapy personnel are employed by some type of organization, whether public or private, or nonprofit or for-profit. By becoming familiar with the range of scholarship, theory, and evidence related to the development and functioning of organizations, occupational therapy managers can become more effective as managers and

as advocates for those they represent. Although health care and community-based organizations are perhaps most commonly described as "open systems," the three perspectives on organizational functioning described in this chapter (rational, natural, and open) each contribute something valuable to our understanding of the internal and external environments in which we operate. Learning to assess how the culture and values of an organization are demonstrated in the everyday behaviors of its employees is a critical skill for the occupational therapy manager that can aid him or her to have increased influence. As more occupational therapists and occupational therapy assistants develop and manage private businesses, it is necessary for these entrepreneurs to become aware of resources to guide them in choosing the most appropriate business structure. Finally, three trends in organizational development and behavior (CQI, operations improvement, and learning organizations) were overviewed. Other aspects of organizational functioning will be discussed in later chapters, but you are encouraged to remain open to the new knowledge that is constantly being generated by a variety of fields that will guide you as you work within various types of organizations.

Additional Resources for Learning More About Organizations

Journals Related to Organizations

JOURNAL OF ORGANIZATIONAL BEHAVIOR

The *Journal of Organizational Behavior* reviews international and multidisciplinary, qualitative and quantitative research. Published articles address both research and theory on a wide range of topics related to occupational organizational behavior. Topics noted for inclusion in the journal include motivation, work performance, equal opportunities at work, job design, career processes, occupational stress, quality of work life, job satisfaction, personnel selection, training, organizational change, research methodology in occupational/organizational behavior, employment, job analysis, behavioral aspects of industrial relations, managerial behavior, organizational structure and climate, leadership and power.

JOURNAL OF OCCUPATIONAL AND ORGANIZATIONAL PSYCHOLOGY

The *Journal of Occupational and Organizational Psychology* publishes empirical research as well as

---

Real-Life Solutions

Kate wondered about theories related to how organizations are structured and how those theories might help her as an occupational therapy clinician and manager. Kate decided to enroll in a master's program in business administration, and she took an introductory course in organizational behavior. She quickly discovered that scholars had been studying how organizations develop and function for decades and that, indeed, there was a range of theories on organizations that she would learn. She also began to see how these theories might be applied within organizations.

She noted that different organizations within the hospital system where she was employed were structured differently. She had previously worked in the system's acute care facility, which was organized in a dual pyramid structure, but now worked in the rehabilitation hospital, which was organized in a product line management structure. In her class, they discussed that all structures had advantages and disadvantages, and she could see now that that was true. She appreciated how easy it seemed to be, in a product line management structure, to solve interdisciplinary problems, but worried whether the new occupational therapists and occupational therapy assistants, who reported to a physical therapist, were getting the clinical supervision they needed.

Kate was most excited about how she was able to apply what she was learning about organizational culture and values to her current job, and could see how knowledge from other fields such as organizational behavior could be helpful in her future as an occupational therapy manager. She had only recently moved to the head injury team and had been confused at first at all of the seemingly "unwritten" rules that all the other staff members seemed to know about. She began to enjoy the idea that, by observing the actions of the other members of her team and how the team members responded to each other, she could not only learn "how things are done" but also gain important insights into the underlying values that were shared among the team members but were not explicitly articulated.

Finally, Kate was impressed with the range of research that she was being exposed to and began to formulate questions about the strength of some of the evidence related to these questions. Although she felt a little overwhelmed at the prospect of all that she could learn to help her succeed as a manager, she also knew that the same evidence-based skills that helped her answer clinical questions could guide her in finding possible answers to questions about organizations and any other aspect of being an occupational therapy manager.

papers addressing theory and emerging issues with the goal of improving readers' understanding of people and organizations. The journal publishes articles that address a variety of contexts and areas of knowledge. Published articles relate to contexts and domains including industrial, organizational, engineering, vocational and personnel psychology, as well as behavioral aspects of industrial relations, ergonomics, human factors, and industrial sociology.

JOURNAL OF ORGANIZATIONAL EXCELLENCE

The *Journal of Organizational Excellence* provides a forum for researchers, organizational leaders and others to share information on emerging techniques and strategies that are being used by organizations around the world. Reports of practices that improve performance and strategies to improve organizational positioning in an increasingly complex and competitive global economy are frequently included.

Professional Organizations and Associations Concerned with the Study of Organizations

THE ACADEMY OF MANAGEMENT

http://www.aomonline.org/
The Academy of Management's central mission is to enhance the profession of management by advancing the scholarship of management and enriching the professional development of its members. The academy is also committed to shaping the future of management research and education. The Academy of Management is a leading professional association for scholars dedicated to creating and disseminating knowledge about management and organizations. Founded in 1936 by two professors, the Academy of Management is the oldest and largest scholarly management association in the world. Today, the academy is the professional home for over 14,000 members from 90 nations.

THE AMERICAN SOCIETY FOR TRAINING AND DEVELOPMENT

http://www.astd.org/astd/
Founded in 1944, the American Society for Training and Development (ASTD) is the world's premier professional association and leading resource on workplace learning and performance issues. The ASTD provides information, research, analysis, and practical information derived from its own research; the knowledge and experience of its members; its conferences, expositions, seminars, and publications; and the coalitions and partnerships it has built through research and policy work. The ASTD's membership includes more than 70,000 people working in the field of workplace performance in 100 countries worldwide. Its leadership and members work in more than 15,000 multinational corporations, small and medium-sized businesses, government agencies, colleges, and universities.

THE SOCIETY FOR ORGANIZATIONAL LEARNING

http://www.solonline.org/
The Society for Organizational Learning (SoL) is an intentional learning community composed of organizations, individuals, and local SoL communities around the world. SoL was created to connect corporations and organizations, researchers, and consultants to generate knowledge about and capacity for fundamental innovation and change by engaging in collaborative action inquiry projects. While bringing together "specialists," the society's goal is more than simple collaboration. The purpose of the SoL is to discover (research), integrate (capacity development), and implement (practice) theories and practices of organizational learning for the interdependent development of people and their institutions and communities such that they continue to increase their capacity to collectively realize their highest aspirations and productively resolve their differences. With this intention, organizations are truly worthy of the commitment of their employees and communities.

U.S. SMALL BUSINESS ADMINISTRATION

http://www.sba.gov/
The mission of the Small Business Administration (SBA) is to maintain and strengthen the nation's economy by aiding, counseling, assisting, and protecting the interests of small businesses and by helping families and businesses recover from national disasters. The SBA provides resources on starting, financing, and managing small businesses, including the basics of developing business plans, applying for loans, and tax issues.

Reference List

Argyris, C. (1997). Double-loop learning in organizations. *Harvard Business Review, 55,* 115–134.

Ellinger, A. D., & Bostrom, R. B. (1999). Managerial coaching behaviors in learning organizations. *Journal of Management Development, 18,* 752–771.

Fennell, M. C. (1980). The effects of environmental characteristics on the structure of hospital clusters. *Administrative Science Quarterly, 29,* 489–510.

Gardiner, P. (1999). Soaring to new heights with learning oriented companies. *Journal of Workplace Learning, 11,* 255–277.

Haines, S. (2002). *What is learning and the learning organization?* San Diego, CA: Center for Strategic Management.

Hall, B. P. (2001). Values development and learning organizations. *Journal of Knowledge Management, 5,* 19–26.

Hall, R. H. (1996). *Organizations: structures, processes and outcomes* (6th ed.). Englewood Cliffs, NJ: Prentice Hall.

Hedberg, B. L., Nystrom, P. C., & Starbuck, W. H. (1976). Camping on seesaws: Prescriptions for a self-designing organization. *Administrative Science Quarterly, 21,* 41–65.

Illinois Hospital Association. (2003). Illinois Hospital Association Homepage. Illinois Hospital Association. Available at *http://www.ihatoday.org*

Jaques, E. (1998). *Requisite organization.* Arlington, VA: Cason Hall.

Kasl, E., Marsick, V. J., & Dechant, K. (1997). A research-based model of team learning. *Journal of Applied Behavioral Science, 33,* 227–246.

Lahteenmaki, S., Toivonen, J., & Mattila, M. (2001). Critical aspects of organizational learning research and proposals for its measurement. *British Academy of Management, 12,* 113–129.

Liebler, J. G., Levine, R. E., & Rothman, J. (1992). *Management principles for health professionals.* Gaithersburg, MD: Aspen.

March, J. G. (1965). *Handbook of organizations.* Chicago: Rand McNally.

McCormack, G. L., Jaffe, E. G., & Frey, W. F. (2003). New organizational perspectives. In G. L. McCormack (Ed.), *The occupational therapy manager* (4th ed., pp. 85–126). Bethesda, MD: AOTA Press.

McGill, M. E., Slocum, J. W., & Lei, D. (1992). Management practices in learning organizations. *Organizational Dynamics, 21,* 5–17.

Mojab, S., & Gorman, R. (2003). Women and consciousness in the "learning organization": Emancipation or exploration. *Adult Education Quarterly, 53,* 228–241.

Mumford, M. D., & Peterson, N. G. (1999). The O*NET content model: Structural considerations in describing jobs. In N. G. Peterson, M. D. Munford, W. C. Borman, P. R. Jeanneret, & E. A. Fleishman (Eds.), *An occupational information system for the 21st century: The development of O*NET* (pp. 21–30). Washington, DC: American Psychological Association.

Peters, T. J., & Waterman, R. H. (1982). *In search of excellence.* New York: Harper & Row.

Rokeach, M. (1973). *The nature of human values.* New York: Free Press.

Scaffa, M. E. (2001). *Occupational therapy in community-based practice settings.* Philadelphia: F. A. Davis.

Schein, E. H. (1992). *Organizational culture and leadership.* New York: Jossey-Bass.

Schermerhorn, J. R., Hunt, J. G., & Osborn, R. N. (1982). *Managing organizational behavior* (5th ed.). New York: John Wiley & Sons.

Scott, W. R. (1992). *Organizations: Rational, natural and open systems* (3rd ed.). Englewood Cliffs, NJ: Prentice Hall.

Senge, P. (1990). *The fifth discipline.* New York: Doubleday.

Small Business Administration (2003). Forms of business ownership. U.S. Small Business Administration. Available at *http://www.sba.gov/starting_business/legal/forms.html*

Starbuck, W. H. (1983). Organizations as action generators. *American Sociological Review, 48,* 91–102.

Sultz, H. A., & Young, K. M. (1997). *Health care USA.* Gaithersburg, MD: Aspen.

von Bertalanffy, L. (1968). *General systems theory: Foundations, development, and application.* New York: Braziller.

Weber, M. (1946). *From Max Weber: Essays in sociology* (Transl. ed.). New York: Oxford University Press.

Weber, M. (1968). *Economy and society: An interpretive sociology.* New York: Bedminister Press.

4

Brent Braveman, Ph.D., OTR/L, FAOTA

Leadership: The Art, Science, and Evidence

Real-Life Management

Jan has been an occupational therapist in an acute care hospital for 6 years. She is commonly recognized as a clinical expert in a number of areas by many of her peers. Recently, Jan's boss, the director of occupational therapy, resigned and Jan was asked to replace her. She is excited about the promotion and the opportunity, but is also nervous about moving into the role of department director. She is questioning her leadership skills because she feels comfortable interacting on a one-on-one basis but is not as comfortable when leading groups.

Jan shared her reservations about taking on a formal leadership role with Carole, the division director who would be her new boss. Carole was empathetic to Jan's concerns and made the commitment to her that, if Jan accepted the position, she would work with Jan to develop her leadership skills. Jan appreciated the offer, but now has the following questions:

1. Can you develop skills as a leader, or are leadership skills something you are either born with or not?
2. What sort of leader does Jan want to be? She respects both Carole and her old boss Steve, but they seem to have very different styles of leadership.
3. If it is possible to develop skills as a leader, what specific steps can she take to do so?

Jan decided to go to the local bookstore to see if there were any resources on leadership skills that would be helpful. She was surprised to find a large number of books that seemed to approach leadership from many different perspectives. After scanning a few books, she also noted that a number of different theories and models were mentioned. She decided to make a visit to the local university library and do some more investigation to find out if any of the theories or models mentioned in the "popular press" books in the bookstore had been validated by research.

Key Issues

- Leadership skills can be developed. Understanding theories of leadership and the existing evidence on these theories can assist in examining one's existing skills and interpersonal tendencies in order to identify areas for development.
- Leadership theories can be classified as "supervisory," or relating to leadership within an organization, or as "strategic," or relating to leadership of an organization.
- Leadership relates closely to traditionally recognized management skills, including planning, organizing, directing, controlling, and problem solving.
- Leadership relates to both management and supervision, but all three of these constructs can be separated, and skills related to each are discussed in this and other chapters.

In writing this book, a number of difficult decisions had to be made regarding the order in which to present the content of the book. These decisions were not immediately evident upon beginning to organize the book. After all, this text is an entry-level book on management. The responsibilities of managers for oversight of the affairs of an organization and the primary functions of managers within organizations are well known. Entry-level texts on management, regardless of the field or discipline in which they are based, often begin by pointing out that managers complete basic functions for organizations that include (1) planning, (2) organizing, (3) directing, and (4) controlling. There are sometimes variations in the presentation because some authors may pull the function of "staffing" out from that of organizing and present five rather than four categories, but, nonetheless, a discussion of the basic functions of management seemed a logical place to begin.

However, as the structure of the book began to evolve, the organization of the content seemed not to be so clear-cut after all. Naturally, occupational therapy managers are involved in the same basic functions as managers in other fields, so it was not a question of whether these functions would be discussed in the book. Rather, the questions became "In what order should concepts be presented?" and "Are there any overarching concepts that should be used to organize others?" For example, it was clear that it was important to include the topics of management, leadership, and supervision, but should management or leadership be defined first? It was not until the writing of a number of the chapters was underway and the challenges of describing these related, but separate topics were encountered that a decision was made on how to structure Chapters 4, 5, and 6.

The overall topic of this book is the management of occupational therapy services. As such, every chapter within the book relates to content, functions, or issues that lie within the domain of concern for occupational therapy managers. The overarching theme for this particular book is how occupational therapy managers can utilize theory and data, information, and other forms of evidence to become more effective. For this reason, particular topics and content have been chosen upon which to focus entire chapters. And so, after much consideration, the decision was made to dedicate

separate chapters specifically to the topics of leadership, the roles and functions of the manager, and the roles and functions of the supervisor. Chapter 4 will review theories and related evidence on leadership. Leadership is a topic that permeates every aspect of management. Whether we are involved in planning a new program, organizing staff for daily work, directing personnel on how to complete their assignments, or controlling output and services by measuring and improving quality, we can function as leaders and have an impact on how others in the organization view the organization and their work. This chapter will also discuss the relationship between leadership and management. Chapter 5 will summarize the roles and functions of a manager, and Chapter 6 will focus on the roles and functions of a supervisor.

Leadership has been a topic of interest and scientific investigation in the fields of sociology, psychology, and business administration and in the popular press for decades. Much of the literature has focused on the qualities of effective leaders, including in-depth explorations of what has made some of our most notable public figures effective as leaders. Examples include biographies of Eleanor Roosevelt and Mahatma Gandhi, and most recently, in the wake of the September 11th attack on the World Trade Center towers, a book on Rudolph Giuliani, the former Mayor of New York City (Gerber & Burns, 2002; Giuliani & Kurson, 2002; Rudolph & Rudolph, 1983).

More recently, leadership has become a topic of interest in health care, although formal exploration of leadership theory through research has not been as common in health care as it has been in other arenas of management. Books on the application of leadership have been written in the fields of nursing, case management, and occupational therapy (Gilkeson, 1997; Grohar-Murray & Dicroce, 2002; Powell, 2000). Thus it is clear that the topic of leadership has warranted much attention, but it is easy to understand that, as an occupational therapy student or entry-level practitioner, you might ask, "Why should I care about leadership at this point in my career? I *just* want to treat my patients!" Although it is easy to appreciate that new practitioners might be most concerned with the patient care issues that they expect to confront on a day-to-day basis, occupational therapy students and new graduates should consider that they will find themselves in both formal and informal leadership roles much sooner than they expect, or perhaps desire.

Health care organizations today are in a constant state of flux and are influenced by perpetually shifting government policy, economic conditions, shrinking reimbursement, increased competition, and heightened scrutiny by consumers who have become more sophisticated in managing their own health care. As a result of managed care and increased competition for both public and private funding, the management structure of most health care organizations, including community-based organizations, has "flattened." The term *flattened* indicates that many managers who used to lead discipline-specific departments have been asked to accept formal supervisory responsibility for other disciplines, and some middle managers have been laid off (Braveman & Fisher, 1997).

The flattening of organizational structure has resulted in day-to-day decision making being pushed to lower levels of managerial hierarchies. The occupational therapy managers of today must have well-developed skills in program development, budgeting, and marketing, and in guiding those whom they supervise in planning, delivering, and evaluating occupational therapy services. In turn, these managers hold higher expectations for staff therapists, including entry-level practitioners, to work independently, solve problems creatively, and work as members of multidisciplinary teams or task forces. As Gilkeson, a leader in the field of occupational therapy, wrote, "Many of today's organizational charts consist of often-shifting project groups that are led by group members possessing the professional background and competencies needed to address the problem assigned to those groups" (Gilkeson, 1997). As noted earlier, you may find yourself in a position of leadership, albeit informal or temporary, sooner than you think.

Management Versus Leadership

It is helpful to begin a practical discussion of leadership by differentiating between the concepts of management and leadership. Most books on management for the entry-level manager will include some discussion of the topic of leadership. One might wonder whether leadership is a function or a subset of managerial responsibilities or a related but separate set of skills and competencies. The two constructs have often been inextricably linked, and it has been sometimes assumed that anyone in a position of authority is essentially in a leadership role. Given the evidence over the past 50 years, this assumption may be a disservice to the novice manager.

One conceptualization of the relationship between management and leadership is that the role of a manager is to maintain stability, whereas a leader guides change. For example, Levey, Hill, and Green (2002) suggested that, whereas management is conservative and maintenance directed, leadership is innovative, change oriented, and informed by vision. Another view suggests that, whereas managers adapt to and cope with change, leaders instigate change and make competitors cope with it (Gilkeson, 1997). Similarly, Beech (2002) suggested that managers tend to rely primarily on strategy, structure, and systems, whereas leaders are inclined to use style, staff, skills, and shared goals to yield desired results.

These conceptualizations of the relationship between management and leadership may be unnecessarily narrow, however. In fact, one may be a manager, a leader, or both. As noted by Schruijer and Vansina (2002), "Such splitting obscures the complexity of life. Leaders often face environmental change and stability simultaneously; organizations may need change in some domains yet stability in others. The concepts of leadership and management are theoretical constructs that are hard to distinguish." Attempting to do so, however, has a functional implication for new managers and is not simply an academic exercise. By thoughtfully distinguishing between the constructs of leadership and management, we may more successfully identify the skills and behaviors associated with each so that they can more easily be practiced and incorporated into our daily behavior.

Managers are often viewed as problem solvers. Leadership differs from routine problem solving in that leaders are often presented with ill-defined problems (Fleishman et al., 1991). Leaders must often begin problem solving by figuring out exactly what problem is to be solved. However, it is when groups face new problems that effective leadership is most needed and is likely to have its greatest impact on the performance of a work group

(Tushman & Anderson, 1986). Another factor that sets leadership apart from more routine problem solving is that leaders must almost always solve problems while considering a broad social context and implement plans while marshaling support, communicating a vision, and motivating others (Mumford, Zaccaro, Harding, Jacobs, & Fleishman, 2000). To be effective, a leader must possess knowledge about the work to be done, who will be involved in doing the work, and the context in which the work will be accomplished.

A definition of leadership is offered in the following section. First, however, for the purpose of this discussion and to distinguish between the constructs of management and leadership, the following definition of management will be used:

> Management is the process of guiding an organization by planning for future work obligations, organizing employees into functional units, directing employees in the process of completing daily work tasks, and controlling work processes and systems to assure adequate quality of work output.

By distinguishing between management and leadership, there is not an intention to downplay the importance of being an effective manager. However, as with any skill set, the more specific that we can be about what is and is not part of the domain of concern, the more likely we will be able to identify matching strategies for developing the skills.

What Is Leadership?

In considering a definition of leadership, it is important to distinguish between the act or process of leading (i.e., leadership) and the individuals who are in the position of guiding others (i.e., leaders). It is problematic to attempt to define and investigate leadership, and in particular strategies for developing skills in the process of leading others, by solely focusing on descriptions of effective leaders. As noted by Barker (2001), "When leadership is defined, the definition usually addresses the nature of the *leader*, and not the nature of *leadership*." To avoid this difficulty, the following definition of leadership is offered:

> Leadership is a process of creating structural change wherein the values, vision, and ethics of individuals are integrated into the culture of a community as a means of achieving sustainable change.

This definition highlights several issues critical to a thoughtful consideration of leadership. First, leadership is a process, and all processes have results. In considering the importance of leadership to occupational therapy personnel, we must therefore consider the desired results of the occupational therapy leader's actions. Second, leadership is a process of change whereby we hope to impact others in some sustainable manner. Leaders, whether functioning within an ongoing management position or as temporary leaders of ad hoc task groups, can have lasting impact on the function of a department or organization. Third, this definition implies that the focus of this process of change is specifically on individuals and that these individuals are part of a larger community. For occupational therapy personnel, this means that, when examining the process of leading, we must consider the impact on individual workers *and* on the larger work community (e.g., the occupational therapy department, our clients, members of other departments in our organization).

Conceptualizations of leadership found in the literature range from narrow to broad—from specific leader behaviors to complex interactions between leaders, followers, and their larger context (Hunt & Conger, 1999). Attempts to develop models of the skills and knowledge required for effective performance (in this case, effective leadership) typically begin with an analysis of the demands being made on people working in a certain area (Mumford & Peterson, 1999). A leader's performance is a function of whether he or she can identify goals, construct viable paths to goal attainment, and direct others along these paths in a volatile and constantly changing environment (Mumford & Connelly, 1991). Leaders must be able to complete the organizing tasks of defining departmental units but must also aptly complete the task of coordinating the actions of others to meet goals related to the organizational mission (Mumford et al., 2000).

Theory and evidence on leadership is still evolving, and much of the existing evidence is descriptive. The majority of research can be found in the business and psychology literature, although some can be found in the health care literature as well. In a review of health and business literature from 1970 to 1999, only 4.4% of 6629 articles reviewed were data based, indicating the continued need for evidence-based research on the topic of leadership effectiveness (Vance & Larson, 2002). House and Aditya (1997) noted that a problem with current leadership study is that it continues to focus almost exclusively on superior-subordinate relationships to the exclusion of organizational and environmental variables, including characteristics of followers, that are crucial to effective leadership performance. New models, theories, and methods of examining leadership continue to be introduced, so much so that not all can be discussed in this chapter. "Mainstream" leadership scholars most consistently agree upon one thing: Leaders are supposed to "motivate" followers to accomplish organizational goals (Barker, 2001). How leaders accomplish this task can be explained, and may depend upon the theory or theories of leadership upon which they base their behavior.

Leadership Theories: An Overview

Early studies of leadership focused on identification of the common traits of effective leaders, or what Thomas Carlyle referred to as "Great Men" or natural leaders (Carlyle, 1907). The assumption behind this form of research was that people could change their personalities and worldviews to adopt the traits of effective leaders in order to become successful leaders themselves (Rost, 2003). Smith and Kreuger (1933) provided an early review of the literature and organized traits into the categories of personality traits (e.g., alertness), social traits (e.g., sociability), and physical traits (e.g., height). Kirkpatrick and Locke (1991) identified six traits that they believe differentiate leaders from other people: drive, motivation, honesty and integrity, self-confidence, cognitive ability, and knowledge of business. The underlying assumptions of trait theories have been challenged in that the traits of an effective leader cannot be differentiated from the traits of an effective manager or person (Barker, 2001). In the last decade or more, little research has been done to validate leadership theory that focuses

exclusively on specific traits of leaders, so these theories will not be addressed further in this chapter.

Early research on leadership also often sought to answer the question "Are great leaders born or made?" Over time, this question appears to have drifted away because evidence now seems to support that many factors may influence the effectiveness of leaders, including skills, knowledge, work experience, and personality. Although we may not be able to change some of our basic personality traits, it seems clear that, over time, we can seek the types of experiences (e.g., practice in solving novel problems and working with different sorts of groups in various environments) that may contribute to becoming a more effective leader. Mumford et al. (2000) suggested that leaders are neither born nor made; rather their inherent potentials are shaped by experiences enabling them to develop the capabilities needed to solve significant social problems. Knowledge and skills may be gained over time, and the problems encountered by leaders often become more complex and long term as they rise higher in organizations, which allows for the existence of leaders at all levels of organizations. Leadership development initiatives often attempt to address intrapersonal competence through efforts that include training in self-awareness (e.g., emotional awareness), self-regulation (e.g., self-control, trustworthiness) and self-motivation (e.g., commitment, initiative, optimism), social awareness (e.g., empathy, service orientation), and social skills (e.g., collaboration and cooperation, conflict management) (Day, 2001; Goleman, 1995).

Boal and Hooijberg (2001) differentiated between what they described as theories about leadership *in* organizations (supervisory leadership theories) and theories about leadership *of* organizations (strategic leadership theories). Supervisory leadership theories, including "path-goal" and "transactional" theories of leadership, draw from expectancy motivation theory. This theory supposes that a subordinate's performance is related to the extent to which he or she believes that his or her actions will lead to specific outcomes. Transactions are, in essence, "Do this, and you will receive that." Strategic leadership theories, including "charismatic," "transformational," and "situational" theories, draw from the study of organizational behavior and the notion that leaders are able to motivate followers to commit to and realize

Table 4-1	Overview of Leadership Theories	
Theory	**Primary Focus**
SUPERVISORY THEORIES OF LEADERSHIP	
Path-goal	Leaders increase personal payoffs for subordinates for goal attainment and make the path to these payoffs easier to travel by reducing obstacles, thereby improving performance.
Transactional	Leaders promise rewards and benefits to subordinates for meeting work goals, and leaders and subordinates agree through transactions on what will lead to reward and how to avoid punishment.
STRATEGIC THEORIES OF LEADERSHIP	
Charismatic	Stresses the personal identification of followers with the leader, who formulates an inspirational vision and impression that the leader's mission is extraordinary.
Transformational	Leaders achieve change by expressing the value associated with outcomes and by articulating a vision of the future resulting in commitment, effort, and improved performance on the part of subordinates.
Situational	Leaders should adopt a leadership style that best fits the developmental level of their subordinates' competence and commitment.

performance that exceeds their own expectations. Leadership within these theories has been likened to the process of "empowerment," in which the end result of leadership is a change in organizational culture that helps subordinates generate a sense of meaning in their work and a desire to challenge themselves to experience success (Bennis & Nanus, 1985). It is interesting to note that, through a focus on transformational leadership, some theorists came to express a deeper appreciation of the value of transactional behavior for both managers and leaders (Lowe & Galen Kroeck, 1996). Table 4–1 provides a brief overview of the classification of the five theories of leadership presented in this chapter and their major foci.

A Few Words About Leadership Theories and Evidence

Before beginning an exploration of the five theories of leadership to be discussed in this chapter and the evidence related to each theory, it will be helpful to make a few comments about the nature of empirical investigations in this area. As noted in Chapter 1, before conducting a search for evidence, one must develop a question to guide selection of evidence. In regard to leadership theory and corresponding behavior of leaders who adopt a particular theory, what we might be *most* interested in knowing is whether behaviors guided by one theory result in more improved performance on the part of subordinates than when a leader uses behavior guided by another theory. This question may be difficult to answer because well-designed empirical investigations of the direct impact of leader behavior on subordinate performance and results are relatively rare. Rather, the question that is most often posed is, "Do behaviors guided by a particular leadership theory result in higher *perceived* effectiveness as measured by indicators of subordinate perception or by organizational measures of leader performance (e.g., peer reviews or performance appraisals)?" This dynamic exists for a number of reasons. First, outside of contrived laboratory situations (i.e., studies of leader behavior with college students who volunteer for a study), relatively few experimental studies examine leaders in real-time and real-life situations. It is easy to appreciate that not many organizations are going to allow their employee leaders to be manipulated (e.g., to change their style of leadership for the purpose of study) because of worry over financial and performance costs to the organizations. Second, when we try to answer the question of whether a particular approach to leadership results in improved *subordinate* performance, things get cloudy very quickly because so many other things besides leadership behavior can influence performance of subordinates, such as the culture of the organization, the skills and experiences of the subordinates, and the relationship of subordinates or work units to other subordinates or work units in the organization.

Recent research on issues such as the mediating effects of subordinate trust in leaders or the congruence of subordinates' values with a leader's value may shed valuable light on why some leaders are effective (Jung & Avolio, 2000). However, such research is not as well developed as that related specifically to direct impact of leader behavior. For this reason, evaluating evidence in regard to leadership theory and behavior may be a sticky situation. However, as a student or new occupational therapy practitioner who may be assuming his or her first leadership role, you may be perfectly happy to find an answer to the question, "If I adopt behaviors guided by a particular leadership theory, am I more likely to *be perceived* as effective?" In the next section of this chapter, four well-established theories of leadership and a less researched but often cited leadership theory will be presented. A summary of a sample of evidence on each theory will be discussed.

Leadership Theories

Path-Goal Theory

The genesis of the path-goal theory of leadership lies in the work of the Institute for Social Research at the University of Michigan. The theory was developed primarily to reconcile prior research findings on the effects of leader-task orientation (the extent to which leaders focused on completing work tasks) and leader-person orientation (the extent to which leaders focused on the emotional and psychological needs of subordinates) on subordinate satisfaction and performance (House, 1996). The initiation of research on the path-goal theory represented a shift in research from a focus on task and person orientation to a focus on leader effectiveness.

Path-goal theory was initially developed as a dyadic theory of supervision concerning relationships between formally appointed supervisors and subordinates in their day-to-day functioning. As such, it did not address leadership of groups, leadership of change, or leadership related to strategic planning or whole organizations, but rather the effect of leader behavior on individuals. However, in 1996, R. J. House presented a "reformulated" theory that he described as a theory of work unit leadership addressing the effects of leaders on the motivation and abilities of immediate subordinates and the effects of leaders on work unit performance. This reformulated theory includes a focus on "unconscious" motives of subordinates and the "valence" of leadership behaviors (i.e., the strength of the attractiveness of outcomes to the followers). The primary propositions of the path-goal theory of leadership are included in Box 4–1.

The function of a leader as explicated in path-goal theory is to increase personal payoffs to subordinates for achieving workplace goals established by management. Leaders make the paths to these payoffs easier to travel by clarifying them and reducing roadblocks to progress and by increasing the opportunities for personal satisfaction en route (House, 1971). Leader behaviors related to clarifying and reducing roadblocks have been referred to as *leader initiating structure*, and leader behaviors related to increasing subordinate satisfaction have been referred to as *leader consideration* (House, 1996). Path-goal theory is basically a "functional" approach to leadership, calling for a diagnosis of functions that need to be fulfilled in subordinates' work environments for them to be motivated, perform at high levels, and be satisfied (Schriesheim & Neider, 1996).

The effective leader as viewed by path-goal theory is one who assists subordinates to navigate the paths that ultimately lead to organizationally desired and individually valued outcomes (Schriesheim & Neider, 1996). House (1996) noted that it is unlikely that any one leader will be effective in all behaviors,

---

Box 4–1: Primary Propositions of Path–Goal Theory of Leadership

- Leader behavior is viewed as positive to the extent that subordinates see the behaviors as an immediate source of satisfaction or key to future satisfaction.
- Leader behavior will improve employee performance to the extent that it
  - Enhances the motivation of members of work units, enhances the relevant abilities of employees, provides guidance, and removes obstacles and provides resources.
  - Makes satisfaction of employee needs and employee rewards contingent on performance, makes work tasks and goal attainment intrinsically satisfying, and

compliments the work environment by providing structure, support, and rewards necessary for good performance.
- Enhances employee work tasks in a way that promotes collaborative working relationships among employees and between employees and the organization, ensures that the requisite resources are available to work units, and enhances the need for the work unit in the eyes of the rest of the organization.
- Serves as a role model for learning relevant task behavior.

Adapted from House, R. J. (1996). Path-goal theory of leadership: Lessons, legacy and a reformulated theory. *Leadership Quarterly, 7*, 323–352.

---

but suggested that, by using shared leadership approaches, leadership may be delegated to others who are skilled in behaviors that the leader is not. The leader only needs to compliment what is missing in a situation to supplement the subordinates' motivation, satisfaction, and performance (Bass, 1990a). As suggested earlier, this may include strategies such as ad hoc work groups or task forces led by disciplinary members who have the right skills for the job at hand. In many settings in which occupational therapy personnel work, this may mean a staff-level therapist with relatively little work experience.

The reformulated 1996 path-goal theory of work unit leadership identifies 10 classes of leader behaviors that are theoretically acceptable, satisfying, and motivational for employees. These behavior classes and examples of each are listed in Table 4–2.

Concern has been expressed that there has been limited recent research on the path-goal theory of leadership and most of the research that has been done addressed the original formulation of the theory. However, it has also been suggested that this theory has a compelling logic that other theories have not achieved (Schriesheim & Neider, 1996). Evans (1996) suggested that, because research has

focused only on limited parts of the theory (e.g., the effect of leader behavior on performance and satisfaction), the theory's major impact may have been its influence on the development of other leadership theories such as charismatic and transformational theories (Bass, 1985; House, 1977).

EVIDENCE FOR THE PATH-GOAL THEORY OF LEADERSHIP

Question: Does the use of leadership behaviors based on the path-goal theory of leadership lead to increased subordinate perception of leader effectiveness?

More than 50 studies have been designed to test the propositions of the path-goal theory, with the results being mixed, some showing support and others failing to support the theory (House, 1996). House noted that a methodological problem with some studies has been that they sometimes used measures that only approximate the constructs of the theory rather than developing and validating measures specifically designed to test the theory.

Most investigations of path-goal theory have explored relationships between leadership behaviors and outcome measures (e.g., satisfaction) while studying the impact of different moderator variables

Table 4-2	Classes and Examples of Leadership Behavior According to Path-Goal Leadership Theory
Leader Behavior	**Examples**
Clarifying	• Setting clear performance goals and how to achieve them • Setting clear standards for performance in job descriptions and everyday assignments • Clarifying from whom the employee should and should not take direction • Using rewards and punishment with restraint and only in response to work performance
Supportive	• Expressing concern about the welfare of employees • Creating a friendly work environment • Listening to employees' complaints
Participative	• Asking for suggestions on how to proceed • Including employees in decision making using formal and informal means
Achievement oriented	• Setting challenging goals • Showing confidence in the ability of employees to perform well • Emphasizing excellence in performance
Work facilitation	• Planning, scheduling, and organizing work tasks effectively to promote employee performance • Mentoring, guiding, and coaching employees • Assisting employees to develop needed knowledge and skills
Interaction facilitation	• Assisting employees to resolve conflicts • Assuring that minority opinions are heard • Using team-building activities to promote close and satisfying relationships
Group-oriented decision process	• Encouraging all members of the work unit to participate in discussions • Preventing individuals from dominating discussions • Waiting to select options until the entire team has had the opportunity to give input.
Representation & networking	• Advocating for the work unit throughout the organization • Presenting a positive view of the work unit to superiors • Obtaining resources to facilitate work • Participating in organization-wide social functions
Value-based behavior	• Use of "envisioning" activities with employees • Showing passion and self-sacrifice to achieve a described vision • Frequent positive evaluation of employees as a group • Communicating high performance expectations and confidence in employee ability to meet the expectations
Shared leadership	• Promoting interdependence among employees • Delegating leadership visibly to various employees for different tasks

Adapted from House, R. J. (1996). Path-goal theory of leadership: Lessons, legacy and a reformulated theory. *Leadership Quarterly, 7,* 323–352.

such as task structure (Bass, 1990a). Evidence for performance as an outcome variable has not been positive and may account for removal of subordinate performance from the most recent statement of the theory. As mentioned earlier, studies in regard to leader behavior and this theory have focused on *perceptions* of leader effectiveness.

Indvik (1986) completed a meta-analysis including more than 40 studies that found support for the basic propositions of path-goal theory, including strong support for the role that leaders may play in developing organizational structures that promote goal attainment by employees. Other meta-analyses were conducted by Wofford and Liska (1993) and Fisher and Edwards (1988), who found an overall positive relationship between leader consideration and subordinate job satisfaction. Table 4–3 summarizes selected evidence on the path-goal theory of leadership.

Transactional Theory

The transactional theory of leadership is based on examining the transactions or exchanges between a leader and his or her subordinates. A transaction occurs whenever the leader promises rewards and benefits to subordinates for their fulfillment of agreements and their contributions to goal achievement (Bass, 1990b). Ideally, the leader and his or her subordinates agree on what the subordinates need to do to get rewards or to avoid punishment. There is not a focus on changing the subordinates' values or the need to establish a particular type of relationship between the transactional leader and his or her subordinates. As such, although the transactional leader may be effective in reaching short-term managerial objectives, there is not necessarily a commitment to the personal development of subordinates by the leader. The transactional leader has been characterized as one who operates within the existing culture, attends to time constraints, focuses on processes to maintain control of situations, and avoids risks.

Transactional leadership consists primarily of two factors or sets of strategies—managing by exception, and providing contingent rewards (Bass, 1985). *Managing by exception* is when leaders avoid intervening or giving directions if the old ways of doing things are working and allow subordinates to continue in their jobs as always if performance

Table 4-3	Summary of Selected Evidence on Path-Goal Theory of Leadership			
Author	Study Type	N	Level of Evidence	Results
Wofford & Liska (1993)	Meta-analysis	120 studies	Strong	Positive relationship between leader consideration (behaviors aimed at increasing subordinate job satisfaction) and job satisfaction.
Fisher & Edwards (1988)	Meta-analysis	12 studies	Strong	Positive relationship between leader consideration and job satisfaction.
Indvik (1986)	Meta-analysis	48 studies with 11,862 respondents	Strong	Analyzed prior "mixed" results and found overall sufficient support for basic propositions of the theory to warrant continued investigation.
Schriesheim & Schriesheim (1980)	Cross-sectional questionnaire	290 managerial and clerical employees	Good	63% of variance in employee satisfaction explained by supportive leadership.

goals are met. A leader who utilizes managing by exception may fall into the background at times when things are going well and only asserts his or her presence when there is a need to intervene and provide specific direction to subordinates on how to change their behaviors so that organizational goals might be more effectively met.

Contingent rewards are rewards and recognition exchanged for accomplishment of assigned work duties or reaching organizational objectives. The more directly that a reward or recognition is tied to a specific behavior, the more impact the reward is likely to have on promoting the desired behavior. The leader who uses contingent rewards approaches subordinates with an eye to exchanging one thing for another. For example, a leader may make it clear that high levels of productivity are necessary to be considered for an average or above-average merit increase in salary. Another example of a contingent reward might be recognizing staff with praise and friendly interaction when duties such as documentation are completed in a timely manner and meet expectations for completeness and accuracy, but withholding such interaction with staff members who are not performing up to par.

EVIDENCE FOR THE TRANSACTIONAL THEORY OF LEADERSHIP

Question: Does the use of the leadership behaviors of management by exception and contingent rewards result in improved subordinate perception of leader effectiveness?

Studies on the impact of the two primary factors identified by the transactional theory of leadership (management by exception and use of contingent rewards) have generally shown positive effects on subordinate performance, although it has been hypothesized in some studies that these effects were mediated by other variables such as the trust placed in the leader by subordinates. A review of the literature shows that contingent rewards appear to have been studied more than the behavior of managing by exception, perhaps because it is easier to introduce a new behavior in organizations and measure the direct impact of rewards and recognition.

Jung and Avolio (2000) found that transactional leadership had only indirect effects on performance when mediated through followers' trust and value congruence. These results were contradicted by those of Podsakoff, MacKenzie, Moorman, and Fetter (1990), who found a direct positive effect of transactional leadership on organizational citizenship behaviors. Other studies, such as that by Gellis (2002), also found direct correlations between contingent rewards and measures of leader effectiveness as perceived by subordinate satisfaction and the willingness of subordinates to extend extra effort to achieve organizational goals. Lowe and Galen Kroeck (1996) conducted a meta-analysis of 23 studies and found that contingent rewards had a positive association with subordinate perception of leader effectiveness, and that management by exception had a low positive correlation with subordinate perception of leader effectiveness but only in studies conducted in public rather than private organizations. Table 4–4 includes a summary of selected evidence on transactional leadership theory.

Transformational Theory

Burns (1978) argued that some leaders, who he described as "transforming," build more effective relationships with their subordinates and express the importance and values associated with desired outcomes in ways that are easily understood by those they lead. He viewed the transformational leader as distinct from the transactional leader and as one who participated in leadership actions not easily explained by the way traditional workplace exchanges had been defined. Bass (1985) introduced the view that transactional and transformational leadership are not contradictory styles but instead are complimentary, and this view has been widely accepted in most recent research. Many studies have investigated both transactional leadership and transformational leadership and found that both can be effective, and that a leader can exhibit both transformational and transactional qualities simultaneously. In fact, it is now usually suggested that a leader who adopts solely a transformational style is unlikely to be successful in the complete absence of transactional relations with his or her subordinates (Bass, Avolio, & Goodheim, 1987).

The transformational leader has been characterized as one who articulates a vision of the future that can be shared with peers and subordinates, intellectually stimulates subordinates, and pays high attention to individual differences among people

Table 4-4	Summary of Selected Evidence on Transactional Leadership Theory				
Author	Study Type	N	Level of Evidence	Results
Gellis (2002)	Cross-sectional questionnaire	187 social workers	Good	Contingent rewards (rewards based upon meeting certain conditions) were significantly correlated with the leader outcomes of effectiveness, satisfaction, and extra effort by subordinates.
MacKenzie, Podsakoff, & Rich (2001)	Cross-sectional correlational	477 sales agents	Good	Although both transformational and transactional leader behaviors were effective, transformational behaviors were more effective than transactional behaviors in influencing extra effort.
Jung & Avolio (2000)	Experimental with randomization	194 students	Strong	Indirect effects on followers' performance were mediated through followers' trust and value congruence.
Podsakoff et al. (1990)	Cross-sectional survey matched with supervisor evaluation of behavior	988 exempt employees	Good	Indirect influence on followers' organizational citizenship behavior was mediated by level of trust in the leader.
Atwater, Dionne, Camobreco, Avolio, & Lau (1998)	Surveys on randomly selected leaders	225 male cadets	Good	Punishment contingent upon performance contributed to higher evaluation of leader effectiveness by subordinates.
Lowe & Galen Kroeck (1996)	Meta-analysis	23 studies	Strong	Contingent rewards have a generally positive association with subordinate perception of leader effectiveness. Management by exception was found to have a low positive association with subordinate perception of leader effectiveness, but only in public organizations.

(Yammarino & Bass, 1990). The transformational leader realizes that the goals of the group are expected to transcend the individuals who comprise it and to result in the achievement of significant change in team effectiveness. Transformational leaders seek new ways of working, seek opportunities in the face of risk, prefer effective answers to efficient answers, and are less likely to support the status quo (Avolio & Bass, 1988). The ability of the transformational leader to make tasks and the mission of the work group outcomes appealing to followers generates commitment, effort, and greater performance on the part of followers (Conger, 1999).

Bass and Avolio (1994) initially identified four classifications of behaviors associated with trans-

Box 4–2: **Characteristics of Transformational Leaders**

- **Charisma:** Instills pride, faith, and respect in subordinates by transmitting a sense of mission that is effectively articulated
- **Individualized consideration:** Delegates projects to stimulate the learning and growth of employees, coaches and teaches employees, and treats each employee with respect
- **Intellectual stimulation:** Arouses followers to think in new ways and emphasizes problem solving and the use of reason before acting

formational leaders: inspirational motivation, individualized consideration, intellectual stimulation, and idealized influence. They developed a measure (the Multifactor Leadership Questionnaire [MLQ]) for the complimentary elements of transactional leadership (e.g., management by exception and contingent rewards) and the primary elements of transformational leadership. Factor analysis indicated that the four characteristics of transformational leaders could be measured by three scales (Box 4–2) that had acceptable reliabilities, resulting in inspirational motivation and idealized influence being combined into a single construct of "charisma."

EVIDENCE FOR THE TRANSFORMATIONAL
THEORY OF LEADERSHIP

Question: Does the use of charisma, individualized consideration, and intellectual stimulation behaviors lead to improved subordinate performance and perception of leader effectiveness?

Research on the impact of transformational leadership has included studies that examine the impact of transformational leader behavior both on subordinate perception of leader effectiveness and subordinate satisfaction, *and* on subordinates' objective performance. Many of these studies have used the MLQ as a measure of leader behavior. In general, evidence supports that the transformational leader behaviors of charisma, individualized

consideration, and intellectual stimulation promote higher levels of subordinate satisfaction, higher perceptions of leader effectiveness, and in some cases higher levels of subordinate performance. A number of studies investigated the impact of transformational leader behaviors above and beyond transactional leader behaviors and found that both sets of behaviors were positively correlated with increased satisfaction and perception of leader effectiveness, providing support for the assertion previously presented that these theories are in fact complimentary.

A study by Elenkov (2002) showed that transformational leader behavior had a direct impact on the performance of Russian companies and positively influenced group cohesiveness. In an experimental study, Levy, Cober, and Miller (2002) documented that transformational leader behavior correlated with feedback-seeking behavior of subordinates so that subordinates were more likely to seek feedback on their performance, facilitating behavior change and improved performance. Other studies by McColl-Kennedy and Anderson (2002), Gellis (2002), and Dvir, Eden, Avolio, and Shamir (2002) found positive but varying levels of relationships between transformational leader behavior and subordinate performance, extra effort by subordinates, and perceived satisfaction. A meta-analysis completed by Lowe and Galen Kroeck (1996) demonstrated that mixed evidence has been found on the correlation of the characteristics of transformational leadership and perception of effectiveness by subordinates, with some studies showing high correlation and other studies showing low correlation. Table 4–5 provides a summary of selected evidence on transformational leadership.

Charismatic Theory

When considering leadership, hearing the word *charisma* brings to mind famous leaders such as President John F. Kennedy, Lee Iacocca of the Chrysler Corporation, and even Adolph Hitler. Charismatic leaders have been portrayed as those who have been able to move followers to overcome great obstacles or to create vision, drive, and enthusiasm among followers in difficult times. The model of charismatic leadership was first introduced by Max Weber in 1946 and has been referred to both as a framework in which more recent theories of

Table 4-5	Summary of Selected Evidence on Transformational Leadership Theory				
Author	Study Type	N	Level of Evidence	Results
Elenkov (2002)	Cross-sectional questionnaire	253 senior managers and 498 immediate subordinates	Good	Transformational leadership directly and positively predicted organizational performance of Russian companies. Group cohesiveness was positively related to the ratings of transformational leaders.
Levy et al. (2002)	Experimental laboratory with randomization	132 students	Strong	Transformational leadership style was significantly related to feedback-seeking behavior.
McColl-Kennedy & Anderson (2002)	Cross-sectional questionnaire	121 sales representatives	Good	Significant but indirect effect of transformational leadership on subordinate performance mediated by the emotions of frustration and optimism.
Gellis (2002)	Cross-sectional survey	187 social workers	Good	Using the MLQ, all transformational leadership factors were significantly correlated with leader outcomes of effectiveness, satisfaction, and extra effort.
Dvir et al. (2002)	Randomized field	54 military leaders, 90 direct followers and 724 indirect followers	Strong	Transformational leadership enhanced by training had a more positive impact on direct followers' development and on indirect followers' performance versus the control group.
MacKenzie et al. (2001)	Cross-sectional questionnaires (2 measures)	477 sales agents	Good	Analysis of objective sales data validated that transformational leadership has stronger direct and indirect impact on sales performance and organizational citizenship behavior than does transactional leadership behavior.
Lowe & Galen Kroeck (1996)	Meta-analysis	23 studies	Strong	Found mixed results for the 3 transformational scales ranging from $r = .19$ to $r = .91$ for charisma, from $r = .21$ to $r = .77$ for individualized consideration, and from $r = .24$ to $r = .74$ for intellectual stimulation.

leadership may be placed (Jones, 2003) and as an element of transformational leadership (Jacobsen & House, 2001). Fiol, Harris, and House (1999) suggested that charismatic leadership theory and other theories that have been described as "strategic" in this chapter (e.g., transformational) share a common paradigm and have more elements in common than different.

Charismatic leaders are those who are successful in tying the self-concepts of subordinates to the goals and experiences associated with their missions so that the latter become valued aspects of the subordinates' self-concepts (Shamir, House, & Arthur, 1993). As a result, subordinates are likely to develop a stronger identification with the group, strengthening behavioral norms, values, and beliefs and enabling a unified effort to achieve the mission's goals. Charismatic leaders also provide a strong vision for the future by providing direction and meaning, communicate high expectations for subordinate performance, and focus on building the self-confidence and personal development of subordinates.

It is hypothesized that charismatic leaders transform subordinate self-concepts through at least four mechanisms (Conger, 1999). These mechanisms are listed in Box 4–3. If this hypothesis is accurate, it then may be assumed that leader behaviors that result in subordinates being more likely to examine their values or beliefs, or that "access" their self-concepts, may correspond with

higher perceptions of leader effectiveness; in fact, this has been a focus of recent research (Conger, Kanugo, & Menon, 2000; Paul, Costley, Howell, Dorfman, & Trafimow, 2001).

Jacobsen and House (2001) noted that the process of charismatic leadership involves three interacting elements: (1) the leader who possesses certain characteristics that have come to be identified with charisma, (2) the constituency from which subordinates respond to the leader, and (3) the social structure in which the leader and the subordinates interact. As previously described, charismatic leaders are those who articulate strong visions, set high expectations, take risks, and model the closely held values of the organization. Subordinates who may be most likely to respond to a charismatic leader are those who are unhappy in their current situation but have been unable to identify mechanisms to take control and change that situation. Charismatic leaders may step to the forefront and be successful in difficult or unstable times within organizations, especially when organization members are distressed because their values are threatened, the path to goal attainment is unclear, and it seems that extraordinary effort may be required to resolve the situation and return the organization to a stable, functional state. However, the situation just described does not guarantee that a charismatic leader is waiting in the wings to step forward.

As with each of the theories presented in this chapter, specific strategies or leader behaviors can be identified that flow from the primary premises of the theory. Examples of the primary strategies most often used by charismatic leaders are summarized in Box 4–4.

EVIDENCE FOR THE CHARISMATIC THEORY OF LEADERSHIP

Question: Do the charismatic leader behaviors of articulating a clear, strong vision, communicating high expectations, taking risks, and setting personal examples of closely held values lead to improved perception of leader effectiveness?

It has been hypothesized that charismatic leadership produces higher performance levels among subordinates as well as more motivated and satis-

---

Box 4–3: **Mechanisms by Which Charismatic Leaders Transform Follower Self-Concepts**

- Change the perceptions of the work itself
- Offer a positive future vision
- Develop a strong collective identity among all followers
- Heighten individual and group self-efficacy

Adapted from Conger, J. A. (1999). Charismatic and transformational leadership in organizations: An insider's perspective on these developing streams of research. *Leadership Quarterly, 10*, 145–169.

Box 4–4: Strategies of Charismatic Leaders

- Help subordinates "reframe" behavior and expectations so that they begin to question the status quo by challenging current social conventions
- Engage the self-concept of subordinates so that it becomes cognitively difficult for them to act in ways that do not support the mission of the organization
- Role-model innovation by taking risks and trying new strategies and approaches while maintaining a willingness to change course based upon results
- Use inclusive language (i.e., "we," "us") to build an association between hesitant subordinates and those who are on board with a new vision

fied subordinates (Bass, 1985). A review of empirical investigations of charismatic leadership found that charismatic leadership was positively correlated with subordinates' performance and satisfaction (Shamir et al., 1993). As with other theories of leadership, the empirical evidence related to charisma includes laboratory studies of perceived effectiveness of charismatic leaders or the correlation between charismatic leader behavior and subordinate traits such as openness to accessing their self-concept when responding to a charismatic leader. These studies have sometimes been conducted with college students, who may be responding to tapes of speakers or to trained actors portraying various leadership styles and behaviors, or reading a prepared manuscript. These types of studies have inherent limitations associated with their design and biases that may come with utilizing college students as subjects. However, there have been field studies in which superiors or subordinates of leaders rated characteristics of leaders in question, and these ratings were correlated with perceived effectiveness of the leaders. Although there is a range of findings from relatively weak to strong, evidence overall suggests that leaders who show higher levels of charisma are perceived as more effective than less charismatic leaders and

may be more effective in contexts in which subordinates are particularly demoralized or where there has been a lack of prior vision or strong leadership.

Although research does indicate a correlation between charismatic behavior and perceived effectiveness, the relationship between charisma and other leadership theories presented in this chapter should be remembered. Charisma has often been associated with historical figures who are especially memorable. The evidence on charismatic leadership should not be mistaken to mean that *only* leaders with charisma are effective. Rather, the evidence on transformational leadership suggests that strategies such as delegating projects to stimulate the learning and growth of employees, personal coaching of employees, and emphasizing problem solving and the use of reason before acting are leader behaviors that may be used by those who feel "less outgoing." Table 4–6 summarizes selected evidence on the charismatic theory of leadership.

There has not been any large-scale exploration of succession of charismatic leaders (what happens when such a leader leaves). However, there has been some inquiry because succession is thought to be more problematic from the perspective of this theory than with respect to other theories discussed within this chapter because it is unlikely that another charismatic leader will be found to replace the leader who is leaving. Conger and Kanungo (1998) followed up on a study of charismatic leaders in organizations conducted in 1989 and found that all of the leaders studied had left their organizations for various reasons (retirement, changing organizations, etc.) and that there was little routinization of charisma. Similarly, Conger (1993) reported, in a study of charismatic leaders acting as change agents in large bureaucratic organizations, that the charismatic leaders had practically no long-term impact on institutionalizing their charisma.

Situational Leadership

As with other theories, a *leadership theory* provides an explanation of how or why a particular phenomenon (in this case, leading others) occurs and how that phenomenon might be influenced. Theories are often composed of both general concepts that refer to larger segments of reality and

Table 4-6	Summary of Selected Evidence on Charismatic Leadership Theory				
Author	Study Type	N	Level of Evidence	Results
Sosik, Avolio, & Jung (2002)	Multisource field data	83 managers, 249 subordinates	Good	Charismatic leadership predicted manager and work unit performance.
De Cremer (2002)	Experimental laboratory (with students)	183 students	Strong	Self-sacrificing leaders were perceived as more charismatic and were able to motivate decision makers to cooperate more.
Conger et al. (2000)	Questionnaire analyzed by structural equation modeling	252 managers	Good	Reverence for a leader, followers' collective identity, and follower perception of group task performance had a direct relationship with charismatic leadership.
Fiol et al. (1999)	Semiotic analysis of presidential speeches	14 (all 20th century, through Reagan)	Good	Charismatic leaders used more inclusive language than non-charismatic leaders and used "reframing" language more often earlier in their terms of office.
Paul et al. (2001)	Laboratory, read statements in a hypothetical situation	379 students	Good	Charismatic and integrative leadership messages from a leader resulted in higher follower collective self-concept accessibilities than did routinized messages.
Shamir, Zakay, Breinin, & Popper (1998)	Cross-sectional questionnaire (2 measures) and data collection from performance appraisals	1642 soldiers (50 company leaders, 42 superiors, 353 staff members, and 1197 soldiers)	Good	The effects of charismatic behaviors on superiors' assessments of leaders' performance also was examined. The findings provide only very partial support that charismatic leadership improves perceived performance.
Lowe & Galen Kroeck (1996)	Meta-analysis	32 studies	Strong	Demonstrated a mean correlation of .35 between leader charisma as measured by the MLQ and ratings of leader effectiveness.
Thor (1996)	A biodata instrument and a temperament inventory	2044 first-line civilian supervisors	Good	Results indicate that charisma is a strong predictor of leader performance and follower satisfaction.

specific concepts that refer to the factors that make up these segments. Thus the key element of a theory is explanation—that is, giving a plausible account for how something works (Kielhofner, 2004). In contrast, *leadership style* refers to the elements of leading, such as the ordering and temporal spacing of leadership behaviors, and can be defined as "a pattern of emphases, indexed by the frequency or intensity of specific leadership behaviors or attitudes placed on different leadership functions" (Casimir, 2001). It has been suggested most recently that effective leaders vary their style because different situations may require different styles.

The situational theory of leadership presented by Hersey, Blanchard, and Johnson (1996) suggests that the most effective leaders are those capable of using different leadership styles and behaviors in response to the demands of the situation and the fluctuating maturity levels of their subordinates. The four styles of leadership identified by this theory are directing, coaching, supporting, and delegating (Box 4–5).

According to the situational leadership theory, the most effective leadership style will depend very much on the person being led, or the follower. The model has been extended to include the developmental level of the follower. According to the model, the leader's style should be driven by the competence and commitment of the follower, and four developmental levels are provided to describe these developmental levels (Table 4–7).

The developmental levels are also situational. A subordinate might be generally skilled, confident, and motivated in his or her job, but might drop to a lower developmental level when faced with a task requiring skills that he or she does not possess. For example, a subordinate who normally functions at a higher developmental level when dealing with day-to-day familiar tasks might drop to the lowest level when confronting an ethical issue that over-challenges his or her comfort level and for which he or she lacks the skill and motivation to rise to the challenge.

EVIDENCE FOR THE SITUATIONAL THEORY OF LEADERSHIP

There has been limited research to establish the credibility of this model; in fact it has been described as one of the most widely known yet least researched views of managerial effectiveness (Vecchio, 1997). Still, Silverthorne and Wang (2001) found moderate but not statistically consistent support for the hypotheses that highly adaptive leaders are more successful than less adaptive peers and that nonadaptive leaders are generally less successful. They found a clear relationship between being more adaptive in leadership style and higher employee productivity.

Lee-Kelly (2002) examined the leadership style of program managers responsible for projects with changing project boundaries and multiple interfaces with other projects. Observations and conclusions of the study that were useful to the project sponsor as well as the project manager were that they might seek either to select situations that would best match the project manager's inclination or style or to avoid projects that were likely to present him or her with situations that are counter to his or her preferred style.

The applicability of the situational theory of leadership to leaders from different cultures has been questioned, because managers in some cultures may wish to avoid a particular leadership style, especially the directive style, even after receiv-

---

Box 4–5: The Four Styles of Situational Leadership

- **Directing** leaders define the roles and tasks of the followers and supervise them closely. Decisions are made by the leader and announced, so communication is largely one-way.
- **Coaching** leaders define roles and tasks but seek ideas and suggestions from the followers. Decisions remain the leader's prerogative, but communication is much more two-way.
- **Supporting** leaders pass day-to-day decisions, such as task allocation and processes, to the followers. The leader facilitates and takes part in decisions, but control is with the followers.
- **Delegating** leaders are still involved in decision making and problem solving, but control is with the followers. The followers decide when and how the leader will be involved.

Table 4-7	Developmental Levels of the Situational Leadership Theory	
Level	Mix of Competence and Commitment	Follower Characteristics
4	High competence, high commitment	Experienced at the job, and comfortable with their own ability to do it well. May even be more skilled than the leader.
3	High competence, variable commitment	Experienced and capable, but may lack the confidence to go it alone, or the motivation to do it well and/or quickly.
2	Some competence, low commitment	May have some relevant skills, but won't be able to do the job without help. The task or the situation may be new to them.
1	Low competence, low commitment	Generally lack the specific skills required for the job at hand, and lack any confidence and/or motivation to tackle it.

ing training and stating that they saw the relevance and usefulness of all four leadership styles. It should also be noted that several authors have questioned the internal consistency of concepts included in the situational leadership theory (Avery & Ryan, 2002). A summary of selected evidence on situational leadership theory is presented in Table 4–8.

Gender and Leadership

There has been considerable study of the relationship between gender, leadership style, and perceived leadership effectiveness. Although not related to any specific theory of leadership, this body of evidence may be of particular interest to new practitioners in the profession of occupational therapy, a profession still dominated by women. In its 2000 Member Compensation Survey, the American Occupational Therapy Association (AOTA) noted that the ratio of women to men in occupational therapy positions has remained substantially unchanged since 1990, with about 94% of the membership being women and 6% men. The percentage of male occupational therapy assistants continued to decrease from 8.2% in 1990 to 6.6% in 1997 and 4.1% in 2000 (AOTA, 2000).

Some have hypothesized that, because of the interaction between role expectations of leaders in organizations and gender roles in society, men and women may be perceived differently even when using the same style or leadership approach. This belief has survived, if not thrived, despite evidence that suggests that, when women are given the opportunity to lead, they tend to employ leadership styles similar to those used by men (Eagly & Johnson, 1990). Although traits, characteristics, and behaviors may vary among members of a particular gender and be shared across gender lines, gender itself may be considered an *institutionalized system* of social practices that has historically resulted in organized inequalities (Ridgeway & Smith-Lovin, 1999). Further, gender has been associated with beliefs regarding status in society and within organizations.

Various leadership styles and behaviors have been characterized as being associated with "masculine" or "feminine" characteristics. The stereotypical feminine leadership style has been characterized by nurturing of interpersonal relationships, whereas the stereotypical male leadership style has been characterized by a focus on task completion and goal attainment (Eagly & Johannesen-Schmidt, 2001; van Engen, van der Leeden, & Willemsen, 2001). These stereotypes may be explained by examining research related to how leadership traits

Table 4-8	Summary of Selected Evidence on Situational Leadership Theory				
Author	Study Type	N	Level of Evidence	Results
York (2003)	Cross-sectional survey	250 social workers in leadership and clinical positions	Good	Found support for propositions of the theory related to "delegation" but not to "support," and these differences were not related to performance ratings, suggesting only partial support of the theory.
Avery & Ryan (2002)	Cross-sectional survey	17 trainees in situational leadership	Good	Subjects did not find it difficult to assess subordinate developmental level, found situational leadership easy to apply, but were more apt to be supportive and wished to avoid directive leadership.
Silverthorne & Wang (2001)	Cross-sectional questionnaire	79 managers and 234 subordinates	Good	The more adaptive that leaders were in style, the more productive the organization was likely to be.

have been "gendered" (associated with the male or female gender). Research has shown that traditional managerial roles are gendered as masculine, meaning that characteristics deemed necessary to be a successful manager have so far been stereotypically associated with men (Kawakami, White, & Langer, 2000). Hackman, Hills, Paterson, and Furniss (1993) demonstrated that subordinates perceived traits and behaviors that they described as masculine—whether utilized by male or female leaders—as effective. In contrast, when subordinates perceived that female leaders displayed traits and behaviors that they characterized as feminine, they saw these traits and behaviors as not as effective.

Stereotypes of male and female leadership styles have been challenged, however, since the feminist movement began, particularly in the last two decades as the role of women in the workforce has continued to change and women have become more visible in leadership roles in the full range of contexts in Western society. Notable female leaders of the past two decades include Supreme Court Justices Sandra Day O'Connor and Ruth Bader Ginsberg, current Secretary of State Condoleeza Rice, and former Secretary of State Madeline Albright, who all assumed leadership roles in labor

functions not typically associated with women. Gender-specific orientations toward perceptions of behavior may be heavily influenced by the gendered division of labor, meaning that the primary base for women's and men's different experiences and different orientations is the fact that men and women have historically carried out and to some degree still carry out radically different tasks in the family and labor markets (Billing & Alvesson, 2000).

More recently, it has been suggested that, indeed, women may demonstrate characteristics and styles previously stereotyped as "masculine" without being perceived negatively (Kawakami et al., 2000). The very notion of what is masculine and what is feminine is in a constant state of flux. Masculinity and femininity are not fixed once and for all, but are constantly changing and are culturally and historically dependent on the meanings we ascribe to them (Billing & Alvesson, 2000).

Kawakami et al. (2000) noted that women can use leader behaviors that have been stereotyped as "masculine" while still being perceived as genuine and not as incongruent with gender expectations. Their suggestion is that women can increase the extent to which they are perceived as effective leaders by using what they refer to as "mindfulness." Mindfulness refers to approaching communication in a thoughtful and conscious manner in each interaction and avoiding the appearance that communication and leader behavior have become routine. By assuming a conscious approach to communication and behavior, it is assumed that others will perceive the speaker or leader as acting in a genuine and novel way, so less attention will be paid to whether behavior is consistent with behaviors stereotypically associated with the gender of the speaker. Although it is unfortunate, in today's world, in which our standards and expectations have been influenced primarily by male role models, a female leader may have to exert effort beyond that of her male counterparts to be conscious of how she is perceived when demonstrating the same behavior. Initial research suggests that a "mindful" approach may indeed allow a woman to use a wider range of leader behaviors while remaining effective.

A review of recent texts that include a discussion of leadership, gender, and health care management reveals a set of recommendations that may be based on outmoded characterizations of gender. For example, Gilkeson (1997) provided suggestions for women on communicating across gender lines that include statements such as "men often will not say that they need help or that they do not understand" and that "men may not particularly care for working with a female manager." Similarly, Drafke (2002) provided suggestions for sending messages to men and women that include statements such as "Ask; do not order men to do things" because it makes them feel "subordinate," and "Soften orders and directions to women who communicate less directly and often generalize." Neither of these authors provides detailed discussion of the strength of the evidence used in forming these recommendations, if indeed any evidence exists to support them.

As we move forward in the 21st century, researchers will need to continue to examine the assumption that leader behaviors can be either masculine or feminine in the context of changing gender roles, especially the worker role, in our society. As noted by Billing and Alvesson (2000), we need to be very careful in labeling leadership as masculine or feminine because conventional ideas may create a misleading impression of women's orientation to leadership and may reproduce stereotypes and the traditional gender division of labor.

Evidence on Leadership and Gender

Question: Do gender and leadership behavior interact so that women should adopt specific approaches to leadership simply because they are female?

Evidence on gender and leadership presents some contradictions. Kawakami et al. (2000) noted that the apparent contradictions in evidence may place female leaders in what they describe as a "double bind." The double bind is that effective leadership has been associated with characteristics that are stereotypically associated with maleness, yet women acting outside of the stereotypical feminine gender role have often been evaluated unfavorably. Billing and Alvesson (2000) noted that there is considerable evidence, including comparative studies of men and women, concluding that there are modest if any differences between male and female leaders who are perceived as effective. The one noted difference is that in the study by Eagly and Johnson (1990), cited previously in this chapter, in which some support for differences is found, with women being more participation oriented than men.

Although the research conducted to date does appear to support the notion that, if women adopt behaviors that are stereotypically perceived as masculine, they may be perceived as less effective, we must also examine the context of this evidence. Much of the evidence that has suggested that women should adopt leader behaviors that are different from those effective for men was produced during the same time frame during which dramatic shifts in the roles of women in the workplace and in our larger society have occurred. Although most would likely agree that workplace discrimination based on gender and concepts such as a "glass ceiling" for women in many fields are still relevant, progress has been made. There is no doubt that the roles of women in the workforce and in other public leadership arenas, including politics, is evolving, albeit slowly. For example, according to the U.S. Census Bureau, the gap between wages earned by men and women for full-time work is narrowing and was the smallest it has been in 2001, with the female-to-male earnings ratio climbing to 0.76:1 from a previous high of 0.74:1 in 1996 (*http://www.census.gov/Press-Release/www/2002/cb02-124.html*). As such, evidence on gender and leadership

Table 4-9	Summary of Selected Evidence on Gender and Leadership			
Author	Study Type	N	Level of Evidence	Results
Kawakami et al. (2000)	Laboratory, view of videotape	42 male business leaders	Good	Male businessmen perceived a woman who chose a "mindfully adopted" style typically associated with men to be a better leader than a woman who did not.
Eagly, Karau, & Makhijani (1995)	Meta-analysis	76 studies	Strong	Men were substantially more likely than women to be assessed as effective in male-dominated contexts (e.g., military), but women were moderately more likely to be assessed as effective in contexts including education, government, and service domains.
Eagly, Makhijani, & Klonsky (1992)	Meta-analysis	114 studies	Strong	Female leaders who were perceived as having stereotypically masculine styles were less positively evaluated and seen as more threatening than male leaders.

may begin to show different results over the next decades as women achieve true equality in the workplace. Table 4–9 provides a summary of selected evidence on gender and leadership.

Chapter Summary

This chapter has provided an introduction to leadership, including a definition of leadership and the relationship between leadership and management. The development of leadership theory was reviewed and five common theories of leadership were discussed. Evidence on each of the theories of leadership was presented, as were methods for translating the tenets of each theory into behavior. Because of the large percentage of women within the profession of occupational therapy and because of the dramatic shift in women's roles in the workplace, evidence related to gender and leadership was also reviewed.

Although the evidence on each of the leadership theories continues to evolve, it seems clear that leaders who adopt behaviors based on multiple theories and who choose strategies and behaviors to fit the situation may be most effective. More importantly, the limited amount of research on personality traits of effective leaders in the last few decades suggests that effective leadership behavior can be *adopted* or *learned* and that novice managers would benefit from conscious evaluation of their leadership skills in order to pursue strategies for becoming more effective leaders.

Resources for Learning More About Leadership

Journals That Often Address Leadership

LEADERSHIP QUARTERLY

This journal brings together a focus on leadership for scholars, consultants, practicing managers, executives, and administrators, as well as those numerous university faculty members across the world who teach leadership as a college course. It provides timely publication of leadership research

Real-Life Solutions

Jan visited her local university library and conducted a review of the theories and evidence related to leadership. The readings and the evidence clarified several issues for Jan. Based on her review of the literature, Jan decided that, with conscious effort and perhaps some training and experience, she could improve her leadership skills and abilities and could take actions to be perceived as a more effective leader. Using what she had learned by reviewing the evidence, Jan decided to accept the position of department director and to do the following:

- Implement strategies based on multiple theories because evidence provides at least partial support for each of the theories of leadership, suggesting that the use of more than one leadership approach may be effective.
- Structure work assignments and tasks to establish a clear connection between performance and rewards to influence subordinates' perceptions of work goals and make the paths to goal attainment clearer.

- Combine the use of transactions to set expectations and establish the relationships between behavior and reward and punishment with methods such as delegating projects to stimulate the growth of employees.
- Help subordinates reframe behavior and expectations by modeling innovation, by taking risks, by trying new strategies and approaches, and by using inclusive language to build an association with a new vision.
- Adopting a "mindful" approach to communication, especially in times of high stress or conflict, but not avoiding any specific behavior just because it has typically been stereotyped as masculine.

Jan also decided to continue to observe other leaders in her organization closely to identify the strategies that they adopted in different situations and how others in the organization perceived these behaviors. After her review of the theories and evidence on leadership, Jan felt more encouraged about taking on the new challenge of accepting the position as director of occupational therapy.

and applications and has a global reach. It also focuses on yearly reviews of a broad range of leadership topics on a rotating basis and emphasizes cutting-edge areas through special issues.

JOURNAL OF MANAGEMENT DEVELOPMENT

The *Journal of Management Development* covers a broad range of topics in its field including: competence-based management development, developing leadership skills, developing women for management, global management, the new technology of management development, team building, organizational development and change, and performance appraisal.

JOURNAL OF LEADERSHIP AND ORGANIZATIONAL STUDIES

The *Journal of Leadership and Organizational Studies* is published quarterly for all who teach, study, or practice leadership. The journal is intended as a forum for the expression of current thought and research (although not for the presen-

tation of empirical research data). The stated goal of the journal is to bring together a recurring reference work designed to appeal to a national base of individuals seeking the latest materials, thoughts, sources, and networking opportunities in leadership education.

JOURNAL OF ORGANIZATIONAL BEHAVIOR

The *Journal of Organizational Behavior* is dedicated to the study of how organizations impact people and how people shape organizations, and publishes information on worldwide work-related issues, including leadership and leadership development. The editorial staff encourages both theoretical and empirical inquiry from a diversity of perspectives, methods, and national cultures.

JOURNAL OF APPLIED PSYCHOLOGY

http://www.apa.org/journals/apl.html

The *Journal of Applied Psychology*, published by the American Psychological Association (APA), emphasizes the publication of original investigations that contribute new knowledge and understanding to fields of applied psychology. The journal's focus is on empirical and theoretical investigations of interest to psychologists doing research that fosters an understanding of the psychological and behavioral phenomena of individuals, groups, or organizations in settings such as education/training, business, government, health, or service institutions, and that may be in the private or public sector, or for-profit or nonprofit.

Associations That Are Concerned with Leadership

The American Society of Association Executives

http://www.asaenet.org/

The American Society of Association Executives, known as the "association of associations," is considered the advocate for the nonprofit sector. The primary mission of this association is to advance the value of voluntary associations to society and to support the professionalism of the individuals who lead them.

The Center for Creative Leadership

http://www.ccl.org/

The mission of the Center for Creative Leadership is to advance the understanding, practice, and development of leadership for the benefit of society worldwide. The center's stated role is to help address the leadership component of both business and organizational challenges. The center was founded 30 years ago in Greensboro, North Carolina, and is today one of the largest institutions in the world focusing solely on leadership. It seeks to generate and disseminate knowledge about leadership and leadership development.

Useful Web Sites on Leadership

Psychology.Com

http://psychology.about.com/cs/lead/

Resources links include: leadership article assessment tools, studies, styles, theory, training/consulting services, development programs, book reviews, student leadership, and world-famous leaders.

The Fastcompany

http://www.fastcompany.com/online/resources/leadership.html

This is an online leadership magazine entitled *Fast Company*.

Darwin Executive Guides

http://guide.darwinmag.com/career/education/leadership/

This Web resource includes an online journal, newsletter, research reports, discussion boards, and executive guide, as well as book reviews.

INQ7.Net

http://www.inq7.net/nwsbrk/2002/aug/09/nbk_4-1.htm

This is a useful online journal on leadership and management.

Academy of Leadership, University of Maryland

http://www.academy.umd.edu/publications/LeadershipReconsidered/chart.htm

This is a publication on what constitutes effective leadership. A chart that can be downloaded from this site lists group qualities as well as individual qualities that are most beneficial for one to be an effective leader.

Fortune Management

http://www.fortunemgmt.com/peak3.html

This site lists six qualities of effective leadership: belief, vision, communication, relationships, integrity, and growth.

Reference List

American Occupational Therapy Association. (2000). *Member compensation survey*. Bethesda, MD: American Occupational Therapy Association.

Atwater, L., Dionne, S. D., Camobreco, J. F., Avolio, B. J., & Lau, A. (1998). Individual attributes and leadership style: Predicting the use of punishment and its effects. *Journal of Organizational Behavior, 19*, 559–576.

Avery, J. C., & Ryan, J. (2002). Applying situational leadership in Australia. *Journal of Management Development, 21*, 242–262.

Avolio, B. J., & Bass, B. M. (1988). Transformational leadership, charisma and beyond. In J. G. Hunt, B. R. Baglia, H. P.

Dachler, & C. A. Schriesheim (Eds.), *Emerging leadership vistas* (pp. 185–201). Lexington, MA: Lexington Books.

Barker, R. A. (2001). The nature of leadership. *Human Relations, 54*, 469–494.

Bass, B. (1985). *Leadership and performance beyond expectations.* New York: Free Press.

Bass, B. M. (1990a). *Bass & Stogdill's handbook of leadership* (3rd ed.). New York: Free Press.

Bass, B. M. (1990b). *Transformational leadership: Theory, research, and managerial applications.* New York: Free Press.

Bass, B. M., & Avolio, B. J. (1994). *Improving organizational effectiveness through transformational leadership.* Thousand Oaks, CA: Sage.

Bass, B. M., Avolio, B. J., & Goodheim, L. (1987). Biography and the assessment of transformational leadership at the world class level. *Journal of Management, 13*, 7–19.

Beech, M. (2002). Leaders of managers: The drive for effective leadership. *Nursing Standard, 16*, 35–36.

Bennis, W. G., & Nanus, B. (1985). *Leaders: The strategies for taking charge.* New York: Harper & Row.

Billing, Y. D., & Alvesson, M. (2000). Questioning the notion of feminine leadership: A critical perspective on the gender labeling of leadership. *Gender, Work and Organization, 7*, 144–157.

Boal, K. B., & Hooijberg, R. (2001). Strategic leadership research: Moving on. *Leadership Quarterly, 11*, 515–549.

Braveman, B., & Fisher, G. S. (1997). Managed care: Survival skills for the future. *Occupational Therapy in Health Care, 10*, 13–31.

Burns, J. M. (1978). *Leadership.* New York: Harper & Row.

Carlyle, T. (1907). *On heroes and hero worship.* Cambridge, MA: Houghton Mifflin.

Casimir, G. (2001). Combinative aspects of leadership style: The ordering and temporal spacing of leadership behaviors. *Leadership Quarterly, 12*, 245–278.

Conger, J. A. (1993). Max Weber's conceptualization of charismatic authority: Its influence on organizational research. *Leadership Quarterly, 4*, 277–288.

Conger, J. A. (1999). Charismatic and transformational leadership in organizations: An insider's perspective on these developing streams of research. *Leadership Quarterly, 10*, 145–169.

Conger, J. A., & Kanungo, R. N. (1998). *Charismatic leadership in organizations.* Thousand Oaks, CA: Sage.

Conger, J. A., Kanungo, R. N., & Menon, S. T. (2000). Charismatic leadership and follower effects. *Journal of Organizational Behavior, 21*, 747–767.

Day, D. V. (2001). Leadership development: A review in context. *Leadership Quarterly, 11*, 581–613.

De Cremer, D. (2002). Charismatic leadership and cooperation in social dilemmas: A matter of transforming motives? *Journal of Applied Social Psychology, 32*, 997–1016.

Drafke, M. W. (2002). *Working in health care: What you need to know to succeed.* Philadelphia: F.A. Davis.

Dvir, T., Eden, D., Avolio, B. J., & Shamir, B. (2002). Impact of transformational leadership on follower development and performance: A field experiment. *Academy of Management Journal, 45*, 735–744.

Eagly, A. H., & Johannesen-Schmidt, M. C. (2001). The leadership styles of women and men. *Journal of Social Issues, 57*, 781–797.

Eagly, A. H., & Johnson, B. T. (1990). Gender and leadership style: A meta-analysis. *Psychological Bulletin, 108*, 233–256.

Eagly, A. H., Karau, S. J., & Makhijani, M. G. (1995). Gender and the effectiveness of leaders: A meta-analysis. *Psychological Bulletin, 117*, 125–145.

Eagly, A. H., Makhijani, M., & Klonsky, B. (1992). Gender and the evaluation of leaders: A meta-analysis. *Psychological Bulletin, 111*, 3–22.

Elenkov, D. S. (2002). Effects of leadership on organizational performance in Russian companies. *Journal of Business Research, 55*, 467–480.

Evans, M. G. (1996). R. J. House's "A path-goal theory of leader effectiveness." *Leadership Quarterly, 7*, 305–309.

Fiol, C. M., Harris, D., & House, R. (1999). Charismatic leadership: Strategies for effecting social change. *Leadership Quarterly, 10*, 449–482.

Fisher, A. C., & Edwards, I. E. (1988). Consideration and initiating structure and their relationships with leader effectiveness: A meta-analysis. In *Best papers: Proceedings of the Academy of Management meeting* (pp. 201–205). Briarcliff Manor, NY: Academy of Management.

Fleishman, E. A., Mumford, M. D., Zaccaro, S. J., Levin, K. Y., Korotkin, A. L., & Hein, M. B. (1991). Taxonomic efforts in the description of leader behavior: A synthesis and functional interpretation. *Leadership Quarterly, 2*, 245–287.

Gellis, Z. D. (2002). Social work perceptions of transformational and transactional leadership in health care. *Social Work Research, 25*, 17–26.

Gerber, R., & Burns, J. M. (2002). *Leadership the Eleanor Roosevelt way: Strategies from the first lady of courage.* Upper Saddle River, NJ: Prentice Hall.

Gilkeson, G. E. (1997). *Occupational therapy leadership: Marketing yourself, your profession, and your organization.* Philadelphia: F. A. Davis.

Giuliani, R., & Kurson, K. (2002). *Leadership.* New York: Hyperion.

Goleman, D. (1995). *Emotional intelligence.* New York: Bantam Books.

Grohar-Murray, M. E., & Dicroce, H. R. (2002). *Leadership and management in nursing* (3rd ed.). Upper Saddle River, NJ: Prentice Hall.

Hackman, M. Z., Hills, M. J., Paterson, T. J., & Furniss, A. H. (1993). Leaders' gender-role as a correlate of subordinates' perceptions of effectiveness and satisfaction. *Perceptual and Motor Skills, 77*, 671–674.

Hersey, P., Blanchard, K., & Johnson, D. E. (1996). *Management of organizational behavior: Utilizing human resources* (7th ed.). Englewood Cliffs, NJ: Prentice-Hall.

House, R. J. (1971). A path-goal theory of leadership effectiveness. *Administrative Science Quarterly, 16*, 321–328.

House, R. J. (1977). A 1976 theory of charismatic leadership. In J. G. Hunt & L. L. Larson (Eds.), *Leadership: The cutting edge* (pp. 115–145). Carbondale: Southern Illinois University Press.

House, R. J. (1996). Path-goal theory of leadership: Lessons, legacy and a reformulated theory. *Leadership Quarterly, 7*, 323–352.

House, R. J., & Aditya, R. M. (1997). The social scientific study of leadership. *Leadership Quarterly, 23,* 409–464.

Hunt, J. G., & Conger, J. A. (1999). Overview. Charismatic and transformational leadership: Taking stock of the present and future (Part II). *Leadership Quarterly, 10,* 331–334.

Indvik, J. (1986). Path-goal theory of leadership: A meta-analysis. In *Best papers: Proceedings of the Academy of Management meeting* (pp. 189–192). Briarcliff Manor, NY: Academy of Management.

Jacobsen, C., & House, R. J. (2001). Dynamics of charismatic leadership: A process theory, simulation model and tests. *Leadership Quarterly, 12,* 75–112.

Jones, H. B. (2003). Magic, meaning and leadership: Weber's model and the empirical literature. *Human Relations, 54,* 753–771.

Jung, D. I., & Avolio, B. J. (2000). Opening the black box: An experimental investigation of the mediating effects of trust and value congruence on transformational and transactional leadership. *Journal of Organizational Behavior, 21,* 949–964.

Kawakami, C., White, J. B., & Langer, E. J. (2000). Mindful and masculine: Freeing women leaders from the constraints of gender roles. *Journal of Social Issues, 56,* 49–63.

Kielhofner, G. (2004). *Conceptual foundations of occupational therapy* (3rd ed.). Philadelphia: F. A. Davis.

Kirkpatrick, S. A., & Locke, E. A. (1991). Leadership: Do traits matter? *Academy of Management Executive, 5,* 48–60.

Lee-Kelly, L. (2002). Situational leadership: Managing the virtual project team. *Journal of Management Development, 21,* 461–476.

Levey, S., Hill, J., & Green, B. (2002). Leadership in health care and the leadership literature. *Journal of Advanced Nursing, 25,* 68–74.

Levy, P. E., Cober, R. T., & Miller, T. (2002). The effect of transformational and transactional leadership perceptions on feedback-seeking intentions. *Journal of Applied Social Psychology, 32,* 1703–1720.

Lowe, K. B., & Galen Kroeck, K. (1996). Effectiveness correlates of transformational and transactional leadership: A meta-analytic review of the MLQ literature. *Leadership Quarterly, 7,* 385–425.

MacKenzie, S. B., Podsakoff, P. M., & Rich, G. A. (2001). Transformational and transactional leadership and salesperson performance. *Journal of the Academy of Marketing Science, 29,* 115–134.

McColl-Kennedy, J. R., & Anderson, R. D. (2002). Impact of leadership style and emotions on subordinate performance. *Leadership Quarterly, 13,* 545–559.

Mumford, M. D., & Connelly, M. S. (1991). Leaders as creators: Leader performance and problem solving in dynamic systems. *Leadership Quarterly, 2,* 289–315.

Mumford, M. D., & Peterson, N. G. (1999). The O*NET content model: Structural considerations in describing jobs. In N. G. Peterson, M. D. Munford, W. C. Borman, P. R. Jeanneret, & E. A. Fleishman (Eds.), *An occupational information system for the 21st century: The development of O*NET* (pp. 21–30). Washington, DC: American Psychological Association.

Mumford, M. D., Zaccaro, S. J., Harding, F. D., Jacobs, T. O., & Fleishman, E. A. (2000). Leadership skills for a changing world: Solving complex social problems. *Leadership Quarterly, 11,* 11–35.

Paul, J., Costley, D. L., Howell, J. P., Dorfman, P. W., & Trafimow, D. (2001). The effects of charismatic leadership on followers' self-concept accessibility. *Journal of Applied Social Psychology, 31,* 1821–1844.

Podsakoff, P., MacKenzie, S., Moorman, R., & Fetter, R. (1990). Transformational leader behaviors and their effects on followers' trust in leader, satisfaction, and organizational citizenship behaviors. *Leadership Quarterly, 1,* 107–142.

Powell, S. K. (2000). *Case management: A practical guide to success in managed care.* (2nd ed.) Baltimore: Lippincott Williams & Wilkins.

Ridgeway, C. L., & Smith-Lovin, L. (1999). The gender system and interaction. *Annual Review of Sociology, 25,* 191–216.

Rost, J. C. (2003). Leadership development in the new millennium. *Journal of Leadership Studies, 1,* 92–110.

Rudolph, S. H., & Rudolph, L. I. (1983). *Gandhi: The traditional roots of charisma.* Chicago: University of Chicago Press.

Schriesheim, C. A., & Neider, L. L. (1996). Path-goal leadership theory: The long and winding road. *Leadership Quarterly, 7,* 317–321.

Schriesheim, J. F., & Schriesheim, C. A. (1980). A test of the path-goal theory of leadership and some suggested directions for future research. *Personnel Psychology, 33,* 349–370.

Schruijer, S. G., & Vansina, L. S. (2002). Leader, leadership and leading: From individual characteristics to relating in context. *Journal of Organizational Behavior, 21,* 869–874.

Shamir, B., House, R. J., & Arthur, M. B. (1993). The motivation effects of charismatic leadership: A self-concept based theory. *Organization Science, 4,* 584.

Shamir, B., Zakay, E., Breinin, E., & Popper, M. (1998). Correlates of charismatic leader behavior in military units: Subordinates' attitudes, unit characteristics, and superiors' appraisals of leader performance. *Academy of Management Journal, 41,* 387–409.

Silverthorne, C., & Wang, T. H. (2001). Situational leadership style as a predictor of success and productivity among Taiwanese business organizations. *Journal of Psychology, 135,* 399–412.

Smith, H. L., & Kreuger, L. M. (1933, Spring). A brief summary of the literature on leadership. *Bulletin of the School on Education,* 3–80.

Sosik, J., Avolio, B. J., & Jung, D. I. (2002). Beneath the mask: Examining the relationship of self-presentation attributes and impression management to charismatic leadership. *Leadership Quarterly, 13,* 217–242.

Thor, K. K. (1996). Charisma and power orientation: Effects on leader performance and follower satisfaction. *Dissertation Abstracts International, B. The Physical Sciences and Engineering, 56,* 8B.

Tushman, M., & Anderson, P. (1986). Technological discontinuities and organizational environments. *Administrative Science Quarterly, 31,* 439–465.

Vance, C., & Larson, E. (2002). Leadership research in business and health care. *Journal of Nursing Scholarship, 34*, 165–171.

van Engen, M. L., van der Leeden, R., & Willemsen, T. M. (2001). Gender, context and leadership styles: A field study. *Journal of Occupational and Organizational Psychology, 74*, 581–598.

Vecchio, R. P. (1997). Situational leadership theory: An examination of a prescriptive theory. In R. P. Vecchio (Ed.), *Leadership: Understanding the dynamics of power and influence in organizations* (pp. 334–350). Notre Dame, IN: University of Notre Dame Press.

Wofford, J. C., & Liska, L. Z. (1993). Path-goal theories of leadership: A meta analysis. *Leadership Quarterly, 19*, 857–876.

Yammarino, F. J., & Bass, B. M. (1990). Long-term forecasting of transformational leadership and its effects among naval officers: Some preliminary findings. In K. E. Clark & M. B. Clark (Eds.), *Measures of leadership* (pp. 151–169). West Orange, NY: Leadership Library of America.

York, R. O. (2003). Adherence to situational leadership theory among social workers. *Clinical Supervisor, 14*, 5–24.

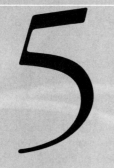

5

Brent Braveman, Ph.D., OTR/L, FAOTA

Roles and Functions of Managers

Real-Life Management

Marty was recently hired as Director of Occupational Therapy Services for a small occupational therapy department. He is excited about this new opportunity and confident in his leadership skills. However, Marty has only been practicing as an occupational therapist for a few years. He thinks that he began to develop solid skills as a supervisor in his last position through experiences supervising fieldwork students and several occupational therapy assistants. In addition, he had some prior experience supervising staff in an earlier career as a director of marketing for a community-based agency. However, he is concerned that he may be getting himself in over his head. Marty has always been a self-directed learner and is confident that, if he can identify the new tasks that he will have to perform, he can seek out information and resources to help him in his new job. As a place to start, he begins to conduct information interviews with other occupational therapy managers in his local area to identify the most common roles and functions that they perform in their daily work. To help make his interviews more effective, he develops the following questions:

1. What are the most common functions that you serve for your organization in your role as a manager?
2. What are some of the specific skills I will need to learn to run and manage my department?
3. What do I need to learn to help the employees that I supervise grow and develop as occupational therapy professionals?

Key Issues

- Four commonly identified functions of managers are planning, organizing and staffing, directing, and controlling.
- All management tasks, including recruitment, hiring, discipline, and financial and information management, can be categorized in one of the four management functions.
- Managers are involved in a variety of activities, such as financial and facility planning, recruitment, employee discipline, and mentoring, that require the development of a wide range of skill sets.
- A key difference between management and supervision is that managers should have "requisite managerial authority," a level of authority often not extended to many supervisors.

Chapter 4 introduced the topic of leadership, and reviewed the primary theories related to leadership and evidence on each theory. The relationship between leadership and management was discussed and the four functions of a manager (i.e., planning, organizing and staffing, directing, and controlling) were briefly introduced. Chapters 5 and 6 will provide an overview of what managers and supervisors "do" as well as a sample of theories and evidence that can be used to guide the work of a manager or supervisor. Chapter 5 will explore key areas of each of the managerial functions in more depth. Chapter 6 will focus specifically on the roles and functions of managers as supervisors. As you read these two chapters, you should keep in mind that the roles and functions of managers and supervisors are closely related. Later, in Chapter 10, some of the key concepts presented in these two chapters will be applied to promoting evidence-based and occupation-based practice within a *community of practitioners*.

Managers by their very nature supervise the work of others; however, in many of the settings in which occupational therapists are employed, it is not always true that those asked to assume supervisory responsibilities have full managerial control. An important difference that distinguishes a manager from a supervisor is that of *requisite managerial authority*. Elliot Jaques (1998) defined requisite managerial authority as the level of control and discretion that a manager must have to be fairly held responsible for the outcomes of work groups. Requisite managerial authority includes the authority to hire and fire employees, an authority that many supervisors do not possess.

Managers are usually concerned with solving problems with long-range implications and planning for the future of a work unit, such as a department or an organization. It is commonly said that, "Management is the art of getting things done through other people." Although this may be what managers often do, it is through the process of supervision that managers interact with employees who "get things done." Peter Drucker encouraged us to define management and supervision by emphasizing the contribution that managers and supervisors make to organizations and not the amount of responsibility and control they have (Drucker, 1974). By doing so, we place the empha-

> ### Box 5–1: Commonly Identified Functions of Management
>
> - **Planning:** The process of deciding what to do by setting performance objectives and identifying the activities needed to accomplish these activities
> - **Organizing and staffing:** Designing workable units, determining lines of authority and communication, and developing and managing patterns of coordination
> - **Directing:** Providing guidance and leadership so that the work performed is goal oriented
> - **Controlling:** Establishing performance standards and measuring, evaluating, and correcting performance

sis for the manager and supervisor on the goals of management and supervision rather than on the subordinate, and this prevents the supervisor from becoming a controller rather than a leader.

When considering management and supervision, it is important to recognize that there are overlaps between the two functions, but that certainly the focus of top management in most organizations is different from that of first-line supervisors. Lyles and Joiner (1986) compared the focus of top management and first-line supervision for common management functions (Table 5–1). These functions (i.e., planning, organizing and staffing, directing, and controlling) are briefly defined in Box 5–1. These common management functions will help set the stage for understanding the roles and functions of the manager and will be explored in more depth in subsequent sections of this chapter.

Planning

Planning is the process of establishing short-term and long-term goals, measurable objectives, and action plans related to the mission of the organization. Goals are usually distinguished from objectives in terms of the scope of the accomplishment.

Table 5-1	Functions of Management: Comparison of Focus of Top Management Versus First-Line Supervisors	
Function	**Focus of Top Management**	**Focus of First-Line Supervisors**
PLANNING Forecasting Budgeting Establishing objectives Scheduling Developing policies	• Long range • Growth • Capital procurement • Service mix • Initiating • Overall financial	• Short range • Day-to-day • Week-to-week • Converting "what" to "how to" • Activities lists • Scheduling tasks and facilities
ORGANIZING Designing the organization Establishing work relationships Work flow Delegating	• Overall structure • Establishing lines of responsibility and authority • Determining line and staff relationships	• Coordination of people, equipment, and supplies to accomplish results • More concerned with relationships between things and specific activities than with overall structure
STAFFING Recruiting Hiring Promotion Training Development	• Developing personnel policies • Providing total training system to support • Negotiating union contracts	• Hiring good staff • Training and developing workers • Assessing staff needs
DIRECTING Motivating Leading	• Modeling good behavior • Developing and promoting a positive overall approach to leadership • Providing a good image in the community	• Leading in such a way as to create a positive climate in which workers operate with optimum efficiency and professionalism
CONTROLLING Establishing standards Measuring, evaluating, and correcting performance	• Monitoring total organizational results • Setting standards and goals	• Tracking work in progress • Appraising work and results • Correcting performance

From Lyles, R. I., & Joiner, C. (1986). *Supervision in health care organizations*. New York: John Wiley & Sons, with permission.

Objectives are measurable steps that are taken to reach a goal that is a major accomplishment related to the output of the organization or system. In addition to establishing goals and objectives, planning includes determining the needs for the human resources, materials, supplies, facilities, and equipment required to meet goals and objectives. Writing the policies and procedures that guide the use of materials, supplies, facilities, and equipment and that guide staff in daily activities is also commonly considered a component of planning, as is the financial planning involved in developing and managing a department budget. Some simple guidelines for effective planning are included in Box 5–2.

Box 5–2: Guidelines for Effective Planning

- Make plans specific and measurable, avoiding vague indicators or terminology.
- Be neither too idealistic nor too practical and limited.
- Avoid underplanning by recognizing potential roadblocks and developing contingency plans, and overplanning by not being too rigid or detailed to allow flexibility.
- Communicate plans consistently and concisely to those above and below you in the organization and ensure two-way communication.
- Assign clear responsibilities for completing plan activities and monitoring progress on goals and objectives.
- Troubleshoot plans prior to their implementation.

Strategic Planning

It is common to distinguish between *strategic* or long-range planning and planning as a day-to-day management function. Strategic planning is the process of determining the long-term goals of an organization as a means of formulating strategies to accomplish these goals (Liebler, Levine, & Rothman, 1992). Over the last several decades, strategic planning has come in and out of favor as organizations have struggled to keep up with the almost frenetic changes in technology and the economy. And yet, operating in an environment fraught with change may be when long-term planning, especially the processes of *mission review* and of *visioning*, becomes most important.

Given the demands for high productivity in most of today's workplaces, it is sometimes difficult to convince managers and staff members to take time from their busy schedules to think creatively about the future. A precursor to beginning or revising a strategic plan should be to spend some time reviewing and perhaps revising a department's mission and vision statements. A mission statement is a setting forth of an organization's or department's purpose, including definition, products, and serv-ices. A vision statement expresses the aspirational and inspirational messages about what a department or organization would like to become as it seeks to fulfill its mission (Hoyle, 1995).

MISSION STATEMENTS

Mission statements are typically established by an organization's founders and usually remain fairly stable over time, although, as discussed in Chapter 3, they can sometimes become diluted or lose focus as organizations age and come to serve not only the purpose for which they were created, but also the practical purpose of providing a source of income for their employees. Although most organizations have established mission statements, many individual departments do not. The process of writing a departmental mission statement can help to refocus and re-energize staff members by helping them better understand the role they serve within an organization and the beliefs and values they hold in common. These beliefs and values are what hold them together as a *community of practitioners*. The concept of a community of practitioners will be explored in more depth in Chapter 10.

Mission statements often communicate the answer to four questions that provide an organization's internal and external publics with an understanding of the role of the organization in society:

1. Why does the organization exist?
2. What function does the organization perform?
3. For whom does the organization perform this function or who are the primary beneficiaries?
4. How does the organization go about filling this function?

There is a wide variety in the length and style of mission statements for different organizations. Some mission statements can be as short as a single sentence and may only imply the answer to some of the questions listed here, whereas others can be relatively lengthy and provide additional information.

As an example, the mission statement of the Department of Occupational Therapy at the University of Illinois Medical Center in Chicago is presented. When I began as Director of Clinical Services for occupational therapy at the medical center in 1992, there was no existing departmental mission statement for occupational therapy. The department had been essentially "deconstructed" as a result of a decision 2 years earlier to close the medical center. This decision was then reversed and plans were made to re-energize the hospital. Many of the staff members had resigned, however, and the morale of those who remained was understandably low. I was hired to rebuild the department, and my first step toward re-energizing the staff was working with the staff to develop the following mission statement:

> "The mission of the Department of Occupational Therapy at the University of Illinois Medical Center at Chicago is to continuously strive to define, develop, implement, and evaluate Models of Best Practice in Occupational Therapy. This mission will be attained within an environment that: fosters professional growth, facilitates open communication, promotes the expression of ideas, and encompasses the values of interactive challenge, clinical reasoning, and the highest ethical standards. The delivery of clinical services is our primary role. Further, we acknowledge the mutual interdependence of education, research, and clinical practice. Education and research are supported through the adoption of active roles in teaching and research efforts."

From this mission statement, you can tell something about the nature of this particular occupational therapy department. It not only indicates the reason for existence of the department and its primary functions but also provides the reader with an indication of how *this* department of occupational therapy is different from departments of occupational therapy at other medical centers. For example, an occupational therapy department that provides similar clinical services but that is located in a small acute care medical center not affiliated with a university might not have the missions of teaching and research.

Whether at the level of the organization or at the level of the department, a mission statement should be thought of as a *management tool*. Too often mission statements are simply a page in a policies and procedures manual or are hung on the wall without having real impact on the day-to-day work of employees. Instead, mission statements can be used as evaluation criteria that help you make decisions about how to prioritize work and the use of resources. In other words, if activities do not relate to your mission (e.g., your reason for existing), why

should you spend your time and the organization's human and financial resources on these activities? A basic economic principle is that of *opportunity costs*, or the idea that, whenever you invest resources, the opportunity cost is the next best thing that is given up because you no longer have enough resources to invest. Using your mission statement as a management tool helps you to minimize opportunity costs.

When writing a department mission statement, you may want to follow the steps suggested in Box 5–3.

Box 5–3: Suggested Steps in Writing a Departmental Mission Statement

1. Inform your boss of your intention and ask for his or her support, assistance, and blessing on taking your department through this process.
2. Gather all relevant documents, including your organization's mission and vision statements and the organization's strategic plan, and distribute these to your staff.
3. Ask someone from the organization's leadership to come and speak to the staff about the organization's mission, his or her vision of the future, and where your department fits in that future.
4. Distribute a list of questions to your staff and have your staff identify key concepts to be represented in your mission statement. You may want to use *nominal group technique* (described in Chapter 11) to share responses.
5. Consider asking another department director or someone from the human resources department to facilitate group discussions for you so you can participate as a member.
6. Ask for a small group of volunteers to write draft statements based on group discussions. Set ground rules for sharing feedback and share all drafts with your boss and other important leaders (e.g., other department directors with whom you work closely).

VISION STATEMENTS

The process of "visioning" can be a fun, creative, and motivating process that communicates the valuable role that employees can play in helping a department or organization to survive and thrive. At the same time, it is important for the person leading employees in a visioning exercise to set clear and appropriate boundaries for the exercise so employees do not become frustrated or waste time. An effective vision statement reflects a vision or dream of a future state that is both sufficiently clear and powerful to arouse and sustain the actions necessary for that dream to become a reality. However, it could be said that a vision that is not based in reality is a *mirage*. Sample portions of vision statements are listed in Box 5–4, and the steps for leading employees of an occupational therapy department through a visioning process are listed in Box 5–5. The process of developing a vision statement may take a number of meetings and a number of weeks or even months if done in a thoughtful manner.

Box 5–4: Sample Portions of Vision Statements

- To become the health care provider and employer of choice in the city of Boston.
- To be a leader in innovation in providing high-quality, cost-effective service.
- To become a national model for provision of creative and highly effective fieldwork education.

Once a vision for your department is clear, a plan of action to bring that vision about is necessary. The process of developing a plan to achieve a vision is the process of strategic planning. As the pace of information exchange and technological development has increased, the very definition of "long term" has changed. At one point in time it was not unusual for organizations to have strategic plans spanning up to 10 years. Given the current

---

Box 5–5: Steps in a Visioning Process for Members of an Occupational Therapy Department

1. Set the boundaries for the visioning exercise (e.g., "Assuming similar levels of staffing as we have today, what is the best that you can imagine for our department in five years?"; "What is your dream for what you hope we can accomplish over the next five years?").
2. Explain the steps of nominal group technique:
   a. Clarify the group objective.
   b. Individually list as many ideas as possible (or you may want to set a limit of two to three ideas per person).
   c. Go around the group and have each member state one idea on his or her list. Individuals may pass if they have an idea that has already been stated.
   d. Record each idea on a flip chart.
   e. After all ideas are listed, clarify each idea and eliminate exact duplicates.
   f. Identify and eliminate items that do not fit the purpose of the exercise or those

   that may not be realistic within the agreed-upon time frame.
3. Identify common themes in the ideas that were presented through facilitated discussion (consider getting a manager from another department to lead the exercise so that you as a manager may participate in the exercise on an equal level with other members of the department).
4. Have a subgroup representing different types of employees volunteer to form a statement of a few sentences in length that represents the vision of the group.
5. Distribute the draft statement to members of the department and key external stakeholders (e.g., managers from other departments, organizational leadership, customers) for feedback.
6. Continue review and revision of the vision statement until consensus is reached that the statement reflects a clear, powerful, and realistic goal for the future of the department.

> **Box 5–6: Key Components of an Effective Strategic Plan**
>
> 1. A mission statement that clearly identifies the reason the organization exists and the primary beneficiary of the organization's efforts
> 2. A definition of major goals or accomplishments related to the primary outputs of the organization
> 3. An action plan including specific objectives detailing how the organization's goals will be achieved
> 4. A description of the human, material, and financial resources needed to meet the identified goals and objectives
> 5. A procedure for monitoring performance and identifying deviations from expected performance so alterations in the action plan can be made
> 6. An evaluation system to determine if goals have been met

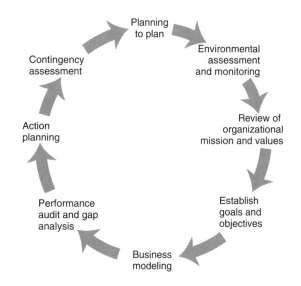

Figure 5–1   The eight steps of a strategic planning process. (Adapted from Goodstein, L. D. [1992]. *Applied strategic planning*. San Diego, CA: Pfeiffer & Company.)

pace of change, it is difficult for many organizations to look a decade into the future, and many strategic plans today cover periods of 3 to 5 years. The key components of an effective strategic plan are listed in Box 5–6.

These key components are reflected in the steps of the strategic planning process as identified by Goodstein (1992). The eight steps of strategic planning are represented in Figure 5–1. It should be noted that the steps involved in planning, whether long-term strategic or for day-to-day activities, are typically not completed for the purpose of planning alone. The information gathered on the environments that influence an organization, the analysis of the needs of clients and customers, and assessment of the internal environment of the organization are also useful for the management functions of marketing and program development, which are discussed in other chapters of this book.

THE EIGHT STEPS OF A STRATEGIC PLANNING PROCESS

Although the phrase might sound odd, one of the most important steps in strategic planning is *planning to plan*. Planning to plan includes consideration of who needs to be involved in the planning process, establishing or discovering communication mechanisms for keeping key stakeholders informed, and identifying constraints or roadblocks to the planning process that may be encountered so that alternatives or *contingencies* may be established. Most importantly, you must identify who might create roadblocks or sabotage your plan if they are not included in the planning process and establish communication systems with them to determine how they wish to be involved.

An evaluation of the internal and external environments of the organization, or *environmental assessment and monitoring*, should be an ongoing step in planning. The internal environment is monitored for changes such as increases or decreases in resources, loss of key personnel, changes in programming, or other changes that might support or detract from the organization's ability to pursue its goals. The external environment is monitored for changes in policies or laws that affect reimbursement or practice, the addition or loss of competitors, changes related to key populations served, or new technological developments that again will support or detract from the organization's pursuit of its mission.

A common strategy for completing organizational and environmental assessments is referred to as a *SWOT analysis*. The acronym SWOT stands for *strengths, weaknesses, opportunities, and threats*. If you have planned sufficiently and have the necessary stakeholders involved in the planning process, conducting a SWOT analysis can be relatively easy, can produce invaluable information, and can also be a reaffirming process to the participants. A SWOT analysis can be conducted by combining a review of key documents or reports (financial reports, outcome statistics, program evaluation, or accreditation reports) with staff interviews, discussions, or a structured brainstorming exercise as described in Chapter 11. Examples of strengths, weaknesses, opportunities, and threats that might be identified for an occupational therapy department are presented in Box 5–7. In real life, the results of a SWOT analysis would most likely be longer and the items would be presented in more detail. Also, a single item might be listed as both a weakness and an opportunity, and this would indicate an important point for discussion among you, your staff, and others involved in planning for the department's future.

A *review of the organizational mission and values* may help to identify potential mismatches between the organization's leadership and the line supervisors and employees responsible for doing the work needed to complete goals and objectives. As noted earlier, an organization's mission typically remains stable over time, but a review of the mission may provide the opportunity to identify "pet projects," or projects that have been started by someone in the organization that are consuming vital resources but are not centrally related to the mission of the organization. It is important to remember that the mission statement may be used as a management tool or "yardstick" against which to measure activities of the organization rather than just an abstract statement of philosophy.

Establishing short-term and long-term goals and objectives related to the mission of the organization is the next step of strategic planning. It should be recognized that involvement in planning (e.g., analyzing the factors influencing a situation and identifying a range of possible future actions that are appropriate and contribute toward achievement of organizational objectives) is not the same at all levels of the organization. It has been suggested that the persons who are involved in planning and daily decision making should vary according to the type

---

Box 5–7: Results of a Sample SWOT Analysis for an Occupational Therapy Department

Strengths

- Highly skilled and stable staff
- Strong department leadership
- Effective working relationship with other departments

Weaknesses

- Lack of experience in areas of new programming recently initiated by the organization
- Set in our ways and less flexible than we could be when responding to organizational needs
- Inadequate space and equipment to increase our volume

Opportunities

- New referral sources and new areas of programming in which we are not currently involved
- Invitation by an academic department of occupational therapy to establish a collaborative relationship on program development and research

Threats

- Salaries have not stayed competitive and we are in danger of losing staff
- Encroachment of other disciplines on areas traditionally addressed by occupational therapy because of our limited staffing and ability to respond quickly to referrals

---

of work being accomplished by those involved. Delegation of authority to personnel at lower levels of the organization has gained increased favor in recent decades and may be effective at times, especially in areas of the organization in which work processes and technologies remain fairly stable. However, concern has been expressed that overdelegation of authority in areas of the organization calling for creativity or in which work processes must continually be revised can result in "the best designers, researchers, explorers, and creators being pulled from what they do best to become involved in the management of an organization or department" (Jaques, 1998). Careful consideration of whom to involve means balancing concern over leaving people out of the process with inappropriately pulling people from critical work assignments.

Once goals and objectives are established, the current or possible structures for staffing and for lines of authority and accountability are examined. This process is referred to as *business modeling*. In many situations, occupational therapy managers may feel as if the structures of an organization are well established and therefore might tend to overlook this step of the strategic planning process. However, remaining open to change and examining new ways of organizing to support goal obtainment is critical. Establishing cross-functional teams, hiring part-time or per diem (as needed) employees, or creating a new product line (moving staff from various disciplines into a single cost center) may be options supported by top administration if managers can show that significant cost savings or revenue enhancements may occur. In the case of a new business, department, or service, business modeling is a critical step beyond the scope of an introductory text on management. New managers who find themselves faced with the opportunity to create a new service should seek consultation with managers in the organization with experience in business planning or seek other resources. For example, the American Occupational Therapy Association (AOTA) has groups of practitioners referred to as "Special Interest Sections" (SISs) (see *http://www.aota.org/*). One SIS, the Administration and Management Special Interest Section, has a subsection specifically for private practitioners and entrepreneurs. This subsection and all the SISs have Listservs available to all AOTA members that allow for the sharing of resources and dialogue about challenges faced.

Once goals and objectives with quantifiable or measurable targets are established and you know where you want to be in the future, you need to establish where you are at present by conducting an audit of current performance. A *performance audit* is conducted by comparing your current performance against measurable quantitative and qualitative outcome indicators of success related to the departmental or organizational mission. The outcome of the performance audit is the identification of the gap between the current and desired indicators of performance.

Action planning is the stage of planning that involves deciding exactly what you are going to do to get to where you want to be and to attain the goals and objectives established earlier in the planning process. As with the first step of "planning to plan," and in fact in each step of the process, developing an action plan that has a high chance of success is more likely if the right people are involved. Engaging in careful consideration of the key stakeholders in processes central to your plan and effectively communicating plans to those who can play roles in supporting or obstructing progress can make the difference between success and failure. A thorough action plan will include specific steps to achieve goals and objectives but will also include target dates for completion and will identify who is responsible for each action. Identifying dates to review progress on the action plan and who will be involved in these reviews is also recommended.

Finally, an assessment of all those things that might reasonably be anticipated to go wrong and the impact of these events is conducted as part of a *contingency assessment*. In other words, this is the phase of planning in which as many of the "What ifs?" are identified as possible. A critical element of this step is imagining any event that, if it occurred, would result in having to abandon key goals and objectives. This is not as complicated or as abstract as it may sound. Often some of our key fears are about those things we know might happen but we might want to otherwise avoid. For example, at one facility I started a hand therapy program and hired a Certified Hand Therapist (CHT), who quickly helped to develop a robust program. Knowing that the CHT had specialized skills that other staff members did not have, I soon began to worry about what would happen if the therapist left the facility or needed to take a leave of absence. By making the contingency assessment a formal and visible step in the planning process, I was able to involve key stakeholders such as referring physicians in the hand therapy program, and gain support and financial resources to train additional staff in treating hand injuries. As a result, a second therapist eventually became a CHT. This not only solved the "What if the CHT leaves?" problem, but also helped to retain a second valued staff member who was looking for a new challenge.

The management function of planning, whether strategic or short term, can be complicated and should not be underestimated by the new manager. A full discussion of strategic planning is beyond the scope of this book, but some resources for further investigation are provided at the end of this chapter, and readers and new managers are encouraged to seek assistance and mentorship when first involved in formal planning activities.

Policies and Procedures

Writing the policies and procedures that guide staff members in their daily work and in the use of materials, supplies, facilities, and equipment is a specific aspect of planning that typically rests with a department manager. Policies are statements of values that are consistent with the mission and frame the reasons for boundaries governing the services provided. Policies set parameters for making decisions about day-to-day operations (Burkhardt & Gentile, 2001). Most organizations have a standard format that is followed to guide managers in deciding what to include in a specific policy and procedure and in knowing which policies should be included in general in a department's policies and procedures manual. For business owners or new managers who do not find existing resources within their organizations, numerous resources are available for purchase that can be found by conducting an Internet search. These products include preformatted tables of contents and policy and procedure forms that can be customized to your department or business. Networking with other managers or business owners can help you in the process of choosing a product appropriate to your practice setting and customizing your policies and procedures manual to your setting. The basic components of a policy and procedure are included in Box 5–8.

Like mission statements, policies and procedures are most useful if they are highly visible to both management and staff. Policies and procedures should be frequently reviewed and updated as needed, and copies should be easily accessible to staff. Effective managers must not only be able to identify a policy and procedure but also be able to clearly articulate its necessity and underlying logic.

Box 5–8: Basic Components of a Policy and Procedure

- **Policy statement:** A brief statement of the guiding principle to be communicated
- **Purpose statement:** A brief statement outlining the reason for inclusion of the policy and procedure
- **Applicability:** Lists the employee groups to which the policy and procedure applies (e.g., all occupational therapy department staff members)
- **Procedures:** Statements outlining the specific actions to be taken by the identified employee groups and criteria for determining adherence to the policy
- **Responsibility:** Names the persons responsible for oversight of the policy and procedure (e.g., all occupational therapy team leaders)
- **Review period:** Lists the date of the last review and update of the policy and procedure (typically policies and procedures are reviewed on an annual basis)

Financial Planning

One of the most important functions of many managers is the development and oversight of a department budget. Budgeting is both a planning and a controlling function. Budgets are typically planned for a calendar year or *fiscal* year (e.g., many organizations operate on a fiscal year that runs from July 1st to June 30th). Developing and managing a budget is a complex process, and occupational therapy practitioners who have the goal of becoming a manager or director of an occupational therapy department are encouraged to attend a course on financial planning and management. In addition to other concepts, planning and managing a budget that can easily exceed $1 million in revenue and expenses in larger departments requires a working knowledge of

- Health care systems, including city, county, state, and national systems
- Payment and reimbursement structures such as Medicare, Medicaid, Worker's Compensation,

private insurance, and grant and foundation support
- Human resources systems and costs, including salary and benefit administration, training and educational costs and systems, and recruitment and retention structures
- Equipment and materials purchasing and management, including medical supplies such as splinting or assistive and adaptive equipment and office and other supportive supplies
- Facilities management and improvement systems, including cleaning and maintenance of physical plant structures

Many budgets include both revenue and expense budgets, although it is not uncommon in settings such as a community-based organization for a manager to have oversight of only expenses with no direct sources of revenue. Revenues may include third-party payment for services from private and public insurers, grants from government agencies or private foundations, and gifts from individuals or foundations. Expenses typically include costs associated with personnel, supplies, facilities management, and equipment. Some key concepts related to revenues and expenses are defined in Box 5–9.

Budgeting is often categorized as a planning function because it is necessary to plan or budget both your projected revenues and expenses. Planning revenues and expenses for new programs can be surprisingly complicated. Occupational therapy managers who assume responsibility for existing services may rely on historical data to help them with the process of projecting work volume, revenue, and expenses. However, when planning a new program, you may have to gather data and information from outside sources and peers.

Planning revenue requires that you project total work volume and then multiply by the gross charge associated with all *units of care* (e.g., 15-minute

---

Box 5–9: Key Concepts Related to Revenues and Expenses

- **Cost centers:** A manner of referring to the grouped costs associated with a set of activities within the organizational structure (e.g., the occupational therapy department, the behavioral health day treatment program, or the human resources department).
- **Gross revenues:** The aggregate, cumulative, or total sum of revenue before any deductions (e.g., the total work volume multiplied by billed charges before any deductions are made).
- **Allowances or deductions:** A percentage of fees that is negotiated with a payer to be deducted or discounted from the gross charge for services.
- **Net revenues:** The amount of revenue that you expect to collect after deductions, such as discounts for managed care payers, are applied.
- **Net profit:** The amount of revenue that remains after deduction of all expenses, deductions, and allowances.
- **Direct expenses:** Costs such as salaries, services, contracts, and equipment directly related to operation of a department.
- **Indirect expenses** *(sometimes called operating expenses):* Costs associated with running an organization that may be spread across departments according to a predetermined rate or formula and that are not influenced by work volume, such as secretarial support, or overhead costs, such as electricity.
- **Cost per unit of care:** The ratio of all expenses to total work volume such that the cost to produce one unit of care (e.g., 15-minute work unit, day of care) is represented and can be tracked over time or compared to costs of other programs or organizations.
- **Full-time equivalent (FTE):** The number of hours paid to a full-time employee during a designated time period, including payment of vacation or other benefit time. For example, payment for a typical 40-hour workweek multiplied by 52 weeks is 2080 hours.
- **Capital equipment:** Nonconsumable equipment with a cost and life span over an amount set by the organization (e.g., any single piece of equipment costing more than $500 and with a life span of greater than 12 months).

work unit, a group, a single visit, or a day of care). There often are different charges associated with different types of units of care. For example, a unit of activities of daily living intervention in a hospital setting may be charged at a set rate such as $32 per 15 minutes of intervention, whereas group intervention on a mental health unit may be charged at a "per group" rate such as $90 per group attended. Combining the number of the total of individual and group intervention units allows you to identify both total volume and subsequently gross revenue. The *net revenue* is then calculated by deducting any discounts or allowances and expenses (e.g., revenue after expenses). There is variation in whether and how discounts are included in departmental budgets in various organizations. For example, a discount of 8% may be uniformly applied to all categories of revenue if the organization discounts an average 8% across all payers. Other organizations may not apply discounts to departmental budgets but may apply the discounts when the budgets of multiple cost centers are "rolled up" into a summary report for a division or group of related cost centers. An example of the calculation of total volume and gross revenue for a given period is provided in Box 5–10.

Planning expenses requires that you project the volume for all types of costs charged to your cost center. The types of expenses charged to your budget will also vary from organization to organization. Expenses typically will include all direct and indirect expenses that can be isolated and applied to the costs of running your department. Other expenses related to the cost of doing business may not

be reflected in a departmental budget even if they are influenced by changes in your work volume. For example, many hospitals have separate transportation departments responsible for moving patients from one location to another in the facility. The salary and equipment costs for this service are directly influenced by the work volume of departments such as occupational therapy or physical therapy but may not reflected in those department's budgets. It is *critically* important that you remain aware of such budgeting and accounting practices so that you do not make any claims or assertions that damage your credibility as a manager. For example, it could be possible to mistakenly talk about your department's "profit" when, after applying discounts and associated costs such as transportation or reception salaries not reflected in your budget, your department actually operates at a loss. Another common mistake might be not recognizing that it is your organization's practice to not account for services paid on a per-stay basis, such as those covered under Medicare Diagnosis-Related Groups (DRGs) (see Chapter 2), within departmental budgets. Boasting that you have intensified services, resulting in increased profits, when these patients are paid under a Medicare DRG would be an embarrassing mistake because you have in fact increased costs to your organization by intensifying services to this group of patients. Naturally, if you could show that intensified occupational therapy services contributed to shorter lengths of stay for patients covered under a DRG, you might be able to show a positive financial impact because expenses would decrease even though there was no change in revenues.

Projection of salary expenses is completed by multiplying the number of *full-time equivalent (FTE)* employees required by your work volume by each employee's hourly rate of salary. Calculating the work that an FTE can handle requires that you identify both the number of hours per year that a typical employee devotes to provision of care during an identified period (often 1 work day) and the number of days that each employee will work. The number 2080 is commonly recognized as equivalent to one FTE (40 hours per week $\times$ 52 weeks per year). Obviously, employees do not work 5 days a week year round. Rather, you must deduct expected vacation leave, sick leave, holiday leave, and other

---

Box 5–10: Sample Calculation of Total Volume and Revenue

Total individual units of care (15 minutes) = 13,240
Total group units of care (1 hour) = 2,210
Charge per 15-minute individual unit of care = $32
Charge per 1-hour group intervention = $90

Total Gross Revenue = (13,240 $\times$ $32) + (2,210 $\times$ $90) = $622,580

planned time for which the employee will be paid but not expected to produce work (e.g., paid leave for continuing education).

A sample calculation of the expected number of *paid and worked hours* for an occupational therapist is included in Box 5–11. To identify the number of FTEs needed to handle the work volume shown in Box 5–10, you would begin by dividing the total number of hours of care by the total number of worked hours shown in Box 5–11:

13,240/4 = 3310 hours of direct care

3310 hours of direct care + 2210 group hours = 5520 hours of care

5520 hours of care/1824 worked hours per FTE = 3.02 FTEs

The 3.02 FTE figure does not mean that you would only need to plan to hire three occupational therapy practitioners (FTEs), however, because this number assumes that all 8 hours worked per day are *productive* or spent in activities for which you can charge. In fact, there are numerous aspects of the workday for which you cannot charge (assuming you work in a setting that charges for services at all). These activities include meetings, such as staff meetings, team or family conferences, or meetings of continuous quality improvement teams. Time spent waiting for inpatients who are late or for outpatients who do not keep their appointments, or the time wasted traveling to a patient's room only to find that he or she is off the patient care unit for a test, is *non-billable or unproductive* time, which is experienced in all organizations. Determining the

number of FTEs necessary to provide your projected volume of care requires that you determine a level of expected *productivity* for each category of employee. Productivity levels are commonly expressed as percentages, such that an expectation of 75% productivity means that each FTE is expected to spend 6 hours of each 8-hour day performing activities that are billable or otherwise defined as productive by the department.

Applied to the earlier example, a productivity expectation of 75% means that, in order to provide 5520 hours of care, we must expect to pay employees for 7360 hours. This means that, rather than 3 FTEs, we require 3.5 FTEs (7360/2080) to handle the work volume used in our example. In real life this can only be an estimate, however, because other factors such as an uneven pattern of referrals or whether or not it is an accepted, responsible, and ethical practice to "double up," or treat more than one patient at a time, in your setting must be considered.

It is also worth noting that employees may be classified as *exempt* or *nonexempt* from U.S. Department of Labor laws regarding payment of overtime. An employee who is exempt from these laws can be required to work longer than 8 hours on a given day without being paid a special rate for the extra hours worked. Nonexempt employees must be paid overtime according to Department of Labor requirements. Many occupational therapists are classified as exempt employees, whereas it is not uncommon for occupational therapy assistants to be classified as nonexempt. Planning on exempt employees to constantly work beyond 8 hours is a risky practice, however, because it may contribute to employee turnover and the associated costs. Determining expectations for productivity levels is a common topic of discussion among occupational therapy managers at conferences and on professional Listservs.

Nonpersonnel expenses must also be projected and include both *fixed* and *variable* expenses. Fixed expenses are those costs that are not directly influenced by changes in volume, such as expenses budgeted for employee continuing education. Variable expenses are those expenses that are directly influenced by changes in volume, such as some types of office supplies or food used for meal preparation activities. Although there may not always be a

---

Box 5–11: Sample Calculation of Paid and Worked Hours for an Occupational Therapist

CATEGORY OF PAY	NUMBER OF HOURS PER YEAR
Paid hours	2080
Vacation (3 weeks used)	−120
Sick days (4 days used)	−32
Paid holidays (11 days)	−88
Paid CE leave (2 days)	−16
Worked hours	1824

CE, continuing education.

direct correlation, over time you will be able to es-timate how an increase or decrease in volume might affect these categories of expenses. An abbre-viated sample of a calculation of expenses is in-cluded in Box 5–12.

Two other important concepts in regard to budget planning are those of budget periods and of variance. It is common practice to spread a yearly budget across 12 months and to be asked to project volume, revenue, and expenses for the year and to also project each of these figures for each month of the fiscal year. In most organizations, you will re-ceive a monthly budget summary or report that compares the *actual* volume, revenue, and expenses to the *projected or budgeted* volume, revenue, and expenses. The difference between the actual and projected or budgeted figures is the *variance*, and the variance can either be positive or negative. A positive variance for volume or revenue means that the actual figures are higher than projected or budgeted and a positive variance for expenses means that the actual figures are lower than pro-jected or budgeted. A negative variance indicates just the opposite relationships. This might sound confusing at first, but simply think in terms of your own personal budget. A variance that means you end up with more money than expected (either because more money came in or you spent less than expected) is a positive variance. On the con-trary, if you earned less money than expected or spent more than you had budgeted, it is a negative variance.

Small variances are expected, because it is sel-dom possible to precisely predict volume for any single budget period. However, large variances in either direction may be an indication of a problem. It is easy to understand why a large negative vari-ance in volume, revenue, or expenses would be of concern to organizational leaders, but you should recognize that the ability to *accurately* plan a budget is what will be rewarded most often, and consis-tently underestimating volume or revenue or over-estimating expenses will likely been seen as indicative of poor management skills.

A simplified budget sheet for one budget period is shown in Table 5–2. For the sake of simplicity, this table assumes that all volume, revenue, and expenses are spread evenly across the 12 budget periods. In real life this is hardly ever the case, and experienced managers will plan for increases and decreases based on historical patterns. For example, in an acute care hospital you might expect December to be a lower month for volume because fewer people will schedule elective surgeries near the holidays. In a pediatric private practice, you might expect volume to drop during the summer months when families commonly take vacations and in-crease in September when school is in session again.

When you review Table 5–2, the following points should be noted:

- This report is for the month of March, which would be the third budget period for an organi-zation that uses the calendar year as its fiscal year.

Box 5–12: **An Abbreviated Sample of Calculation of Expenses**	
CATEGORY OF EXPENSE	TOTAL COST
DIRECT EXPENSES	
Salaries (3.5 FTE × $48,000 average salary)	$168,000
Medical Supplies (average $1.74 per hour of care)	$9,604
Office Supplies (average 50.7 cents per hour of care)	$2,800
Food Supplies (7 cents per hour of care)	$400
INDIRECT EXPENSES	
Phones (16.3 cents per hour of care)	$900
Postage (3 cents per hour of care)	$200
Equipment Repair and Service Contracts	$2,200
Continuing Education ($600/employee)	$2,100
TOTAL EXPENSES	**$188,904**

Table 5-2	Sample Budget Report for Budget Period 3—March							
Budget Activity	Actual	Budget	Variance	% Variance	YTD Actual	YTD Budget	Variance	% Variance
Revenue								
Individual Treatment	33,344	35,306	(1,962)	−5.56	109,184	105,918	3,226	3.08
Group Treatment	15,390	16,575	(1,185)	−7.15	43,830	49,725	(5,895)	−11.86
Total Revenue	48,374	51,881	(3,507)	−6.76	153,104	155,643	(2,629)	−1.69
Direct Expenses								
Salaries	14,883	14,000	883	6.31	36,000	42,000	(6,000)	14.29
Medical Supplies	615	800	(185)	23.13	2,000	2,400	(400)	16.67
Office Supplies	187	233	(46)	19.74	600	699	(99)	14.16
Food	31	33	(2)	6.06	80	99	(19)	19.19
Indirect Expenses								
Phones	75	75	0	0	220	225	(5)	2.22
Postage	14	17	(3)	17.65	47	51	(4)	7.84
Equipment Contracts	183	183	0	0	549	549	0	0
Continuing Education	0	150	(150)	0	200	450	(250)	55.55
Total Expenses	15,988	15,491	386	3.21	39,696	46,473	(6,777)	14.58
Net Revenue Before Allowances	32,386	36,390	(4,004)	−11.00	113,408	109,170	4,238	3.88

The report indicates figures for both the budget period and the *year to date (YTD)*, or the sum of all activity for the months of January, February, and March combined.

- When a figure in the variance column indicates that the *actual amount* is lower than the *projected or budgeted amount*, it is presented in parentheses (e.g., "(1,962)" under "Variance") whether the variance is positive or negative. This is a common practice in many organizations.
- The figures in the "% Variance" columns indicate the relationship between *actual amounts* and *projected or budgeted amounts*, so a positive or negative number can represent a positive or negative variance depending upon whether you are discussing a revenue item or an expense item.

Finally, new managers must become familiar with the process of planning for a *capital equipment* budget. Capital equipment is often requested during a planning and budgeting process that occurs separately but concurrently with the planning and submission for approval of departmental budgets. The definition of capital equipment is determined by the organization, but typically includes a minimum cost (e.g., single items over $500) and a minimum life span (e.g., nonconsumable equipment with a life span of over 12 months). Sometimes *capital improvements*, or improvements in facilities costing more than a pre-established cost limit, are considered in the same process.

Depending on the nature of the equipment being requested, its cost, and the financial health of the organization, obtaining approval for a capital equipment request can be easy or very difficult. Items that are critically important to the provision of intervention or daily work, such as a refrigerator for storage of patient food used in meal preparation activities or an ultrasound machine used in treating persons with hand injuries, may be more easily justified. Equipment that may result in increased revenue or contributes to bringing new referrals and business to an organization may also be more likely to be approved if you can write a sufficient justification showing that the initial outlay of resources is warranted given the increased net revenue (the change needs to be a real increase in *net* revenue and not just in non-reimbursed charges). Examples of such equipment would include a work simulator used in intervention with persons with various types of physical impairments or a driving simulator used to evaluate the capacity of persons with various types of disabilities to return to driving.

In writing a justification for a piece of capital equipment, the following points might be considered:

- Initial cost of purchase
- Cost of supplies and maintenance associated with the equipment's use (paper, parts, repairs, routine calibration, etc.)
- Space required for operation and installation costs
- Revenue associated with direct charge for use of the equipment or with intervention facilitated by purchase of the equipment
- Estimated life of the equipment
- Training costs for employees to learn to use the equipment
- Potential liabilities or safety issues in use of the equipment

Facility Planning

Planning for new facilities and space is an aspect of planning that occupational therapy managers sometimes face but that can be daunting if you are poorly prepared for the task. Although the accreditation standards for occupational therapy educational programs include a standard related to maintaining and organizing treatment areas, equipment, and supply inventories, few programs include detailed content related to planning and designing treatment areas. A full discussion of the process is beyond the scope of this chapter; however, it is important that you know that resources are available if needed, and that finding yourself in the position of having to guide development of an occupational therapy clinic is not unimaginable. Twice in my career as an occupational therapy department director, I have found myself responsible for planning new spaces. In both instances, it was because the hospitals in which I worked were building new outpatient centers and chose to move re-

habilitation services into a new facility. In addition, some therapists choose to open private practices or businesses that require planning for space and materials. Nosse, Friberg, and Kovacek (1999) outlined nine steps in the process of designing and planning a therapy facility (Table 5–3). You are encouraged to consult this and additional resources on planning facilities for additional information. In addition, you might consider these simple steps to better prepare you:

- Visit other facilities to get ideas for planning and look at the space used by multiple disciplines.
- Ask other managers in your facility and at others what they like best about their space and, more importantly, what mistake were made in its design.
- Have staff brainstorm a "wish list" for use of space.
- Put a blank sheet of paper on the wall in each room and have staff members make notations of problems or suggestions for new space as they think of them.

Table 5-3	Overview of the Stages and Steps for Planning Facilities
Stage	**Step**
Predesign	1. Planning team selection for those involved in facility planning 2. Preplanning
Design development	3. Detailed planning 4. Final planning 5. Keeping track of the project
Construction	6. Construction and equipment procurement
Preoperations	7. Final checkout
Occupancy/Startup	8. Occupancy 9. Revisions and critique

From Nosse, L. J., Friberg, D. G., & Kovacek, P. R. (1999). *Managerial and supervisory principles for physical therapists.* Baltimore: Lippincott, Williams & Wilkins, with permission.

Organizing and Staffing

Organizing is the process of designing workable units, determining lines of authority and communication, and developing and managing patterns of coordination. Organizing involves creating the most effective grouping of activities together with the necessary guidelines and coordinating systems so that the organization's goals can be achieved as efficiently as possible. If carried out properly, organizing will provide clear identification of

- Who is responsible for work tasks and outputs of critical work processes
- Who has the authority to make decisions
- The functional separation of work activities
- Expected levels of performance for individuals and groups

Organizing as a management function was discussed in depth in Chapter 3, but will be reviewed briefly here as well. Organizing is more often associated with mid-level or upper management rather than first-line supervisors. However, all levels of managers and supervisors are involved in overseeing and supporting organizational structures on a daily basis. First-line supervisors often can provide valuable input into the effectiveness of or problems with existing organizational forms. The basic steps of organizing are listed in Box 5–13.

Staffing is the process of assuring that the right person is completing the right tasks within predetermined work units and that these persons have the necessary skills to do the job. Staffing is the management function that ensures that the organization will have sufficient quantity and quality of personnel to achieve its mission and goals. Staffing is an ongoing process that accounts for recruiting, hiring, training, firing, and replacing personnel as necessary. The primary activities associated with staffing are described in Box 5–14 (Lyles & Joiner, 1986).

Human Resources Planning

Developing a staffing plan includes identifying the number, type, and qualifications of staff needed to meet the needs of a department and its customers.

Box 5–14: Primary Activities Associated with Staffing

- **Human resources planning:** Collaborating with management and supervisors at all levels of the organization to forecast the short-term and long-term personnel needs of the organization based on the organizational mission, leadership vision, and strategic plans.
- **Recruitment:** Seeking out and attracting adequate numbers of qualified personnel to meet the organizational needs on an ongoing basis, including contingencies such as resignations and leaves of absence.
- **Hiring:** Selecting the appropriate personnel for vacant positions, and associated activities such as benefits counseling, background, and reference checks.
- **Orientation:** Introducing the new employee to organizational policies, procedures, values, personnel, and environments.
- **Training and development:** Meeting the short- and long-term education and professional development needs of employees at all levels of the organization.
- **Separation:** Terminating the employment of personnel because of resignation, inadequate job performance, or a decrease in organizational resources. Disciplinary activities may preclude separation as necessary.

Box 5–13: Basic Steps of Organizing

1. Recognize organizational goals and objectives.
2. Review the internal and external organizational environments.
3. Determine the organizational and departmental structures needed to reach the goal.
4. Determine the authority of relationships, and develop organizational charts and job descriptions.

Staffing plans must account for the expected work volume, including fluctuations for various days of the week or seasons, and the length of time spent with each client, including the full range of billable and nonbillable services (an example of service that is often not billable to a third-party payer or to the client is a team conference). Defining the *skill mix*, or the appropriate ratio of occupational therapists, occupational therapy assistants, and service extenders or aides needed to provide care that is effective but also cost efficient, is also part of developing a staffing plan. Finally, staffing plans must consider the skills of staff members within an employee classification. For example, in a hospital setting in which policies state that occupational therapists provide services in a neonatal intensive care unit on a 7-day-a-week basis, the staffing plan must accommodate the need for a therapist who has demonstrated age-specific competencies to be available each and every day.

Recruitment and Hiring

Recruiting new employees can be fun and rewarding, but it may also be a difficult, confusing, and sometimes frustrating responsibility. It is one of the most important functions that managers perform, however, and must be approached with the utmost care and attention. Recruitment of an employee includes identification of the type of employee needed based on an established staffing plan, advertising for candidates, and screening and interviewing candidates to identify a candidate who is a good match for the vacant position.

Typically the process of identifying the type of employee needed begins by reviewing the job description for the position for which you are recruiting. More information on job descriptions is provided in Chapter 10. Often you may hire the same type of employee with skills similar to those of the last person who held the now vacant position, but it is important to recognize that, over time, the nature of a department's work can change with shifts in referrals sources or the addition or deletion of programs. Because there can be a wide variation in the salaries of an occupational therapist, an occupational therapy assistant, and an occupational therapy aide, comparing the work to be done against current job descriptions can help to assure that you are hiring the right type of employee and making the most effective use of resources. For example, a salary of $52,000 that was paid to an experienced occupational therapist leaving an organization might cover the salary of both an occupational therapy assistant and an occupational therapy aide. However, in making the decision to hire an occupational therapy assistant or aide, you would need to be sure that you would still have a sufficient number of occupational therapists to complete the evaluation and intervention planning tasks not appropriate for an occupational therapy assistant or aide. You should also consider whether the employee you are hiring needs to have prior experience or if you might be able to hire a new graduate or a therapist with less experience. At times you may need to take advantage of the increased independence and lowered supervision needs of an experienced therapist, whereas at other times the enthusiasm and fresh outlook that many new graduates bring, along with lower salary expectations, may justify the increased costs for training and supervision necessary for new graduates.

Advertising includes writing and placing an ad or announcement in a newspaper, professional magazine, or journal or on a Web site or Listserv or working with a professional recruiter. The best way to decide what to put in your ad is to spend time reviewing ads placed by other organizations both within and outside of health care. Advertising can be very expensive (more than $1000 for a small ad in a single edition of some professional magazines), and you need to be sure that your advertising contains all of the necessary information to attract the sort of candidates you hope to reach while being concise and attractive or "eye catching" to the reader. The AOTA (*http://www.aota.org/*) has both a professional magazine (*OT Practice*) and an Internet-based service ("OTJobLink") that sell space for employment advertisements. *Advance for Occupational Therapy Practitioners* is a private publication that is also a popular medium for advertising for new employees (*http://www.advanceforot.com/*). The advantage of the services just mentioned is that they allow you to recruit on a regional or national basis. This allows you to reach a broader net of potential candidates, but also means that you may have to consider negotiating expenses for interviews or for relocation if you hire someone who is not local. Advertising in local papers or on a state occupational therapy association Listserv or Web site or buying mailing labels (also available from the AOTA and some state occupational therapy associations) allows you to narrow your recruitment to a smaller geographic area, but in return you may not reach as many potential candidates.

A different alternative for recruiting is using a professional health care recruiter who will identify potential candidates for you and help to arrange interviews. In some ways, this saves you time and may save the expense of advertising; however, professional recruiters or "headhunters" can charge high fees if they successfully place a candidate in your organization. Often there is no fee charged unless you hire a candidate referred by the recruiter, but, if successful, the recruiter may charge a fee equal to a large portion of the employee's annual salary, so it can be an expensive method of recruitment. A disadvantage is that some therapists are reticent to use recruiters and you will only reach the candidate pool with which the recruiter has contact. In addition, you may waste valuable time if the recruiter is unsuccessful and end up spending money on advertising anyway. In times when there are shortages of available therapists, you may have to consider using recruitment alternatives such as health care recruiters or "sign-on bonuses" that you would not otherwise use. Developing and maintaining a peer network will allow you to keep up with trends in recruitment practices as they change and allow you to remain competitive.

Screening employees is the process of reviewing applicants' basic qualifications and experience to determine if they meet the pre-established criteria for hiring. This is done so that you only offer interviews to candidates who might be a match for your work setting. Pre-established criteria may include

factors such as whether candidates are licensed or eligible for licensure in your state, if they have the level and type of experience matching your needs, if there are large gaps in their employment history that cannot be explained, or if they can demonstrate specialized competencies related to a patient population or program (e.g., Sensory Integration certification). In addition, you may screen candidates out of the interview process because of concerns over professionalism that arise as a result of poorly written cover letters or résumés. Using criteria that are pre-established is important and particularly helpful when you receive a large number of résumés. When this happens, an intermediate step between screening résumés and conducting face-to-face interviews can be conducting telephone interviews. Interviewing is essentially a process of finding the best match between potential employees and both the open position *and* the culture of your department and organization.

An effective method of interviewing that helps to match an employee to both the job and the culture of the department and organization is *attribute-based interviewing*. In this approach, the attributes of the desired employee are identified and described in writing, and then open-ended questions are developed that allow the interviewer to get a sense of how closely the potential employee matches the desired attributes. Examples of attributes that might be desirable in a new occupational therapy team leader and sample open-ended questions are provided in Table 5–4. It is important also to consider who will be involved in an interview process and the extent to which those persons will be involved in selecting a preferred candidate. There may be value in including subordinates, peers both

Table 5-4 Sample Attributes and Open-Ended Interview Questions

Attribute	Open-Ended Question
Direct style of conflict management	Tell me about a time that you had to give someone you supervised some difficult feedback and how you went about doing it.
Committed to maintaining a role in patient care	If you could design your perfect job, what would be the mix of supervisory duties and patient care responsibilities?
Creative problem solver	Tell me about a time that you faced a complex problem and how you led your team in the process of solving it.

from within the occupational therapy department and from other departments, or other key supervisory and managerial personnel in the interviews.

Hiring a new employee includes checking references and negotiating salary, benefits (including relocation expenses), and the date the employee will begin work. A full history of previous employment, including the start and end dates, the title of the position held by the candidate, the reason for leaving the job, and the names of supervisors, should be obtained. All previous employers should be contacted to verify that the information is correct. You should be aware that, because of fear of liability in litigation, some employers will only verify factual information and may not comment on the employee's skills or performance. Only after references are checked should a formal written offer be extended. Two copies of an offer letter stating the rate of compensation, benefits, and starting date, along with a job description, should be mailed to the candidate, who should sign both copies indicating acceptance of the position and return one to you and keep the other for himself or herself.

Orientation

McNamara (2003) provided a helpful list of suggestions for beginning the process of orienting an employee to a new position in a manner that both provides information and makes the new employee feel welcome in his or her new organization. These suggestions include

- Send a letter of welcome before the employee begins, providing him or her with a contact number if he or she has questions.
- Meet with the employee the first day, even if just for a few moments, before he or she reports to the human resources department, if required to do so.
- Give the employee a tour of the facilities, including basics such as the location of lockers and bathrooms, kitchen and telephone use, and the location of the cafeteria, if one is present.
- Provide a schedule for the first few days.
- Assign a fellow employee as a buddy to answer questions and to have lunch with the new employee on the first day. Join them for lunch if possible.
- Meet with the employee at the end of the first day.

- Meet on at least a weekly basis for the first few weeks.

Before orientation begins, you should start a departmental personnel file in which you keep copies of important documents such as the signed letter of offer and job description; a copy of the employee's license, if applicable; and a checklist of all activities completed during orientation.

Bacal (2003) noted that there are two related kinds of orientation. He referred to the first as "overview orientation," which deals with the basic information an employee will need to understand the broader system he or she works in and is often conducted by the human resources department. Overview orientation includes helping employees understand

- The system in which the organization functions in general (e.g., schools, community, medical model)
- Important policies and general procedures (non–job specific)
- Information about compensation and benefits
- Safety and accident prevention issues
- Employee and union issues (rights, responsibilities)
- Physical facilities

Bacal named the second type of orientation "job-specific orientation," which is the process that is used to help employees understand

- The function of the organization, and how the employee fits in
- Job responsibilities, expectations, and duties of the employee
- Policies, procedures, rules, and regulations
- Layout of the workplace

An important part of the orientation process for occupational therapists is the assessment of competencies. Competencies are specific statements of an individual's ability to perform a specific skill or activity in a particular situation. Assessment of competencies is discussed in more depth in Chapter 7. Although some competencies should be assessed on an annual basis, especially in organizations subject to accreditation by bodies such as the Joint Commission on Accreditation of Healthcare Organizations, others may only be assessed at the time of initial orientation. For example, an employee's understanding of procedures related to electrical or fire safety or to blood-borne pathogens should be assessed on an annual basis. Other competencies, such as the ability to safely transfer a patient or to fabricate a common splint, might only be assessed as part of the orientation process.

Training, Education, and Development

McNamara (2003) identified a variety of reasons for organizations to provide for the training and development of employees. These reasons include

- When a performance appraisal indicates performance improvement is needed
- To "benchmark" the status of improvement so far in a performance improvement effort
- As part of an overall professional development program
- As part of succession planning to help an employee be eligible for a planned change in role in the organization
- To train about a specific topic to meet customer service or other needs of the department or organization

Schein (1992) differentiated the functions of training, education, and development. The differences in these functions relate to the focus of the learning activity and when it will be applied in an employee's professional development. Briefly, these functions can be described as follows:

- *Training activities* are related to improving an employee's capacity to perform his or her current job, such as learning a new treatment technique related to a patient population that he or she currently treats.
- *Education activities* are related to improving an employee's capacity for a specific but future job, such as a staff therapist taking an introductory course on supervising others.
- *Development activities* are related to overall capacities that may be used in any job, such as time management or communication skills.

The manager of a department is typically responsible for integrating information from multiple systems to identify and meet the training, education, and development needs of staff. These systems include employee performance appraisals, competency assessment systems, strategic plans,

program evaluation results, and staffing plans, among others. Meeting the training, education, and development needs of staff is accomplished through a variety of strategies, including department in-service education, sending staff members to outside continuing education programs, and individual supervision.

Discipline and Separation

Managers (along with supervisors) are responsible for overseeing performance and providing feedback and guidance to employees to correct inappropriate behavior (such as tardiness to the workplace) and to improve the quality and quantity of performance if it does not meet minimal standards. Feedback for minor concerns or feedback focused on helping employees develop as persons and professionals is routinely delivered as part of an ongoing performance appraisal system. Performance appraisal systems will be discussed in more detail in Chapter 6.

When a manager must provide feedback on unacceptable or substandard performance, he or she must utilize a formal disciplinary process. Such a process typically consists of several steps. The specific action to be taken depends on the seriousness of the behavior or problem being addressed, whether the employee has received feedback before, and the length of time since the employee last exhibited the behavior. The steps of a sample disciplinary process applied to the problem of an employee who is tardy to work are provided in Box 5–15.

Although often difficult for the manager or supervisor, disciplinary procedures are beneficial and necessary for the safety and well-being of those the organization serves as well as the health and survival of an organization. In the long run, these procedures are also in the best interest of the employee who experiences difficulty meeting the performance or behavioral expectations of his or her job.

Although the word *discipline* likely conjures up negative thoughts, the first steps of an effective disciplinary procedure focus on providing the employee (or fieldwork student) with the information and skills to bring his or her behavior and performance into compliance with organizational expectations. Progressive disciplinary systems provide multiple opportunities for the employee to correct deficiencies by providing progressively more stern feedback and increasingly severe conse-

---

Box 5–15: A Sample Disciplinary Process Applied to Tardiness to Work

- **Step 1–Remind/Reinstruct:** On a first instance of unexcused tardiness, the behavior is brought to the employee's attention and he or she is reminded of the importance of being on time, the problems that being late causes, and that it is always necessary to call in to a supervisor if he or she is going to be late.
- **Step 2–Verbal Warning:** On a second instance of unexcused tardiness within a short period of time in relation to the first, the behavior, problems associated with the behavior, the policy or expectation, and that this is the second (or more) instance of the unacceptable behavior is brought to the employee's attention.

  A second reminder of the necessary behavior is provided and the possible ramifications of continued unacceptable behavior are pointed out. A dated notation is placed in the employee's personnel file.
- **Step 3–Written Warning:** On a third instance of unexcused tardiness within a short period of time in relation to the second, the actions in Step 2 are repeated. This time the employee should be invited to a formal meeting to discuss the behavior, the resulting problems, and what the manager might do to assist the employee to prevent the behavior from continuing, and to problem solve with the employee. A referral to an employee assistance program (EAP) is made.* The seriousness of the situation and the possible implications for the employee are stressed, and again a dated notation is placed in the employee's personnel file. The human resources department may need to be consulted or informed at this point.
- **Step 4–Suspension:** On the next instance of unexcused tardiness within a short period of time in relation to prior instances, and after consulting with human resources, the employee is suspended from work without pay for a period of time (1 day to 1 week depending on the seriousness of the behavior). Offers of assistance to help prevent the behavior are made, a second referral to an EAP is made, the fact that the employee may be headed for termination is stressed, and all facts and conversations are documented in the personnel file.
- **Step 5–Termination:** On the next instance of unexcused tardiness within a short period of time of returning from suspension, the employee will be terminated. Immediately upon noticing the behavior, the human resources department is contacted and a plan is developed. The employee's manager and a representative from human resources meet with the employee, review briefly the cause for termination, and stay with the employee until he or she gathers personal belongings and leaves the building. All facts and conversations are carefully documented in the personnel file.

*Many large organizations have employee assistance programs (EAPs) that aid employees with a range of personal problems that might affect performance, including stress management, substance abuse, and a range of other issues. Such services are typically provided in a confidential manner to the employee and are often free of charge.

---

quences. Such systems should also provide multiple opportunities for the manager to offer assistance and to ask the employee what the manager or organization could do to help the employee overcome the difficulty he or she is experiencing. Most often employees are able to correct the problem behavior or bring performance up to standards, and it is not necessary to continue to termination.

Terminating an employee is undoubtedly one of the most difficult things a manager must do. Although it will not eliminate the discomfort, you should know that no manager should act alone when terminating an employee. In large organizations, someone from personnel or human resources should always be involved, and in private businesses where the manager is also the owner, legal counsel, another business owner, or a supervisor should be involved in the process to provide guidance and support to the manager and to be a witness to the actions taken.

It should be stressed that there is considerable room for sound managerial judgment in the process just presented. Like any staged model, you may skip steps if behavior warrants, or, with the passing of time, steps may be repeated. An employee with a solid performance history who is tardy one day after not having been tardy for a year most likely deserves to be reminded of the importance of being on time and likely does not warrant a verbal warning. Of course, behaviors such as theft, patient abuse, or serious ethics violations may warrant moving directly to termination on the first instance of the behavior. Other than for very serious infractions, you should only move to terminating an employee if you have

- Given the employee clear indication of what you originally expected from him or her via a written job description previously provided to him or her.
- Supplied clearly written personnel policies that specify conditions and directions about firing employees, and the employee initialed a copy of the policy handbook to verify that he or she had read the policies.
- Warned the employee in successive and dated memos that clearly described the continuance of the problem behavior over a specified time despite your specific and recorded offers of assistance and any training.
- Clearly observed the employee still having the performance problem. (You should note that, if the employee is being fired within a probationary period specified in your personnel policies, you may not have to meet all of these conditions.)

Directing

Directing has been defined as "the provision of guidance and leadership so that the work performed is goal oriented. It is the exercise of the manager's influence, the process of teaching, coaching, and motivating workers" (Liebler et al., 1992). Management activities that might be grouped under the function of directing include mentoring or coaching in addition to elements of traditional performance planning and supervision. Typically a department manager is responsible for the creation of an overall staff development plan or program, including support of continuing education and professional development in the department budget, allowing for release time for staff to attend professional development activities. Supervisory approaches and strategies, including appraisal of performance and the creation of individual professional development plans, will be the focus of Chapter 6, so the remainder of this section of this chapter will focus on mentoring.

Mentoring

Mentoring is a process in which a typically older, more experienced professional enters into a formal relationship with a typically younger, less experienced professional focused on guiding the professional development of the younger professional. Mentoring relationships are different and can be much more significant that the typical relationship between a supervisor and supervisee. Mentors (the more experienced professional) and "mentees" (the less experienced professional) may work at the same organization and may also have a supervisor-subordinate relationship, but this is not necessarily the case. Naturally occurring mentoring relationships can be intense for both parties, with the mentor feeling a sense of responsibility for the development of the mentee and the mentee feeling a sense of responsibility to meet the expectations of the mentor. Becoming involved in a mentoring relationship means a commitment of time by both parties. The mentor invests time in meeting with the mentee, looking for opportunities that will promote growth, listening to and meeting with the mentee to discuss concerns and plans for the future, and providing praise for accomplishments. The mentee also invests time in meetings, in communicating regularly with the mentor, in following up on suggestions for activities made by the mentor, and in making himself or herself available by displaying a willingness to learn.

Mentoring relationships sometimes happen naturally when two professionals meet in the course of their work lives and recognize their affinity for each other and begin to commit to a professional relationship that is sustained over time. Mentoring relationships typically include four stages: birth,

Box 5–16: The Four Stages of a Mentoring Relationship

1. **Birth of the relationship** is when the first meeting occurs to define expectations.
2. **Engagement** is task-focused and is when the relationship is strengthened through identifying goals and establishing potential activities to help the mentee achieve his or her goals.
3. **Sustainment** occurs through honest, mutually respectful, and positive interactions. At this stage, the process and outcome of behaviors are co-evaluated, interactive feedback is given to correct problem areas, and positive aspects of the relationship are reinforced.
4. **Transition** is characterized by ending the relationship when goals have been attained or the time commitment is fulfilled.

Adapted from Robertson, S. C., & Savio, M. C. (2003). Mentoring as professional development. American Occupational Therapy Association OT Practice Online. Available at *http://www.aota.org/featured/area2/links/link16h.asp*

engagement, sustainment, and transition. These stages are defined in Box 5–16 (Robertson & Savio, 2003).

As an occupational therapist, I have been fortunate enough to find not one, but two mentors. I met my first mentor as a level II fieldwork student in the Continuing Education Division of the AOTA. My fieldwork supervisor, Susan Robertson, immediately became a professional inspiration and role model for me. Our relationship flourished during my fieldwork experience and continues until this day. For my first decade of practice, Susan served as my mentor. My experience is presented here as a case example of mentoring.

Although the mentoring described so far has been in regard to naturally occurring mentoring relationships, formal mentoring programs in which professionals are paired with each other by the program or employing organization have also been developed. Mentoring in general has been connected in the human resources literature with positive organizational outcomes, including more promotions (Dreher & Ash, 1990; Scandura, 1992), reduced turnover (Victor & Scandura, 1991), and greater career satisfaction (Ostroff, Horton, & Crosby, 1993). Orchestrated mentoring experiences are typically shorter in duration than naturally occurring relationships; are often less intense, with pre-

Case Example: Mentoring

I began my first day of my level II fieldwork experience at the AOTA Division of Continuing Education by meeting with my supervisor, Susan Robertson. Susan's unbridled enthusiasm for educating others was immediately evident. During my fieldwork, I benefited from the opportunities that Susan orchestrated for me, including involvement in a wide range of projects and interaction with leaders in the profession. Some of the specific actions that Susan took were

- To assign me strategically to projects that fit my goals and strengths but that challenged me to grow
- To introduce me to key leaders at meetings

- To call the attention of others to the contributions I made to association projects
- To challenge me to set development goals for myself

As I continued my fieldwork, I began to feel a sense of responsibility to do well on all assignments not only to meet my own performance expectations but to also make Susan proud of me.

After I completed my fieldwork, Susan and I agreed to keep in touch and did so. Over the next few years, I kept Susan informed of my professional activities. Susan followed my career with great interest, not only providing me with praise for accomplishments, but also challenging me to think ahead to my next job

(continued)

and to constantly think strategically about the activities with which I became involved. At Susan's urging, I became involved in state occupational therapy association activities and pursued volunteer leadership experiences that helped me with skill development. Despite being uncomfortable at first, I made presentations at local and national conferences with Susan's support, and these experiences proved valuable to me later in my career when I had to make presentations to other groups. I also furthered my education by obtaining a master's degree.

As my mentoring relationship with Susan matured, the nature of the interactions we had changed and Susan began to share more about how she was working on developing her own career; however, she continued to challenge me to grow. Even as I accumulated years of professional experience and became the director of an occupational therapy department, Susan and I maintained regular contact. For example, each year at the AOTA annual conference, we would have dinner and, after catching up on what was going on in our personal lives, Susan would inevitably shift the conversation to discussing my career and what I should be doing next.

Eventually I reached a point in my career at which I began to primarily seek mentoring from a new boss as I accepted a job in academics and changed the focus of my career. Rather than expressing loss or even jealousy, Susan expressed sincere joy and respect for my accomplishments. Although my maturation as a professional led to the end of our formal mentoring relationship, Susan and I remain close colleagues and friends to this day. This mentoring relationship was effective because of the actions that both Susan and I took to support the relationship.

As a mentor, Susan

- Fostered self-reflection
- Instructed and motivated me to achieve new goals and develop new skills
- Supported my critical thinking and clinical reasoning
- Facilitated problem solving and decision making as I progressed through the first decade of my career
- Encouraged the application of learning to new situations and challenges

As a mentee, I
- Actively reflected on the advice and observations shared by Susan
- Sought self-motivating learning opportunities to build on the suggestions and guidance provided by my mentor
- Engaged in critical thinking, clinical reasoning, and reflective self-examination
- Collaborated actively with Susan to solve problems and make key career decisions
- Related learning to the professional goals that Susan and I identified

---

determined meeting frequency and prescribed activities; and may be limited because the mentors fear the perception of *favoritism* because the relationship may be very public (Blake-Beard, 2001).

The theme of this book is using evidence to guide the management of occupational therapy services. Almost every function of management can be guided by theory and some form of evidence. Presenting the evidence on *every* topic discussed in this text would not be helpful; however, occasional illustrations of the strategies presented in Chapter 1 would be of use. Therefore, the evidence related to orchestrated mentoring will be used as an example. Let's assume that you have become aware of the benefits of mentoring and wonder if it would be a good use of your organization's resources to develop a mentoring program for new managers. Your question then would be

What does the evidence presented in the literature suggest about the effectiveness of formal mentoring programs compared to naturally occurring mentoring relationships?

When searching the literature on mentoring, limiting your search to empirical studies, you would find that there are only a handful of empirical studies that have compared the effectiveness of formal programs to naturally occurring mentoring relationships. Each of these studies found that naturally occurring or "informal" mentoring relationships resulted in greater outcomes for the mentees in terms of career development than did participation in a formal mentoring program. Two of the three studies reported that informal mentees perceived higher levels of psychosocial support. That evidence is summarized in Table 5–5.

	Summary of Selected Evidence on Formal Mentoring Programs				
Author	**Study Type**	**N**	**Level of Evidence**	**Results**	
Ragins & Cotton (1999)	Quantitative analysis of survey	510 informal mentees, 104 formal mentees	Good	Informal mentees rated their mentors as more effective and received higher salaries than mentees with formal mentors. Informal mentees also reported higher levels of psychosocial support.	
Hurley & Fagenson-Eland (1996)	Qualitative interview and survey	16 informal & 30 formal mentees	Good	No difference between groups in the level of career development or role modeling reported, but informal mentees did report higher levels of psychosocial benefit.	
Chao, Walz, & Gardner (1992)	Quantitative analysis of survey	212 informal & 53 formal mentees	Good	Informal mentees reported greater career support and higher salaries than peers in informal relationships, but no support for a hypothesis that informal mentors provide greater levels of psychosocial support.	

Table 5-5

Controlling

Controlling is the process of measuring performance against expectations and taking action to eliminate obstacles to achieving organizational goals. One primary method of controlling everyday functions is through the use of control mechanisms or control indicators. A control mechanism or control indicator is a "check" or measure that is in place to constantly monitor the output or product of a system. When the check indicates that performance falls below a previously established limit, it means there is an unacceptable variation in the system or a problem to be addressed. Control mechanisms can be related either to *outcomes*, or the desired targets for a process, or to *processes* themselves, or controls intended to specify the manner in which tasks will be completed through the use of policies, procedures, and rules.

Common examples of control mechanisms that might be used by an occupational therapy manager would include taking the temperature in a refrigerator that stores patient food each day so action can be taken if the temperature is not sufficiently cool, noting the length of time it takes to respond to a referral after it is received by the occupational therapy department so action can be taken when the time exceeds a predetermined period of time, or checking the cords on all electrical equipment once monthly so action can be taken if a cord is frayed or damaged. Monitoring the productivity level of occupational therapists and occupational therapy assistants by counting the number of units of care that they provide or enter into a computerized billing system to identify when productivity levels drop below minimum standards would also be an example of controlling as a managerial function.

The process of controlling includes three phases: (1) establishing standards, (2) measuring perfor-

---

Box 5–17: Controlling: A Three-Phase Process

- **Establishing Standards:** Determining the specific indicators or quantifiable measures of acceptable work
- **Measuring Performance:** Comparing outputs of processes to established standards
- **Correcting Deviations:** Taking action to improve outputs of processes that do not meet established standards

---

Box 5–19: Characteristics of Adequate Control Mechanisms

- **Timeliness:** The control signifies a problem in a timely manner so corrective action can be taken before serious harm or loss of resources is experienced.
- **Economy:** The control is conducted in a routine manner that does not require significant human or financial costs or resources.
- **Comprehensiveness:** The control measures a sufficient variety and extent of available data so problems are caught and are not inadvertently overlooked.
- **Specificity and appropriateness:** The control is specific to the process being measured so false alarms do not consume time or effort.
- **Objectivity:** The control is easily understood by all personnel and there is no question as to when measures fall below or above pre-established standards.
- **Responsibility:** Responsibility for monitoring the control on an ongoing basis is clear to all personnel so measures are checked regularly according to a predetermined schedule.

---

mance, and (3) correcting deviations (Box 5–17). There are various types of controls (sometimes also referred to as standards) that can be used depending upon the process or mechanism that is being monitored. Controls can relate to physical characteristics of a product or to quantity, quality, or cost. The most common types of controls and brief definitions of each are listed in Box 5–18.

Regardless of the type of control, in order to be effective, the control must be structured so you become aware of the problem in a timely and efficient manner and you receive adequate information to take appropriate action. The characteristics of adequate control mechanisms are listed in Box 5–19.

Box 5–18: Types of Controls

- **Physical:** Standards related to tangible elements of a product or outcome of a process, such as smoothness, texture, or size
- **Quantity:** Amounts or counts that provide a measure of conformance and efficiency, such as the number of units of care provided, or hours billed
- **Quality:** Quantitative measures of quality, such as outcome measures or patient or customer satisfaction
- **Cost:** The cost of a process, such as the cost per unit of service provided, or the cost of materials associated with a process, such as fabricating a splint

---

Information Management

With improved technology, the amount of data and information that managers receive on a daily basis can be overwhelming. The ability to transmit large amounts of information to a person in another department or across the world in seconds through e-mail, to access millions of Internet sites or search multiple databases for current evidence, or to have statistics and data automatically collected and reported from documentation or billing systems has clear advantages. There can also be the danger of wasting time sorting through meaningless data. On any single day, an occupational therapy manager may receive reports related to budget, staff productivity, rates of client visits, client charges, equipment usage, continuous quality improvement

Table 5-6	Common Types and Sources of Data and Information, and Possible Uses	
Type of Data	**Source**	**Use**
Demographics (age, sex, educational level, etc.)	• Admissions records • Public data sets	• Program planning • Program evaluation
Revenue (payer source, rates, discounts)	• Accounting • Budget reports	• Budgeting • Program planning
Expense (accounts payable)	• Financial reports • Purchasing records	• Budgeting • Program planning and evaluation
Payroll (salary, benefits, leave usage)	• Accounting • Budget reports	• Staffing plans • Recruitment and retention
Productivity (visits, staff activity)	• Automated charge systems • Department billing records or productivity tracking sheets	• Staffing plans • Performance appraisal • Recruitment
Personnel (licensure, competencies, professional development, performance)	• Human resources • Departmental personnel files • Professional association data sets	• Accreditation visits • Staffing plan development • Professional development plans
Clinical (diagnosis, intervention, outcomes)	• Medical records • Outcome databases	• Continuous quality improvement • Program evaluation
Legal (contracts, leases)	• Legal or grants and contracts department	• Facility planning

efforts, and clinical outcomes. It has been said that *information* is *data* that have been organized so they are useful and can be easily interpreted.

So, if there is the possibility of excess data and information overload, what are the most common types of data and information to which you must attend? Luckily in many larger organizations, some data are organized into useful information for you and often delivered to you automatically in the form of paper or electronic reports. With increasingly sophisticated and automated systems, data and information at the departmental level may also be available in this manner. Other times you may need to collect data yourself, such as when you are in the process of developing new programming for a target population for which your organization does not have an existing data collection mechanism. A simple question to ask yourself before you begin data collection is "What do I want to know and what will this data help me learn in order to improve the performance of my department?" If

you cannot identify the specific use for the data before collecting it, you should re-examine whether it is worth the resources to collect the data in the first place. Turning *data* into *information* requires that you know what question you are seeking to answer before you begin to collect the data. Table 5–6 lists common types and sources of data, information, and other forms of evidence used by managers and a sample of how these can be utilized.

Chapter Summary

This chapter reviewed the commonly identified functions of a manager (planning, organizing and staffing, directing, and controlling) and provided an introduction to some of the key activities associated with each of those functions. It was noted that managers are most often also supervisors, but then many occupational therapy supervisors do not have requisite managerial authority. Hopefully you have begun to get a flavor for the diversity that characterizes what managers "do." Moreover, you have likely begun to appreciate why it is that any introductory text on management typically presents a wide range of topics at a basic level. It is also likely that this chapter left you with many unanswered questions about becoming an occupational therapy manager. Some of those questions will be answered in the remaining chapters. However, for those questions that remain, you should have confidence that, if you master the basic skills of evidence-based practice, you will be able to seek out and identify the most current information to guide your decision making in choosing an effective answer.

At the beginning of this chapter, you were introduced to Marty, who had just accepted a position as the director of occupational therapy. Although he had some experience as an occupational therapy supervisor, he was unsure of what he needed to learn and so conducted a number of information interviews.

Real-Life Solutions

Marty completed a number of information interviews with other local occupational therapy department directors before beginning his new job. Although he was somewhat overwhelmed at the wide range of tasks that these managers completed, he was comforted to hear from most of his interviewees that he should begin by reviewing an introductory text on management. He was surprised to hear repeatedly that he could organize his learning needs and objectives according to the commonly identified management functions of planning, organizing and staffing, directing, and controlling.

Marty began to see that, like the practice of occupational therapy, management is guided by both theories and models that help you to conceptualize how to begin to address a set of responsibilities and by specific skill sets that help you perform discrete management tasks. Similarly, he began to understand that the principles of evidence-based practice could be applied to any type of occupational therapy practice, including management. When Marty considered the different activities that his peers had mentioned (strategic planning, policies and procedures, budgeting, planning facilities, recruitment of staff, discipline, and mentoring), he began to appreciate more how what he had learned about the functioning of health care systems, organizations, and leadership would help him in his new job. He also took solace in how often the directors that he interviewed encouraged him to rely on the expertise of other professionals in his new organization, including those in human resources, finance, continuous quality improvement, information management, and facilities management.

Marty was probably most surprised by how much the directors felt they still had to learn, and the extent to which they noted that they relied on a peer network to find the answers and solutions to their everyday questions and problems. Based on recommendations from his information interviews, Marty decided that he would be wise to do the following to help assure his success in his new role as an occupational therapy manager:

1. Join the SISs in Administration and Management offered by both his state occupational therapy association and the AOTA.
2. Maintain contact with the network of peer managers he began to develop while conducting his information interviews.
3. Immediately establish contacts in the departments responsible for key *staff* functions, including human resources, finance and accounting, continuous quality improvement, and facilities management.
4. Explore learning opportunities offered by his organization, his state occupational therapy association, the AOTA, and a local university, as well as those in the community, to develop skills for completing key management functions such as interviewing and budgeting skills.
5. Continue to read and search the literature from diverse disciplines and journals, including business administration, organizational development, human resources, and psychology, to remain aware of current developments in research and evidence related to his job as an occupational therapy manager.

Resources for Learning More About the Roles and Functions of Managers

Journals That Often Address Management and Management Issues

MANAGEMENT SCIENCE

Management Science is a scholarly journal that scientifically addresses the problems, interests, and concerns of organizational decision makers. Through publication of relevant theory and innovative applications, the journal serves the needs of both academicians and practitioners.

JOURNAL OF MANAGEMENT DEVELOPMENT

The *Journal of Management Development* covers a broad range of topics in its field, including competence-based management development, developing leadership skills, developing women for management, global management, the new technology of management development, team building, organizational development and change, and performance appraisal.

JOURNAL OF MANAGEMENT STUDIES

The journal provides in-depth coverage of organizational problems and organization theory, reports on the latest developments in strategic management and planning, presents cross-cultural comparisons of organizational effectiveness, and includes concise reviews of the latest publications in management studies as well as lively debate on topical and important issues in management.

Associations That Are Concerned with Management and Management Issues

THE AMERICAN OCCUPATIONAL THERAPY ASSOCIATION

http://www.aota.org/

The stated mission of the AOTA advances the quality, availability, use, and support of occupational therapy through standard setting, advocacy, education, and research on behalf of its members and the public. The AOTA provides its members with a variety of resources related to the supervision of occupational therapy personnel, including a number of papers that provide guidelines for the occupational therapy supervisor; access to Special Interest Sections (SISs) that provide Listservs and quarterly newsletters, including the Administration and Management SIS; and continuing education options.

AMERICAN MANAGEMENT ASSOCIATION

http://www.amanet.org/index.htm

The American Management Association (AMA) states that its mission is to provide managers and their organizations worldwide with the knowledge, skills, and tools they need to improve business performance, adapt to a changing workplace, and prosper in a complex and competitive business world. The AMA serves as a forum for the exchange of the latest information, ideas, and insights on management practices and business trends. The AMA disseminates content and information to a worldwide audience through multiple distribution channels and its strategic partners by offering seminars, conferences, current issues forums and briefings, books and publications, research, and online self-study courses, which cover such topics as supervisory skills.

Miscellaneous Resources Related to Management

THE NATIONAL MENTORING PARTNERSHIP

http://www.mentoring.org/index.adp

MENTOR/National Mentoring Partnership is an advocate for the expansion of mentoring and a resource for mentors and mentoring initiatives nationwide. For more than a decade, MENTOR/National Mentoring Partnership has been leading the effort to connect America's young people with caring adult mentors. MENTOR was created in 1990 by financiers and philanthropists Geoff Boisi and Ray Chambers. The Web site includes downloadable resources on mentoring, a list of research on the effectiveness of mentoring, and resources for developing mentoring programs.

Miscellaneous Resources

- Goodstein, L. D., Nolan, T., & Pfeiffer, J. W. (2003). *Applied strategic planning: How to develop a plan that really works.* New York: McGraw-Hill.

Applied Strategic Planning provides information on strategies to effectively communicate a corporate vision, recognize the role of culture in changing strategic direction, integrate your plan into your company's day-to-day operations—both horizontally and vertically, master methods of strategic business modeling, write effective mission statements, use consultants effectively, and create contingency plans. The book uses humorous drawings, anecdotes, and cartoons, many of which come directly from the experiences of top companies before they had a workable strategic plan in effect. There are also numerous charts, diagrams, and checklists that make the book especially easy to apply in your own organization, whatever its size or structure.

Reference List

Bacal, R. (2003). A quick guide to employee orientation. The Work911 Workplace Supersite. Available at *http://www.work911.com/articles/orient.htm*

Blake-Beard, S. D. (2001). Taking a hard look at formal mentoring programs: A consideration of potential challenges facing women. *Journal of Management Development, 20,* 331–345.

Burkhardt, A., & Gentile, P. (2001). Creating policies and procedures that work. *OT Practice, 6*(1), 15–18.

Chao, G. T., Walz, P. M., & Gardner, P. D. (1992). Formal and informal mentorships: A comparison on mentoring functions and contrast with non-mentored counterparts. *Personnel Psychology, 45,* 619–636.

Dreher, G. F., & Ash, R. A. (1990). A comparative study of mentoring among men and women in managerial, professional and technical positions. *Journal of Applied Psychology, 75,* 539–546.

Drucker, P. (1974). *Management: Tasks, responsibilities and practices.* New York: Harper & Row.

Goodstein, L. D. (1992). *Applied strategic planning.* San Diego, CA: Pfeiffer & Company.

Hoyle, J. R. (1995). *Leadership and futuring: Making visions happen.* Thousand Oaks, CA: Corwin Press.

Hurley, A. E., & Fagenson-Eland, E. A. (1996). Challenges in cross-gender mentoring relationships: Psychological intimacy, myths, rumors, innuendoes, and sexual harassment. *Leadership and Organizational Development Journal, 17,* 42–49.

Jaques, E. (1998). *Requisite organization.* Arlington, VA: Cason Hall.

Liebler, J. G., Levine, R. E., & Rothman, J. (1992). *Management principles for health professionals.* Gaithersburg, MD: Aspen.

Lyles, R. I., & Joiner, C. (1986). *Supervision in health care organizations.* New York: John Wiley & Sons.

McNamara, C. (2003). Basics: Definitions (and misperceptions) about management. The Management Assistance Program for Nonprofits. Available at *http://www.mapnp.org/library/mgmnt/ defntion.htm#anchor662641*

Nosse, L. J., Friberg, D. G., & Kovacek, P. R. (1999). *Managerial and supervisory principles for physical therapists.* Baltimore: Lippincott, Williams & Wilkins.

Ostroff, C., Horton, S., & Crosby, F. J. (1993). The role of mentoring in the information gathering process of newcomers during early organizational socialization. *Journal of Vocational Behavior, 33,* 15–37.

Ragins, B. R., & Cotton, J. L. (1999). Mentor functions and outcomes: A comparison of men and women in formal and informal mentoring relationships. *Journal of Applied Psychology, 84,* 529–550.

Robertson, S. C., & Savio, M. C. (2003). Mentoring as professional development. American Occupational Therapy Association OT Practice Online. Available at *http://www.aota.org/featured/area2/links/link16h.asp*

Scandura, T. A. (1992). Mentorship and career mobility: An empirical investigation. *Journal of Organizational Behavior, 13,* 169–174.

Schein, E. H. (1992). *Organizational culture and leadership.* New York: Jossey-Bass.

Victor, R. E., & Scandura, T. A. (1991). A study of mentor-protégé relationships in large public accounting firms. *Accounting Horizons, 5,* 20–30.

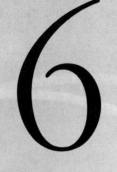

Brent Braveman, Ph.D., OTR/L, FAOTA

Roles and Functions of Supervisors

Real-Life Management

Carlota has worked as an occupational therapist for a school system for 6 years. During this time, she has acted as a clinical resource for other therapists, including occupational therapists, occupational therapy assistants, physical therapists, and speech-language pathologists. Other staff members frequently ask if she can sit in on treatment session for a few minutes to give them advice and seek her out for her opinions. She also has supervised multiple fieldwork students and has found great satisfaction in these experiences.

Recently, a supervisory position as a senior therapist has become available and Carlota's peers have been encouraging her to apply for the position. Carlota has previously passed up opportunities to be promoted into a position with more formal supervisory responsibilities because she has always been nervous about having to be someone's "boss." She thinks that she would enjoy a job where she spent more of her time coaching others and contributing to their professional development but is not as sure about having to give constructive criticism. Carlota also is sure that she is not interested in "moving up the ladder" and becoming a department director. She feels certain that her passions rest in working with clients but also in helping others become better therapists.

Carlota wonders too if she can assume the role of supervisor without also taking on responsibilities such as budgeting and personnel management that seem to be such a source of frustration and conflict for her own boss. She wonders if there is a difference between being a manager and a supervisor and, if so, what those differences might be. Carlota decides to speak to Craig, the District Occupational Therapy Manager, to find out what responsibilities would be included in a job as a senior therapist for the school district.

Key Issues

- Many occupational therapists and occupational therapy assistants become involved in the supervision of other occupational therapists, occupational therapy assistants, fieldwork students, and volunteers without accepting full managerial responsibilities.
- Formal authority is the influence associated with a specific rank or position within an organization, whereas power is the ability to coerce others to act. Power may exist with or without formal authority.
- Models and resources to guide the supervision of others exist within the human resources and the occupational therapy literature.
- There are a number of theories of motivation that are helpful in guiding supervision strategies as well as strategies for rewards and recognition of others.
- Performance appraisal is a key responsibility of many supervisors and is most effective when it is an ongoing and cyclical process that occurs throughout a performance appraisal period.

Chapter 4 introduced leadership as an overarching theme relevant to both management and supervision. Both managers and supervisors are in positions to provide leadership to others regardless of the level of formal power or authority that they hold within an organization. The major theories of leadership were introduced, as was evidence related to the effectiveness of adopting leader behaviors based on each theory. Chapter 5 reviewed the major management functions (planning, organizing and staffing, controlling, and directing) and noted that, although most managers are supervisors, many supervisors do not have what was referred to as *requisite managerial authority*. Chapter 6 will focus on the role and functions of the supervisor in more depth and summarize the common duties of the occupational therapy supervisor. Theory related to the motivation of employees will be introduced and evidence related to a number of key issues of concern to the supervisor will be presented.

Supervision

After reading Chapter 5, you might be asking yourself, "If managers are responsible for the planning, organizing and staffing, directing, and controlling functions in an organization, what do supervisors do?" In that chapter, it was noted that there are many areas of overlap between the management and supervision functions in organizations, but that not all supervisors have requisite managerial authority. Most occupational therapists and some occupational therapy assistants supervise others relatively early in their careers (and without formal training) as they accept fieldwork students, collaborate with and supervise occupational therapy assistants, or utilize volunteers.

Management was previously defined as

The process of guiding an organization by planning for future work obligations, organizing employees into functional units, directing employees in the process of completing daily work tasks, and controlling work processes and systems to assure adequate quality of work output.

Supervision is that aspect of management that relates to directing employees in their daily work tasks and seeks to assure that their performance meets established standards and supports the goals and objectives of the organization. Therefore, supervision is defined as

The control and direction of the work of one or more employees in a manner that promotes improved performance and a higher quality outcome.

According to McNamara (2003), supervisors typically are responsible for the progress and productivity of those employees who directly report to them within an organization. Supervision often includes conducting basic management tasks (decision making, problem solving, planning, delegation, and meeting management), organizing teams, noticing the need for and designing new job roles in the group, training new employees, employee performance management (setting goals, observing and giving feedback, addressing performance issues, etc.), and ensuring conformance to personnel policies and other internal regulations. McNamara also included the tasks of hiring and firing employees. In order to maintain requisite managerial authority and to be fairly held ultimately responsible for the outcomes of work groups, you *must* have authority to hire and fire employees and have full direction over the employees for whose work outcomes you will be held responsible. However, it is typical in health care, school systems, and community settings for occupational therapists to be responsible for supervising others without being responsible for the full range of managerial functions.

The Roles and Functions of Supervisors

Although there are variations in the exact job responsibilities of supervisors from one setting to another, there are also typical functions that most supervisors serve. Salomon (1999), writing for the American Management Association, presented a list of the 10 most common duties of supervisors:

1. Determine priorities.
2. Schedule and distribute work.

3. Coordinate the efforts of others.
4. Observe and evaluate employees' performance.
5. Give accurate and honest performance-based feedback.
6. Coach and train employees.
7. Handle administrative duties and relevant paperwork.
8. Communicate clearly about policies, procedures, and processes.
9. Address problems and conflicts in a timely manner.
10. Look for ways to improve the way work gets done.

These duties can be grouped conceptually into three main supervisory functions: (1) management, (2) education, and (3) support (Nicklin, 1995). The management function of supervisors includes those duties related to monitoring and evaluating the work of others. The education function of supervisors includes those duties related to the development and evaluation of competencies of staff. The support function of supervisors includes duties related to professional development, including promotion of self-awareness and emotional growth.

Supervisors carry out managerial, educational, and support functions within an organizational environment (see Chapter 3), and their jobs and their level of influence on others are heavily influenced by structures within that environment. Two important supervisory concepts influenced by the internal structure of an organization that are important to understand when examining the role and influence of a supervisor are *span of control* and *power or authority*. These concepts will be discussed next.

Span of Control

One structural decision that must be made by management that has a direct impact on the day-to-day life of supervisors is determining the span of control for each supervisor. Span of control is defined as the number of immediate subordinates who report to any one supervisor. If a supervisor's span of control is too large, he or she may be ineffective because of the inability to adequately attend to the needs of individual employees and to monitor the quality of employees' work on a close enough basis.

However, if the span of control of a supervisor is too small, there may be unnecessary labor costs to the organization and time may be wasted as a result of unnecessary layering of the organization and duplication of tasks. Determining the most effective span of control relies on a number of factors related to the size, structure, and history of an organization. The most commonly identified factors influencing span of control are identified in Box 6–1.

Box 6–1: Factors Affecting Span of Control

- **Type of work:** Routine and repetitious work on the part of employees supports a larger span of control, whereas complex or unpredictable work tends to limit span of control.
- **Degree of training:** The presence of highly trained staff supports a larger span of control, whereas less trained staff tend to require more supervision and limit span of control.
- **Organizational stability:** Stable organizations with little change and staff turnover support a larger span of control, whereas constant change and high turnover tend to limit span of control.
- **Geographic location:** The location of staff to be supervised in one or in easily accessed locations supports a larger span of control, whereas supervising staff dispersed in various or hard-to-access locations limits span of control.
- **Flow of work:** Regular and even flow of work in a predictable manner supports a larger span of control, whereas work that flows unevenly or in an unpredictable manner may limit span of control.
- **Supervisor's qualifications:** The presence of more qualified and experienced supervisors supports a larger span of control, whereas less qualified or inexperienced supervisors limit span of control.

(continued)

Box 6–1: **Factors Affecting Span of Control** *(continued)*

- Availability of staff specialists: The availability of specialists to provide consultation in specific areas (e.g., someone who is a specialist in assistive technology) supports a larger span of control, whereas reliance on only formal supervisors limits span of control.
- Values system of organization: Organizations that most highly value minimizing salary expenses paid for supervision, very high productivity, and profit may support a larger span of control, whereas organizations that most highly value close supervision of new staff, fostering employee satisfaction, or staff retention may limit span of control.

Power and Formal Authority

Although different supervisors may use varied supervision styles, all supervisors rely on others to respond to requests or orders to do what they are asked or told to do. Supervisors rely on power or formal authority to achieve compliance by their subordinates with formal commands for action to achieve desired goals and outcomes. Scholars of organizational development and functioning frequently distinguish between the concepts of power (the ability to force compliance to one's wishes through coercion despite resistance) and formal authority (the right to issue orders or direct action by virtue of one's formal position). Formal authority has also been termed *legitimate power* (Liebler, Levine, & Rothman, 1992).

Although power is often associated with positions of authority, it must be recognized that power within organizations comes in many forms. For example, labor unions may hold great power to coerce management to act in ways against its wishes through threats of labor strikes. Even individual employees may hold power over managers or supervisors regardless of rank if they have a great deal of influence among other employees or have some characteristic that brings them power. A common example in occupational therapy may be the power

that a therapist with specialized skills, such as a Certified Hand Therapist, may hold when it is evident that it would be difficult to replace that employee if he or she were to leave the organization.

Formal authority typically is associated with specific positions or ranks within organizations. Liebler et al. (1992) identified several sources of formal authority studied by theorists in the fields of social psychology, management, and political science. These sources are (1) acceptance or consent to authority, (2) formal organizational patterns, (3) cultural expectations, (4) technical competence and expertise, and (5) characteristics of authority holders. The key concepts associated with each of these potential sources of authority are summarized in Table 6–1.

Whetten and Cameron (1998) named the power that is separate from the formal authority associated with an organizational position "personal power." Although a manager or supervisor uses position power to exert influence over those at lower levels in the organization, he or she typically has little or no formal authority to influence persons at higher levels of the organization. In order to influence one's supervisor or organizational leaders, one must rely upon personal power. As a result, anything that a manager or supervisor can do to increase his or her personal power will help in the important types of negotiations that they complete on behalf of their departments (e.g., negotiating yearly budgets or gaining resources to provide training for staff). Personal power may be enhanced through increasing one's knowledge or expertise, by improving one's personal attractiveness, and through demonstration of effort (Box 6–2).

Whetten and Cameron (1998) also provided five general suggested strategies for enhancing one's position power. It is easy to imagine that a cynical person might view these strategies as underhanded or, to use a common phrase, as "kissing up." This might be an accurate characterization for those who only occasionally utilize these strategies and demonstrate limited follow-through. However, those managers and supervisors who use these strategies consistently and with the sincere intent to combine personal success with a contribution to organizational success are likely to find themselves more valuable and central to an organization's functioning. The suggested strategies for increasing position power are outlined in Box 6–3.

Table 6-1	Key Concepts Related to Identified Sources of Formal Authority

Acceptance or Consent to Authority	• Authority involves acceptance of a superior's decision by a subordinate. • Subordinates often accept orders without conscious questioning. • Subordinates seek to act in a manner that is acceptable to the superior even when there has been no explicit order. • Subordinates are part of a psychological contract that includes acceptance of authority in return for appropriate rewards for compliance.
Formal Organizational Patterns	• The rights and duties of members of organizations are consistent with the rules accepted as rational in society in general. • Jurisdictions of authority are reasonably fixed. • Authority rests with a position independent of the individual who fills that position.
Cultural Expectations	• Individuals in a society are culturally induced to accept authority. • Acceptable use of authority is predefined by social structures such as laws or organizational policies. • Acceptance of authority is learned through normal socialization.
Technical Competence or Expertise	• Technical competence carries inherent limited authority to control specified activities. • Authority may vary and move from person to person and is influenced by the demands of the situation in addition to recognized positions.
Characteristics of Authority Holders	• Authority rests in individuals. • The talents and traits of an individual may become the source of authority. • Characteristics that influence authority may relate both to the individual and to the interaction between the individual and the position he or she holds within an organization.

Box 6-2: Strategies for Increasing Personal Power

• **Knowledge and information:** Gaining specialized training and education in areas of need to the organization that other managers do not possess can set you aside from your peers. Examples might be development of advanced expertise in continuous quality improvement, program evaluation, applications of information technology to management functions, or strategies for professional development.

• **Personal attractiveness:** Enhancing your "likeability" can be accomplished by working to portray a friendly and approachable style and by involving yourself in activities in the workplace that provide an opportunity for you to establish personal relationships with others, such as volunteering to help organize a company picnic or holiday event.

• **Demonstration of effort:** Sincere efforts and hard work can be demonstrated by volunteering for special assignments or task forces, meeting deadlines consistently, working extra hours, and contributing to group managerial discussions and events. Persons who are perceived as trying hard may also be perceived as knowledgeable and sought out for advice.

Box 6–3: **Five Strategies for Increasing Position Power**

1. Increase your centrality in the organization by looking for opportunities to include new functions central to the flow of work in your job. Volunteer for new responsibilities during times of staff change or layoffs.
2. Increase the personal discretion and flexibility of your position by replacing routine activities with involvement in new projects and the early stages of decision making.
3. Build difficult-to-evaluate tasks into your job by developing advanced expertise that will be of help to the organization but that most others do not have, so you become the "go to" person for high-profile functions.
4. Increase the visibility of your job performance by developing and nurturing relationships with organizational leadership. Volunteer to make presentations from task groups, offer suggestions and examples when a presenter asks a large group in which you are involved, or volunteer to become a trainer.
5. Increase the relevance of your job tasks to the organization by finding ways to provide services to other departments, becoming a trainer or mentor in organizational procedures, or volunteering to become an organizational representative to an external group.

Box 6–4: **Characteristics of Effective Supervisors**

- Solid foundation of technical knowledge
- Desire to achieve at high levels
- High expectations of achievement from others
- High level of self-confidence
- Ability to instill a sense of value in others
- Ability to communicate effectively

Becoming an Effective Supervisor

Supervisors can have dramatic influence on the quality of daily work life, job satisfaction, and retention of employees. Being effective as a supervisor goes beyond being respected, appreciated, or well liked by employees, however, because the supervisor has responsibilities to both employees and the organization. Although many large organizations provide ongoing training for supervisors and managers, smaller organizations may not have the resources to conduct training, and few occupational therapists receive formal training before becoming a fieldwork supervisor or beginning to supervise an occupational therapy assistant. So what does it mean to be *effective* as a supervisor, and how do you gain these skills? Commonly identified characteristics of effective supervisors are listed in Box 6–4.

One key to becoming an effective supervisor is to clearly understand what is expected of you. A good place to start is to review your job description with *your* supervisor. Before meeting with your supervisor, highlight the formal supervisory functions listed in your job description so that you and your supervisor can review them to be sure that performance expectations for these functions are clear and reasonable. In addition, try to identify any *unwritten* expectations of supervisors by observing others with the same or similar positions and discussing their responsibilities with them. Another helpful strategy is to consider the various *customers* that you serve. Chapter 11 provides an in-depth discussion of *continuous quality improvement*. The primary focus of a continuous quality improvement approach is improving customer satisfaction. All employees (and employee groups) have multiple customers within an organization. An internal customer is anyone who uses or relies on the work of another in order to do his or her job. For supervisors, two key customers are the subordinates who report to them and the supervisor to whom they report. Strategies for identifying the requirements of customers are covered in more depth in Chapter 11, but a simple strategy for the supervisor is to ask his or her subordinates and his or her boss "What is most important to you?" It might be assumed that the answers to this question would be easy to identify, but sometimes the most valued requirements of customers are not among the formal duties listed in job descriptions.

Another key strategy to becoming an effective supervisor is conducting a self-assessment. Self-assessment is a reflective process of identifying the demands and responsibilities of your position and the needs of your customers and objectively comparing them to your ability to satisfy them through your skills and personal characteristics. Self-assessments can be completed in a number of ways. It is recommended that all practitioners, whether clinicians, educators, researchers, or managers, have a professional development plan that is updated on a regular basis.

The first step in developing such a plan is self-assessment. Formal assessment methods such as the Professional Development Tool, available from the American Occupational Therapy Association (AOTA) to its members, provide a structured approach to self-assessment, including the use of peer reviews, assessment of customer satisfaction, and the development of written learning objectives to guide professional growth (Case-Smith, 2003). Maintaining membership in the AOTA and your state occupational therapy association is one of the best strategies for finding resources to become a more effective occupational therapy supervisor.

Another method of self-assessment is completing a self-assessment matrix. Matrices such as the one for Carlota from our introductory case scenario (Table 6–2) are a simple way of planning for any aspect of professional growth. The horizontal axis includes the three commonly identified domains of learning, which are *knowledge*, *skills*, and *attitudes*. The vertical axis includes supervisory duties related to the management, education, and support functions of the supervisor found in your job description. Each cell of the matrix includes a goal, professional activity, or area of growth for the coming year. Completing a self-assessment matrix can be part of the process of planning for participation in your annual performance appraisal. The matrix can be shared with your supervisor so that he or she will be aware of your goals and be able to help you achieve them.

Another approach to self-assessment is to apply an adapted strategic planning process to planning for your professional growth. Such an adaptation is suggested by Harvey and Struzziero (2000). The steps involved in this approach (Figure 6–1) include

Table 6-2	Carlota's Sample Supervisory Self-Assessment Matrix		
	Knowledge	Skills	Attitude
Management	I need to know more about how formal job descriptions are used in the process of giving feedback to those I supervise, so I will attend a workshop on writing job descriptions at the AOTA conference.	I am familiar with the rules for providing effective feedback, but I need to practice giving feedback and maintaining body language and facial expressions that communicate confidence and don't contradict what I am saying verbally. I plan to ask other supervisors to observe me over the coming 2 months and give me feedback on my presentation.	I need to become more comfortable with the concept that giving feedback to staff members as a supervisor is a positive activity that contributes to their growth and to improved quality of service to our clients. By becoming more involved in the planning of the overall staff development program, I may become more comfortable with my role in providing feedback as a supervisor.

(continued)

Table 6-2	Carlota's Sample Supervisory Self-Assessment Matrix *(continued)*		
	Knowledge	**Skills**	**Attitude**
Education	I need increased familiarity with the competencies for the occupational therapy assistant to identify appropriate tasks and activities for delegation in the school system setting. I also require additional information on the various ways to assess competencies. The AOTA has a number of resources on assessment of competencies.	I am interested in improving my presentation skills so that I am more comfortable providing in-service education to staff. I will investigate presenting or co-presenting at our state occupational therapy association conference as an opportunity to plan and deliver an educational presentation.	I need to value more the influence that supervisors can have on the professional development and competency of staff given the shrinking resources in most school systems to support outside continuing education. By developing enhanced skills, I hope to feel more satisfied with my role in competency assessment and skill development of staff.
Support	I am going to complete an evidence-based review on theories of employee motivation in order to increase my understanding of factors that contribute to employee satisfaction and dissatisfaction.	I plan to attend a course offered by the human resources department on conflict resolution to increase my mediation skills so that I can be more effective and perceived as more supportive in helping staff resolve conflicts with other staff, parents, and teachers.	I tend to want to solve problems for employees immediately, when sometimes they just want someone to empathize with them. I need to put more value on taking time to listen to employees and help them solve their own problems so that they feel more emotionally supported.

1. Developing a vision for your personal growth
2. Conducting an internal assessment of strengths and weaknesses and an external assessment of opportunities and threats (e.g., SWOT analysis)
3. Defining a personal mission and establish goals for growth to enable you to achieve your mission
4. Developing a strategic plan, including measurable goals and objectives
5. Developing an action plan, including specific actions you will take and target dates for completing these actions related to each objective
6. Implementing your personal strategic plan
7. Conducting a formative evaluation (Was the plan implemented as intended?) and a summative evaluation (Were results what you expected?)
8. Feeding the evaluation results back into your personal strategic plan to begin the process again and to plan for additional growth

Certainly a large part of becoming an effective supervisor is coming to understand the needs of those you supervise and learning strategies to promote their growth, performance, and motivation. Throughout this book, you are encouraged to recognize the wide range of related knowledge (i.e., knowledge developed by other fields or disciplines not included in the occupational therapy paradigm) that can be used by the occupational therapy manager or supervisor to guide his or her daily work. In the following sections of this chapter, knowledge and evidence related to models of su-

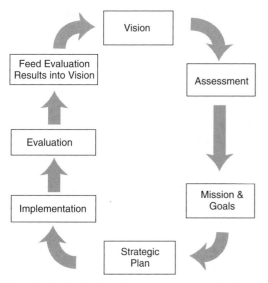

Figure 6–1 Application of strategic planning to development as a supervisor. (Adapted from Harvey, V. S. & Struzziero, J. [2000]. *Effective supervision in school psychology*. Bethesda, MD: National Association of School Psychologists.)

pervising others and to theories of motivating others will be summarized.

Models of Supervision

Much of the supervision provided by occupational therapy supervisors is intended to guide occupational therapists and occupational therapy assistants in intervening with patients and clients. The fields of psychology, education, and social work have produced much of the work that has been completed on developing models of supervision specifically related to the supervision of therapists. The models that have been developed in supervision theory are generally split into four categories: (1) psychotherapy-based models, (2) developmental models, (3) social role models, and (4) eclectic/integrationist models. Each of these models will be briefly reviewed.

Models of Therapist Supervision

Psychotherapy-Based Models

Therapists of any discipline work from an implicit theory of human nature that reflects how the ther-

apist views reality. Psychotherapy-based models of supervision tend to make the same assumptions about the nature of what constitutes an effective supervisor-trainee relationship as they do about what constitutes an effective therapist-client relationship.

The *person-centered supervision model* is based on the client-centered psychotherapy approach of Carl Rogers and tends to transfer client-therapist theory to the supervisee-supervisor relationship. Therefore, the emphasis is on the relationship between the supervisor and supervisee rather than the process of supervision. The most important aspects of supervision are the modeling of the necessary and sufficient conditions of empathy, genuineness, and unconditional positive regard (Kadushin, 1992).

The *cognitive-behavioral model* of supervision applies learning theory to supervision and generally comprises the following five elements: (1) establishing a trusting relationship, (2) skill analysis and assessment, (3) setting goals, (4) construction and implementation of strategies to accomplish goals, and (5) follow-up evaluation. This model of supervision assumes that being an effective therapist is primarily a function of skills, with the purpose of supervision being to teach appropriate therapist behaviors. A professional role is thought to consist of identifiable tasks requiring specific skills, and the supervisor assists the professional in developing skills that can be applied and refined (Patterson, 1986).

Developmental Models

Developmental approaches to supervision became popular in the 1990s. A main concept underlying developmental models of supervision is the notion that we each are continually growing, in fits and starts, in growth spurts and patterns. The object is to maximize and identify growth needed for the future at any given time (Leddick, 2004). Under a developmental model, it is assumed that close supervision is needed for a new therapist but, as the therapist gains experience, his or her need for supervision is lessened and the relationship with the supervisor changes also.

Stoltenberg and Delworth (1987) described a developmental model with three levels of supervisees: beginning, intermediate, and advanced. Within each level, the authors noted a trend to begin in a rigid, shallow, imitative way and move toward more competence, self-assurance, and self-reliance at each level. Particular attention is paid to (1) self- and other awareness, (2) motivation, and (3) autonomy. For example, typical development in beginning supervisees would find them relatively dependent on the supervisor to diagnose clients and establish plans for therapy. Intermediate supervisees would depend on supervisors for an understanding of difficult clients, but would resent suggestions about the types of clients they have treated before. Resistance, avoidance, or conflict is typical of this stage, because supervisee self-concept is easily threatened. Advanced supervisees function independently, seek consultation when appropriate, and feel responsible for their correct and incorrect decisions.

SOCIAL ROLE MODELS

The basic tenets of the social role models are that, as the needs of the supervisee change, the role of the supervisor should change to better meet those needs. For example, at times the supervisor may need to assume more of a role as a teacher and at other times may need to assume the role of counselor or consultant. Under this model, the style of the supervisor is determined by his or her theoretical orientation and the focus of supervision is determined according to the role the supervisor is assuming at any given time (Patterson, 1986).

ECLECTIC/INTEGRATIONIST MODELS

Eclectic or integrationist models blend a number of different supervision theories (i.e., a social role model as well as a developmental approach). The main components of these models include a customized approach, needs assessment, and consideration of the supervisee's developmental level and cognitive style, as well as an assessment and evaluation of the supervisee's skills.

The *discrimination model* combines an attention to three supervisory roles with three areas of focus. Supervisors might take on a role of teacher when they directly lecture, instruct, and inform the supervisee. Supervisors may act as counselors when they assist supervisees in noticing their own "blind spots" or the manner in which they are uncon-

sciously "hooked" by a client's issue. When supervisors relate as colleagues when discussing specific therapeutic cases, they might act in a consultant role. Each of the three roles is task-specific for the purpose of identifying issues in supervision (Bernard & Goodyear, 1992). The discrimination model also highlights three areas of focus for skill building: process, conceptualization, and personalization. Process issues examine how communication is conveyed. For example, is the supervisee reflecting the client's emotions and concerns in how he or she responds, or did the supervisee reframe the situation for the client? Conceptualization issues include how well supervisees can explain their application of a specific theory to a particular case—how well they see the big picture—as well as what reasons supervisees may have for what to do next. Personalization issues pertain to issues related to therapeutic use of the self in therapy to establish an effective interpersonal relationship (Leddick, 2004).

Management Approaches to Supervision

In addition to the models of supervision just described, there are four management approaches supervisors can take to handle operational situations that are commonly identified in the management literature. These approaches are (1) the systematic management approach, (2) the human relations approach, (3) the quantitative approach, and (4) the contingency (or situational) approach. The systematic management approach (also known as the traditional, classic, or scientific approach) relies on measurement and analysis of various tasks and activities that take place in the work environment. This approach to supervision has a greater reliance on established organizational policies and procedures and on prescribed relationships in formal work groups. In the human relations approach, it is assumed that a manager or supervisor who understands people's behaviors will be able to get his or her employees to cooperate and accomplish an organization's goals. This approach to supervision has a greater reliance on participatory techniques and upon individuals and groups to solve operational problems. The next type of approach is the quantitative approach, or systems theory of management, which relies on the use of numbers and statistics, as well as the sciences. This approach to supervision

Box 6–5: **Four Commonly Identified Management Approaches to Supervision**			
SYSTEMATIC	HUMAN RELATIONS	QUANTITATIVE	CONTINGENCY
• Relies on measurement and analysis of tasks	• Relies on participatory techniques	• Relies on numbers, statistics and the scientific approach	• Relies on the manager's judgment to choose the right approach for the situation
• Uses policies, procedures, and formal relationships in work groups	• Uses informal group relations to solve problems	• Uses self-directed and automated programs such as statistical analysis software	• Uses any of the strategies from any approach

has a greater reliance on staff-directed or automatic programs to prescribe operating procedures. The fourth and last approach is the contingency (or situational) approach, which is where a manager's decision and action depend on the particular situation at hand. This approach requires a greater need for sensitivity to deal with different situations, as well as skills and flexibility to apply all the different management approaches. These four approaches are summarized in Box 6–5.

Occupational Therapy Perspectives on Supervision

The supervision models presented in the previous section of the chapter were developed by disciplines other than occupational therapy. Limited theoretical work has been completed specifically related to the supervision of occupational therapy personnel. However, discipline-specific information and resources are available to the occupational therapy supervisor. The focus of these resources tends to be more on the supervisory relationships, responsibilities, and recommended levels of supervision for various categories of occupational therapy personnel (e.g., occupational therapists, occupational therapy assistants, and occupational therapy aides).

For example, the AOTA provides its members with a document entitled "Guidelines for Supervision, Roles, and Responsibilities During the Delivery of Occupational Therapy Services" (AOTA, 2004). This document suggests that the amount of supervision required by an occupational therapy practitioner depends upon a "mutual understanding between the supervisor and supervisee about each other's competence, experience, education, and credentials." The frequency and method of supervision may vary according to the complexity of the clinical situation, the type of practice setting, regulatory requirements, and the number and diversity of clients. These supervision guidelines follow a developmental approach to supervision as was described earlier in this chapter.

The American Physical Therapy Association (2004) provides similar definitions of supervision to guide the level of supervision of physical therapy personnel. It must be noted that the requirements stated in a state licensure law for supervision always supersede any recommendations for supervision made by a professional association. Such licensure laws may change over time, and it is the responsibility of the occupational therapy manager or supervisor to remain aware of requirements for supervision, especially when they may have an impact on staffing or productivity expectations, because it is unlikely that higher level non–occupational therapy managers will be familiar with the licensure laws for individual disciplines.

In addition to the amount of supervision required, a distinction is often made in the *type* of activity to be supervised. One common strategy is to distinguish between supervision of *client-related* and *non–client-related tasks*. This distinction is especially important in regard to the supervision of occupational therapy aides. Client-related tasks include all elements of intervention when the patient or client is present and there is contact between the occupational therapy personnel and the client.

Non–client-related tasks include clerical tasks and preparation of the environment or work area when there is no direct contact with the patient or client. The following conditions should be present when a client-related task is assigned to an occupational therapy aide (AOTA, 1997):

- The anticipated outcome of the intervention is predictable.
- The situation will not require judgment or adaptation by the aide.
- The client has demonstrated some ability to complete the task before and the task process is routine.

A final helpful concept found specifically in the occupational therapy literature related to supervision is that of *service competency*. Service competency is defined as "[t]he process of teaching, training and evaluating through which the occupational therapist determines that the occupational therapy assistant performs tasks in the same way that the occupational therapist would and achieves the same outcomes" (AOTA, 1997). Although the AOTA defines service competency in regard to the supervision of an occupational therapy assistant by an occupational therapist, it is a useful concept in the supervision of occupational therapists and occupational therapy fieldwork students as well. Establishing service competency between two practitioners simply means that, if both persons perform a particular task, they will achieve the same outcome. The process of completing competency checks on a new employee is essentially the process of establishing service competency. Service competency may be established or verified in a number of ways, including

- Observation of a supervisee by a supervisor, comparing performance against a predetermined checklist
- Having two practitioners complete a task independently (i.e., take range of motion measurements) and comparing results
- Use of videotapes or "master cases" in which both practitioners review the tape or case and compare their analyses of problems, goals, or results
- Use of written tests or checklists of performance

In addition to models of supervision, there are a number of theories that seek to explain the levels of motivation and satisfaction of employees and the impact that these have on employee retention. These theories will be reviewed in the next section of this chapter.

Theories of Motivation, Employee Satisfaction, and Retention of Employees

Organizations invest huge sums of money and time in orienting, training, and developing the skills of personnel. Losing a well-trained and productive employee can have numerous negative consequences for an organization, including

- Increased workload and dissatisfaction among the employees who remain
- Lost revenue as a result of lowered production and billing
- Customer dissatisfaction resulting from difficulties meeting customer expectations because of short staffing
- Lost business and referrals resulting from lowered customer satisfaction

Loss of an employee, or employee "turnover," is not uncommon in the health care industry or in community-based organizations. Estimates of the cost of replacing an employee have ranged from 25% to 150% of the employee's annual salary, including hiring and recruiting costs, training costs, lost productivity during the first 6 months of employment, and use of temporary employees during transitions (Bliss, 2001; Keller, 2000). Particularly in the fields of occupational therapy, physical therapy, and nursing, where jobs are often plentiful, changing jobs several times in the first decade of practice is not uncommon. However, although supervisors and managers can do little to lessen turnover driven by personal factors such as the desire to move geographically or enter a new area of practice, you can influence an employee's decision to stay with your organization by understanding theories related to employee motivation and satisfaction.

Motivation

Motivation can be thought of as the level of arousal, direction, and persistence of behavior related to a goal. The simple idea that people have needs continues to be the best explanation for what activates behavior. Satisfaction can be thought of as a consequence of performance in the workplace that is influenced by the types of rewards that individuals receive (both intrinsic and extrinsic rewards) and their connection to performance (Lawler, 1994).

Edward E. Lawler III, Professor of Management and Organization and founding director of the Center for Effective Organizations at the University of Southern California, stated that any theory of motivation must answer three questions:

1. What activates behavior?
2. What directs behavior?
3. What reactions do individuals have to the outcomes that result from their behavior?

Theories of motivation in the workplace can be organized into two basic types: (1) content theories, which stress the analysis of human needs, and (2) process theories, which focus on the thought processes of employees that influence behavior. Not all theories that have been utilized to explain employee motivation and satisfaction address all three of Lawler's questions. The most contemporary of each of these types of theories and the evidence related to their application to the workplace will be briefly reviewed next.

CONTENT THEORIES

Content theories describe the needs, motives, and goals of people, and these theories help us to understand how objects or outcomes become goals for people. Such theories specify why people value some outcomes and the factors that influence the values that people assign to their goals. Content theories are useful for managers because they help them understand what people will and will not value as work rewards or as need satisfiers. Essentially, content theories suggest that managers must

- Understand that different employees have different needs in terms of what they need and desire from work
- Identify how an organization can meet the varying needs of employees
- Create ways that different employees can meet individual needs and simultaneously contribute to the organization

Maslow's Hierarchy of Needs. One content theory with which you are most likely familiar is Abraham Maslow's theory of human motivation (Maslow, 1970). Maslow's hierarchy has been utilized as a framework for considering how factors in the work environment might influence the motivation and satisfaction of employees, and hence the likelihood that they will stay with their employer. Applications of Maslow's theory to work settings emphasize the meaning and significance of human work and focus on the fact that humans are motivated to obtain both intrinsic and extrinsic outcomes. As such, this theory addresses the second two of Lawler's questions (What directs behavior, and what reactions do individuals have to the outcomes that result from their behavior?) but does not provide a clear answer to the question as to why needs originate.

According to Maslow, the behavior of an individual related to meeting basic needs or satisfying primary drives decreases as these needs are satisfied. Basic needs and drives may be viewed as a hierarchy in which higher order needs cannot be pursued unless lower order or more basic needs are already satisfied. The categories of needs in the hierarchy are not completely exclusive, however. In other words, one category of needs does not need to be fully met before an individual may turn his or her attention to other needs higher in the hierarchy. Rather, as one level of need becomes gratified, another begins to emerge.

In regard to motivation, Maslow argued that, unlike motivation based on primary drives, motivation based on growth needs does not decrease as the needs become satisfied. To the contrary, Maslow stated that, as people experience growth and self-actualization, they simply want more. Obtaining growth creates a desire for more growth, whereas obtaining food decreases one's desire for food (Lawler, 1994). Still, the stages may be used as a general framework through which to view the progression of needs. Maslow identified five categories of needs that, in order from lowest to highest, are (1) *physiologic* needs, (2) *safety* needs, (3) social or *affiliation* needs, (4) *esteem* needs, and (5) *self-actualization* needs. These categories of needs are explained further in Box 6–6.

Most persons in Western society are able to meet their most basic needs. Granted, we are all familiar with the plight of the homeless or those who must

---

Box 6–6: Maslow's Hierarchy of Needs

- **Physiologic Needs:** Basic human needs to sustain life itself, such as food, clothing, and shelter, that must be satisfied before a person can focus on other needs or before the pursuit of other needs provides a source of motivation for action
- **Safety Needs:** The need to be free from danger and to seek self-preservation for today and the future
- **Social or Affiliation Needs:** The need to belong and to be accepted by social groups and person of importance to the individual
- **Esteem Needs:** The need to develop positive self-esteem and to gain recognition and acceptance from others
- **Self-Actualization Needs:** The need to maximize one's potential, whatever that might be

---

live in extreme poverty; however, most of those with whom we will interact in the workplace as employees will have found a way to meet these most basic needs. For those individuals, other needs become more central; however, we must understand that, in a turbulent economy, all workers may feel threatened even at the most basic levels when workplaces experience layoffs or downsizing.

When a worker feels that his or her job is safe and that he or she will be able to maintain food and shelter not only for today but also in the future, affiliation needs will begin to surface. Employees will seek mechanisms by which they feel they are accepted as a member of the work group and gain a sense of belonging and will strive to develop meaningful relationships with their peers. Once affiliation needs are met, employees will seek more than just being a member of a group and will hope to gain a sense of satisfaction that is based in self-confidence and the recognition and respect that is gained from others in the workplace. Most employees seek opportunities that provide them with mechanisms to feel useful and competent in their work. In addition, most workers seek opportunities

to gain recognition from their supervisors and peers as well as to be rewarded for their efforts. All of these opportunities help to meet the esteem needs of workers. Finally, once esteem needs begin to be satisfied, employees may seek to become the best at what they do within their work life, or to seek self-actualization. This can mean different things for different workers. For some, it may mean taking on a leadership role within the organization or developing advanced or specialized skills. For others, it may mean becoming involved in other venues within the work environment, such as task forces or committees, through extra volunteer efforts. The employee who is ready for self-actualization is likely to be the employee who stands out in terms of performance and extra effort.

Early research provided strong evidence related to Maslow's hierarchy to establish that, unless existence needs are satisfied, none of the higher order needs will come into play. There is also evidence that, unless security needs are satisfied, people will not be concerned with higher order needs. There is little evidence to support the view that a hierarchy exists above the security level. Thus, functionally using a hierarchy that attempts to do anything beyond grouping the most basic needs together (e.g., existence and security) and grouping all higher order needs together cannot be supported by evidence (Lawler, 1994). Although management would benefit from addressing both security and higher order needs, different employees may experience different higher order needs, with one focusing on autonomy and another focusing more on esteem.

Herzberg's Hygiene/Motivation Theory. Frederick Herzberg's hygiene/motivation theory, developed out of work originally conducted with 200 Pittsburgh engineers and accountants, has become one of the most replicated studies in the field of workplace psychology. According to this theory, employee satisfaction and dissatisfaction at work nearly always arise from different factors, and are not simply opposing reactions to the same factors. Satisfaction and dissatisfaction are not opposite ends of a single continuum, but instead are two separate constructs. An important implication of this theory is that employees can be both very satisfied and very dissatisfied at the same time. If this is true, managers and supervisors must recognize that different factors contribute to employee satisfaction than to dissatisfaction. In other words, employees will not automatically be satisfied if there is an absence of dissatisfiers, nor will employees be automatically satisfied with the presence of satisfiers.

The hygiene/motivation theory states that the primary drive for persons to work is for their own self-satisfaction and contentment, because work or the engagement in healthy occupations contributes to individuals' happiness and satisfaction. Applied to the workplace, this theory identifies two sets of factors related to human needs: *hygiene factors* and *motivation factors*. Examples from these two sets of factors are listed in Box 6–7.

Because hygiene factors and motivation factors are separate constructs, managers and supervisors need to attend to both types of factors to maximize employees' satisfaction with the workplace and to minimize dissatisfaction. It is also important to recognize that the strength of factors may vary and that employees may value different factors to different extents. For example, whereas one employee may place primary importance on salary and be willing to accept the presence of some dissatisfiers if his or her salary is sufficiently high, another employee might highly value recognition from superiors and work that is interesting and satisfying and be willing to accept a lower salary. Hygiene factors and motivating factors cannot be used in an exact formula to assure employee satisfaction, but can be used as a guide to examine the status of the work-

place and to guide managers and supervisors to assess the workplace and make changes that are likely to appeal to a range of employees' values and needs.

Evidence related to this "two-factor" theory is mixed, with some evidence showing support and some providing reasons to question the theory, but neither body of evidence is sufficiently strong to validate or completely reject the theory. Lawler (1994) noted that even proponents of the theory have accepted that some factors may cause both satisfaction and dissatisfaction, and the thought that satisfaction and dissatisfaction are indeed separate constructs has been questioned. He pointed out, however, that simply because some factors can influence both satisfaction and dissatisfaction, this does not mean that they are not on separate continua. Rather, the fact that a single factor may influence both may simply highlight the importance of that factor in a given environment.

McClelland's Acquired Needs Theory. According to the acquired needs theory, three types of human needs are acquired over time as a result of life experiences. These needs result in motivation that is driven by how needs are associated with individual work preferences. The three types of needs are

1. Need for *achievement,* or the desire to do something better or more efficiently and to master more and more complex tasks
2. Need for *affiliation,* or the desire to establish and maintain friendly and warm relations with others in the environment

---

Box 6–7: Hygiene and Motivation Factors

HYGIENE FACTORS	MOTIVATION FACTORS
• Rewards (financial) that are perceived to correlate with performance and the current marketplace • Safe, pleasant, and comfortable working environments • Pleasant and supportive interpersonal relationships with peers and supervisors • Competent and supportive supervision and management • Job security	• Recognition from peers and supervisors for positive contributions to the workplace • Opportunities for promotion and advancement within a career track • Levels of authority, decision making, and responsibility that match one's responsibilities • Work that is satisfactory and matches the psychological contract entered into with the employer • Personal growth and development

3. Need for *power*, or the desire to control others, to influence their behavior, or to be responsible for others

Table 6–3 relates each of these needs to individual work preferences and provides examples of each.

The acquired needs theory is most useful when each need is matched with a set of work preferences specific to a work environment, because the preferences may look very different in various settings, such as a school system, a medical-model setting or hospital, a private business, or a community-based organization. Creating an explicit process of examining the various needs of employees within a setting and including employees in generating statements of work preferences and examples of work forms that meet their needs is a concrete way that this theory can be applied.

There is limited evidence to date to support this theory, but some research has generated interesting questions about the role of culture in influencing the balance of needs in terms of achievement, affiliation, and power. As might be expected, the need for achievement has been shown to be higher in the United States than in some other countries (Miller & Kilpatrick, 1987).

PROCESS THEORIES

Although content theories emphasize what employees need in regard to motivation, they do not address how employees become motivated or why they choose one action over another in the workplace. Process theories place higher emphasis than content theories on "how" to motivate employees.

Vroom's Expectancy Theory. Victor Vroom developed the expectancy theory of motivation that postulates that motivation depends on individuals' expectations about their ability to perform assigned work tasks and receive desired rewards. In simple terms, outcomes have value if they lead to other valued outcomes (Vroom, 1964). The theory does not address the question of what causes people to value particular outcomes nor that about what other outcomes are likely to be valued.

The three main constructs of this theory are *valence*, *expectancy*, and *instrumentality*. Valence is the importance placed upon a specific reward by an employee, recognizing that not all employees equally value the same rewards and experiences. Expectancy is the belief by an employee that his or her efforts are linked to performance or that, if he or she develops increased skills or makes extra

Table 6-3	Work Preferences of Persons High in Need for Achievement, Affiliation, or Power	
Individual Needs	Work Preferences	Example
High need for achievement	Prefers to work alone and accept responsibility, desires challenging targets and goals, and desires specific feedback on performance	Private practitioner who opens her own business providing work injury prevention services with the opportunity to earn based on how successfully she sells her products
High need for affiliation	Prefers to work with others, values team activities and opportunities to communicate and collaborate with others	Senior therapist in a rehabilitation hospital who accepts a role as coordinator of continuing education and collaborates with team supervisors to plan for the professional development of staff
High need for power	Prefers to take charge of work tasks and influence others, seeks attention and recognition for playing a central role	A department director who assumes responsibility for supervision of therapists and volunteers for high-profile task groups within the organization

efforts, this will result in improved performance. Instrumentality is the belief that the quality of performance within a workplace is related to the rewards that are given in return. For example, consider an occupational therapist working as a salesperson for a company that sells assistive and adaptive equipment. The therapist's expectancy is the belief that more sales calls will result in higher sales (performance). The therapist's instrumentality is that higher sales (performance) will result in higher commissions (rewards). Finally, the therapist's valence is the importance attached to the commissions (rewards). These three factors result in motivation. If any one of these factors doesn't exist, then motivation vanishes. If the salesperson does not believe greater effort leads to peformance, then there is no motivation. Similarly, if commissions don't increase with sales, then instrumentality disappears. If commissions are not important to the salesperson, he or she will likely not extend effort even if he or she has high expectancy and instrumentality.

Vroom's motivation theory is often illustrated by the following equation:

$$\text{Motivation} = \text{Expectancy} \times \text{Instrumentality} \times \text{Valence}$$

This equation indicates that motivation is determined in a relationship that is multiplicative, so expected levels of motivation should be very low if any one of these variables is very low; conversely, to expect that motivation will be very high, one must expect that all three variables are very high. For example, if a manager wonders whether a cash bonus program would have any effect on productivity levels, he or she might anticipate that, if an employee feels that if any of the following conditions exist, there is low likelihood that motivation will be positively affected:

- The employee feels he or she cannot meet the performance targets to qualify.
- The person is not confident that a high productivity level will truly be recognized and result in bonuses being distributed.
- The person does not value the reward of a cash bonus.

The implication of this theory for managers and supervisors is that they must focus on increasing all three variables as they relate to employees by fostering employees' sense of competency, drawing concrete relationships between desired work behaviors and the outcomes of those behaviors, and customizing rewards to match individual employee desires to the extent possible.

The evidence relating to expectancy theory has been generally supportive, although research to more specifically articulate aspects of the theory, such as the suggested multiplicative effect, has not been presented (Salancik & Pfeffer, 2003). An aspect of the theory that has been generally supported that is of particular interest to managers and supervisors is that the rewards that are linked to improving performance can vary from employee to employee and from culture to culture. As a result, managers must consider how they may vary rewards for the performance of employees within organizational structures that sometimes prescribe how rewards are provided in very structured manners.

Employee Retention

Retaining valuable employees is of critical importance to organizations, and the impact of rewards and recognition on employee retention is well documented in the literature. Determining monetary rewards in the form of salary increases may be reserved as a function of the manager, but both managers and supervisors can provide praise and recognition to employees in various forms.

REWARDS AND RECOGNITION

Many managers and supervisors pay insufficient attention to providing their subordinates with rewards and recognition outside of the formal performance appraisal meeting that typically occurs once a year. This is unfortunate because, as noted by Liebler et al. (1992), "Calling attention to correct behavior is more effective in promoting self-discipline, cooperation, and improved performance than calling attention to incorrect behavior." Incorporating the provision of genuine praise for a job well done into your daily work can contribute to improving staff morale.

There have been a number of theories related to motivation and retention of employees in organizations. Most theories address two types of rewards that are thought to influence the motivation of employees: (1) *intrinsic rewards*, which are rewards received as a direct consequence of a person's actions, and (2) *extrinsic rewards*, which are rewards given by another person, often a manager or supervisor. Typical examples of each of these types of rewards are presented in Box 6–8.

Assuring that intrinsic rewards become available to employees can be particularly challenging for the manager or supervisor. To facilitate adequate intrinsic rewards, you must balance the needs of the organization and assure that work is completed in an effective and efficient manner while designing work processes and environments with the flexibility to provide for the individual needs and desires of different employees. Planning and specifying job tasks and work settings in which they are accomplished in a way that is motivational for employees is referred to as *job design*. Job design includes four strategies that can be used by managers who seek to provide adequate intrinsic rewards for employees while also facilitating employee satisfaction and organizational productivity. These four strategies are

1. Job *simplification*, or standardization of work procedures and using employees in clearly defined and specialized tasks
2. Job *enlargement*, which includes strategies to increase the breadth of a job by adding to the variety of tasks performed by a worker
3. Job *rotation*, or increasing the variety of tasks completed by periodically shifting workers between jobs and different tasks

4. Job *enrichment*, which is the practice of building motivating factors into job content by expanding job content and adding work functions typically performed by higher level employees, such as planning or supervision functions

When providing extrinsic rewards, careful consideration of the impact that a particular reward may have is warranted. You must also consider if the reward may have consequences that are not anticipated. Unfortunately, managers and supervisors may sometimes assume that employees would appreciate and enjoy the same types of rewards and recognitions that they might, and inadvertently provide a reward that is in fact experienced as punishing or unpleasant. For example, although you might assume that any employee would appreciate being taken out to lunch or dinner, having to stay late in the evening in order to free up the time during the day to attend a lunch or spending hours outside of work with the boss on a usually free evening might *not* be perceived as a reward. Providing an employee with a gift certificate so that he or she might enjoy a meal with a family member or friend might be more rewarding. Similarly, you might assume that recognizing an employee in a public manner, such as presenting him or her with a certificate or plaque as a "thank-you" in front of a large gathering of his or her peers, would be a welcome event. However, for the employee who is fearful of appearing in front of large groups of people, this "reward" might be experienced as punishing or embarrassing. Another unexpected negative impact of providing rewards and recognitions is

---

Box 6–8: Examples of Intrinsic and Extrinsic Rewards

INTRINSIC REWARDS	EXTRINSIC REWARDS
• Gratification for making a contribution to the public good • Positive self-regard that comes with developing new skills • Enjoyment when spending time in pursuits of interest • Feelings of achievement when successfully completing assigned work and overcoming obstacles	• Increased salary and merit raises tied to performance • Public recognition, such as words of praise and thanks • Promotions and increased power and authority • Safety and security that comes with other benefits, such as health and retirement benefits

that often success is a team effort, and providing a reward or recognition to an individual may unintentionally send a message to other employees that their efforts are not appreciated. An employee who volunteers to take on a special project or join a task group such as a continuous quality improvement team may only be able to do so because the employee's peers cover part of his or her workload. Careful consideration of when to reward or recognize an individual and when to reward an entire department or team for achievements will help to avoid sending unwanted messages. Factors to consider in regard to rewards and recognitions are included in Box 6–9.

Providing rewards and recognition to employees does not have to be expensive or difficult. One of the most effective strategies that I have used to recognize employees was to write each employee a personalized thank-you note and attach it to a small bag of homemade cookies during Occupational

Therapy Month. In the note, I thanked the employee for the special contribution that he or she made to the department, such as always being the first person to volunteer when extra work needed to be done or doing a wonderful job as a clinical fieldwork educator. I received feedback from a number of employees indicating that this was the best form of thanks they had ever received, and they especially appreciated that I recognized their individual efforts.

RETENTION OF EMPLOYEES

Retention of valued employees is a major concern for occupational therapy managers and supervisors. As noted earlier, there can be tremendous costs associated with employee turnover, including recruitment expenses, lost revenue, and the need to train a new employee. Traditionally, retention of employees was primarily a human resources function, but responsibility for staff recruitment and retention has shifted over the last few decades to be a responsibility of line managers as organizations have trimmed staff functions such as their human resources departments to save costs. In addition, the knowledge of the disciplinary manager and supervisor about what contributes to satisfaction and dissatisfaction for employees has become highly valued. Although studies on employee retention from various disciplines (e.g., occupational therapy, physical therapy, nursing) reveal that similar factors influence retention regardless of discipline, designing effective strategies to improve retention is easier with discipline-specific input. The most effective way to address recruitment and retention concerns is for the occupational therapy manager to develop a collaborative working relationship with the organization's human resources professionals.

Although it is common for new practitioners to stay in their first jobs for a relatively short time (1 to 3 years) and for some employee turnover to be related to uncontrollable factors such as moving due to a spouse's relocation or choosing to be a stay-at-home parent, there are some factors that contribute to turnover that can be influenced. Nosse, Friberg, and Kovacek (1999) identified factors related to employee turnover and actions that could be taken by managers to limit the impact of

---

Box 6–9: Factors to Consider in Selecting Rewards and Recognitions

- Investigate and consider whether to reward or recognize an individual or a team or department.
- Don't assume that all persons equally value the same types of rewards and recognition.
- Associate the reward or recognition with specific accomplishments rather than general performance.
- Individualize rewards and recognition whenever possible, such as writing individual thank-you notes or choosing rewards related to an employee's personal interests.
- Consider recognition that demonstrates your personal awareness of the employee's contribution to the organization.
- Provide reward and recognition in a timely manner close to the time of achievement.

Table 6-4	Turnover Factors and Management Actions Encouraging Employee Retention
Turnover Factors	**Management Actions Encouraging Retention**
Poorly defined position responsibilities	Clearly define performance expectations.
High-stress position	Remove obstacles that interfere with job performance and provide needed resources.
Work that does not utilize employee skills	• Define job prior to employment. • Match employee skills with job.
Unreasonable performance expectations	Involve employees in the process of setting performance expectations.
Limited growth opportunities	• Create opportunities for growth and development. • Involve employees in the work design process.
Lack of recognition for accomplishments	• Recognize good performance. • Provide opportunity for peer recognition.
Lack of opportunity to express concerns and dissatisfaction	Provide formal mechanisms and encourage employees to express work-related concerns.
Inflexible work conditions	Make allowances for flexible work arrangements whenever possible.
Pay inequities	Use market information to determine wage and benefit programs.
Limited autonomy	Adopt a management style that encourages employee participation and a level of autonomy based on ability.
Open job market	Develop jobs with competitive compensation and challenging content.
Undesirable work conditions	Put in place offsetting conditions that decrease the negative impact of undesirable working conditions.

From Nosse, L. J., Friberg, D. G., & Kovacek, P. R. (1999). *Managerial and supervisory principles for physical therapists.* Baltimore: Lippincott Williams & Wilkins, with permission.

these factors. The factors and suggested managerial actions are presented in Table 6–4. A sample of selected evidence related to the retention of employees is provided in Table 6–5.

Box 6–10 lists the most common factors shown to contribute to employee retention in the occupational therapy, physical therapy, and nursing literature. Although some strategies are beyond the simple control of the occupational therapy manager or supervisor because they require the commitment of organizational resources, there are strategies that can be implemented in the course of your daily work. These strategies are listed in Box 6–11.

Performance Appraisal

Although the process of performance appraisal can be unnerving for both the employee and the unseasoned supervisor, this does not have to be the case. If the supervisor has effectively shared information with employees on a routine basis throughout the performance cycle, the appraisal meeting itself need not be confrontational or unnecessarily unpleasant. However, this assumes that there has been ongoing communication, and unfortunately this is often not the case. All too often, supervisors only provide casual feedback to employees unless there

Table 6-5	**Summary of Selected Evidence on Employee Retention**			
Author	Study Type	N	Level of Evidence	Results
Gowda (1997)	Survey of case managers	218	Good	Active coping, salary, role stress, and opportunity for promotion correlated with burnout and job dissatisfaction.
Irvine & Evans (1995)	Meta-analysis	23	Strong	Work content and work environment had a stronger relationship with job satisfaction than economic or individual difference variables in nursing job satisfaction.
Will (1995)	Survey of paramedics	299	Good	Satisfaction with work and coworkers contributed more than pay or promotion to job satisfaction and retention.
Smith, Schiller, Grant, & Sachs (1995)	Survey of occupational therapy managers	320	Good	The top retention strategies used were fostering interpersonal staff relationships, employee appraisals, and continuing education, although more than 70% used 17 similar strategies.
Kraeger & Walker (1993)	Survey of occupational therapy managers	106	Good	Limited opportunity for advancement was identified as a primary source of turnover. Primary retention strategies used were continuing education, educational benefits, part-time options, and flexible schedules.
Brollier (1986)	Survey of occupational therapy directors and therapists	93 directors and 348 therapists	Good	The department director's ability to influence higher administration was particularly important in affecting staff satisfaction with work.
Brollier (1985)	Survey of occupational therapy directors and therapists	93 directors and 348 therapists	Good	The department director's leadership style had significant influence on staff job satisfaction.

Box 6–10: Factors Shown to Contribute to Employee Retention

- Potential for promotion
- Part-time options
- Autonomy in decision making
- Job security
- Competitive salaries
- Flexible schedules

- Vacation and holiday leave
- Positive staff relationships
- Continuing education
- Health benefits
- Educational reimbursement
- Adequate supervision and feedback

Box 6–11: Everyday Strategies for Retaining Employees

1. Ask employees "What do you think?" on a regular basis.
2. Provide verbal praise and say "Thank you" for a job well done.
3. Follow-up on expressions of concern or dissatisfaction from employees even if you are not sure you can solve the problem.
4. Use ad hoc work groups and committees to solve departmental problems and ask for volunteers.
5. Look for ways to increase flexibility, such as offering to let employees leave early or come in late when work volume is temporarily low.
6. Don't always try to immediately "fix" an employee's problem; sometimes they just want you to listen and understand their daily frustrations.

is a serious problem. This practice results in two types of problems. First, it can result in missed opportunities for professional growth for employees. Second, it can result in the employees feeling as if the feedback is coming as a surprise. If an employee feels surprised in a performance appraisal meeting, even if the appraisal is going better than he or she expected, it can only mean that the supervisor has not done an adequate job in providing supervision.

An effective performance appraisal process is cyclical and can be thought of as occurring in four stages. These four stages of an effective performance appraisal cycle are (1) assessment, (2) performance planning, (3) intermittent review, and (4) accomplishment review. Each of these stages will be reviewed in more detail in this section.

Stage I: Assessment

Assessment occurs at the beginning of a performance cycle, which is typically a 12-month period in most organizations. Assessment is most effective when it is a collaborative process between the employee and his or her immediate supervisor and includes a self-assessment by the employee. A comprehensive self-assessment includes a review of the current job description for any area for which the employee feels he or she could use additional guidance as well as identification of areas for personal and professional growth. Self-assessment can assist with the identification of goals related to training (learning needs for the current job), education (learning needs for future professional opportunities), and development (general learning needs and skills that can apply to any employment situation). The supervisor should guide the self-assessment process so that it also includes identification of any organizationally determined *key result areas*. Key result areas may relate to standard sections of job descriptions or to organizational values such as "customer service," "continuous quality improvement," or "cost-effectiveness." Although assessment of performance is typically included in the human resources policies and procedures of most organizations, structured tools to guide assessment for employees are not always provided. Use of structured tools such as AOTA's Professional Development Tool or a self-assessment matrix similar to that shown in Table 6–2 adapted to a specific job description can make the self-assessment process easier and contribute to the identification of realistic goals. Assessment also includes examination and integration of feedback from one's supervisor on performance for the previous performance period.

Stage II: Performance Planning

Performance planning is the process of identifying mutually agreed upon goals related to programmatic needs and individual desires for growth. It also includes identification of the actions that will be taken by both the employee and his or her supervisor to facilitate the employee reaching established goals. Occupational therapists and occupational therapy assistants are well familiar with the process of setting goals because it is a key part of the occupational therapy process. Setting goals as part of a performance planning process is not so different. Just as when setting goals for a client, when an employee and his or her supervisor collaborate on goals for a performance period, it is important that the goals be (1) specific, (2) measurable, and (3) achievable. Goals should be specific in that a goal should clearly indicate what is and is not to be covered by the goal. Goals should be measurable so that it is possible for both the employee and his or her supervisor to know exactly when the goal has been achieved. Finally, goals should be achievable during the performance period. Employees may have long-term goals that extend over several performance periods, but these should be broken down into short-term goals that can be achieved within a single performance period. This is important because, in most organizations, raises in salary (e.g., merit increases) are typically based upon achievements in one 12-month period.

In addition to establishing specific, measurable and achievable goals, action plans should be developed that clearly identify the steps that will be taken by the employee to reach his or her goals as well as those actions that the supervisor will take to support the employee in goal attainment. It is typical in many organizations that the goals and action plans are documented in writing and signed by both the employee and the supervisor to indicate that they have collaborated on the development of the performance plan.

Stage III: Intermittent Review

During this stage, the supervisor evaluates the performance of employees both in their standard assigned duties and on their progress toward achieving their development goals. One of the most basic and most commonly overlooked principles of the performance appraisal process is that feedback should be *frequent and ongoing*. It is very easy to get caught up in the many responsibilities that most supervisors have in today's organizations, and it can be difficult to sequester the time to prepare and deliver feedback to employees in a timely and constructive manner. It can also be difficult at times to give negative feedback to an employee. Keeping simple rules of feedback in the forefront of one's attention can help a supervisor stay on track with providing intermittent review in an effective manner. A few of these rules for providing feedback are provided in Box 6–12.

Once an action plan is established and the performance period begins, it is important that some planning for contingencies occur as the employee goes about trying to achieve his or her goals. Although it is important to hold employees accountable for diligently working on their development plans, it is also important that, as managers or supervisors, we hold ourselves accountable for providing adequate support to the employee. We must recognize when circumstances within the organiza-

---

Box 6–12: Simple Rules for Making Feedback Constructive

Give feedback in a timely manner.

- *Timely:* "This morning when you snapped at Sharon for asking for your help, it concerned me."
- *Untimely:* "Sometimes you snap at your coworkers when they ask for your help, and it concerns me."

Make feedback objective and descriptive rather than judgmental.

- *Descriptive:* "This morning you seemed intent on people understanding your point of view."
- *Judgmental:* "You were so stubborn in the meeting this morning."

Make feedback specific rather than general.

- *Specific:* "I'm concerned that you were late for the last two meetings."

- *General:* "It bothers me that you're never on time."

Deal only with things that the employee can change, that is, deal with behavior rather than characteristics.

- *Behavior:* "If you spoke a little more slowly, your patients might not feel so overwhelmed."
- *Characteristics:* "You're voice is so high and squeaky."

Consider your motives when giving or receiving feedback.

- *Constructive motives:* "If I share this with Dave, he'll be a better clinician."
- *Destructive motives:* "Dave's such a hotshot, I'll bring him down a notch."

tion interfere with the employee's ability to reach his or her goals. A common example might be when vacancies occur in staffing or budgets are reduced and the supervisor is unable to follow through on commitments to send an employee to a continuing education course. In the case of this or other contingent events that interfere with a performance action plan, alternative actions can be identified, but only if the employee and supervisor are meeting on a regular basis.

Stage IV: Accomplishment Review

The fourth stage in the performance appraisal cycle includes the process of providing feedback to the employee to objectively note the extent to which he or she met or exceeded expectations for the essential functions of the job, other assigned duties, and the extent to which he or she achieved the goals developed at the beginning of the performance cycle. If intermittent reviews have been conducted and the employee has been provided both regular praise and suggestions for improving performance throughout the year, the accomplishment review should be essentially a time to summarize earlier discussions and begin planning for the next appraisal cycle. Whether positive or negative, employees should never be surprised during this step of the performance appraisal process. If employees enter an accomplishment review and feedback does not match what they expect to hear, the manager or supervisor should re-examine how he or she is providing feedback to the employee.

With the exception of new employees, stage IV and stage I are typically completed together. After providing feedback on the past year, it is time to return to the process of reviewing a current self-assessment and establishing goals for the next performance appraisal period.

The traditional supervisory appraisal has been criticized as being heavily influenced by bias and subjectivity (Latham & Wexley, 1994). One strategy to increasing the perceived fairness and objectivity of performance appraisals is by including multiple sources, including peers and managers or supervisors from other departments who are familiar with the performance of the employee being evaluated. Peer reviews often have a high level of worker acceptance and involvement; they tend to be stable, task relevant, and accurate. By helping peers to un-

derstand each other's work and by airing grievances in a nonthreatening manner, peer reviews may also help people to get along better. For the organization, this means higher performance. For the employees, this means a better place to work and less frustration; it may also help employees to concentrate less on politics or working around other people, and to spend more time on their work (or to put in less overtime) (Toolpack Consulting LLC, 2002). A team of evaluators may be assembled to increase the accuracy and completeness of the picture of performance assembled by management (Ewen, 1994). The advantages of such an approach may include the following:

- Feedback on a wider variety of work behaviors may be gathered, including cooperation, planning, delegation, and teamwork.
- Direct reports from multiple sources may be more reliable than supervisory judgments alone.
- There is less chance that feedback will be perceived as discriminatory if peers are involved in providing the feedback, and especially if the employee influences which peers provide feedback.
- Multirater evaluations may do better to empower employees to assume responsibility for their own career development.
- The employee helps to identify those who are involved in the appraisal process, and this increases the perception of fairness.
- The process motivates behavior change as a result of process credibility, accuracy, and validity.

Challenges and limitations to implementing a multisource performance appraisal system include the following:

- There may be perceived threats to the traditional role and authority of the manager and supervisor.
- Feedback on the same skill or behavior may vary from source to source and must be integrated into a single report.
- Feedback from peers may focus on personal characteristics or behaviors not related directly to work performance.
- Staff members may require training in the process of providing objective feedback.
- The process requires additional time and effort to collect information and integrate the information collected.

In Chapter 1, you were introduced to some of

the evidence related to performance appraisals and a critical appraisal matrix summarizing the evidence on strategies to increase the perception of employees that performance appraisals are fair and objective. Research on this topic continues to be conducted both in health care and other industries. If you are responsible for conducting performance appraisals, you are encouraged to review the evolving evidence on a regular basis.

Chapter Summary

This chapter reviewed the major roles and functions of the supervisor. The concepts of power and formal authority were differentiated and strategies for increasing both personal and position power were provided. Several strategies for conducting a self-assessment in order to develop a plan for becoming a more effective supervisor were covered in this chapter, and you are encouraged to take full advantage of the many resources available that are provided both within and outside the profession of occupational therapy. This chapter provided just a sample of the many theories and models that might guide you as a supervisor, and you are reminded that the evidence on these models and theories continues to be developed. Finally, an overview of the processes of performance appraisal and of providing rewards and recognition to employees was provided. Together, Chapters 5 and 6 have provided a solid introduction to the primary roles and functions of the manager and supervisor.

At the beginning of this chapter, you were introduced to Carlota, who was interested in learning more about the roles and functions of a supervisor. She was interested in some aspects of becoming a supervisor but wondered if she could assume supervisory responsibilities without also assuming managerial tasks such as budgeting. Carlota decided to consult with Craig, the District Manager for Occupational Therapy in the school district in which she was employed, to find out what responsibilities might be included in the job of senior therapist.

Resources for Learning More About Supervision

Journals That Often Address Supervision

THE HEALTHCARE MANAGER

The Healthcare Manager provides practical, applied management information for managers in institutional health care settings. This quarterly journal,

---

Real-Life Solutions

After a conversation with Craig, Carlota felt much more comfortable with the idea that there are opportunities to become involved in the supervision of others without also accepting all the typical duties of a manager. Carlota learned that not having "requisite managerial authority" can sometimes be a complicating factor because you do not have control over who reports to you. At the same time, she became excited about the extent of resources available to help her develop as a supervisor.

Craig shared with Carlota that the school system offered occasional courses related to supervision for principals and others who had supervisory roles, and that he had discovered a wealth of information on topics such as conducting performance appraisals, motivating and retaining employees, and providing rewards and recognition in the human resources literature while working on papers for a master's degree in Human Resource Development that he was pursuing. In addition, he shared that, whenever he encountered a new challenge and was unsure of how to proceed, he turned to his network of peers locally and nationally who were available to him through his participation in state and national occupational therapy associations.

Craig encouraged Carlota to become a member of both the state association and the AOTA, as he had done. Finally, he offered to support Carlota by guiding her through the completion of a self-assessment in order to form a professional development plan that included goals related to becoming a supervisor. By the end of their conversation, Carlota was ready to agree to formally interviewing for the position of senior therapist.

written for health care professionals in a managerial or supervisory role, focuses on strengthening management and supervisory skills.

SUPERVISION

This journal, published by the National Research Bureau, features articles aimed at teaching vital facts on minimizing costs and maximizing output for supervisors in industrial relations and operating management; however, many articles address topics relevant for managers and supervisors in any organization. Full-text articles are available online through many university libraries.

MANAGEMENT DECISION

Management Decision, published by Emerald Group Publishing, features articles and commentary on practical applications of theories applied to real situations in organizations for business managers, consultants, teachers, and students concerned with general management and strategy. Full-text articles are available online through many university libraries.

MANAGEMENT TODAY

This journal, published in London by Haymarket Business Publications, features articles, research, commentary, profiles, training, and book reviews on all aspects of business management. Full-text articles are available online through many university libraries.

Associations That Are Concerned with Supervision

AMERICAN MANAGEMENT ASSOCIATION

http://www.amanet.org/index.htm
   The American Management Association (AMA) states that its mission is to provide managers and their organizations worldwide with the knowledge, skills, and tools they need to improve business performance, adapt to a changing workplace, and prosper in a complex and competitive business world. The AMA serves as a forum for the exchange of the latest information, ideas, and insights on management practices and business trends. The AMA disseminates content and information to a worldwide audience through multiple distribution channels and its strategic partners by offering seminars, conferences, current issues forums and briefings, books and publications, research, and online self-study courses that cover such topics as supervisory skills.

NATIONAL ASSOCIATION FOR EMPLOYEE RECOGNITION

http://www.recognition.org/
   The National Association for Employee Recognition is dedicated to the enhancement of employee performance through recognition, including its strategies and related initiatives. The association provides a forum for information and best practices sharing as well as education to foster the use, excitement, effectiveness, and enthusiasm of recognition.

THE AMERICAN OCCUPATIONAL THERAPY ASSOCIATION

http://www.aota.org/
   The stated mission of the AOTA advances the quality, availability, use, and support of occupational therapy through standard setting, advocacy, education, and research on behalf of its members and the public. The AOTA provides its members with a variety of resources related to the supervision of occupational therapy personnel, including a number of papers that provide guidelines for the occupational therapy supervisor; access to Special Interest Sections (SISs) that provide Listservs and quarterly newsletters, including the Administration and Management SIS; and continuing education options.

Miscellaneous Resources
WORK911

http://www.work911.com
   Work911 is a commercial Web site operated by Bacal & Associates in Ontario, Canada. In addition to commercial products, there is a wide range of free-access features, including articles on topics related to supervision, management, and organizational development.

THE SUPERVISION NEWSLETTER

The SuperVision Newsletter is produced by the Office of Human Resources for managers and supervisors at the University of California, Berkeley. A range of articles written in an easy-to-use and easy-to-apply style are available and can be downloaded in a .pdf format.

Reference List

American Occupational Therapy Association. (1997). *Guide for supervision of occupational therapy personnel in the delivery of occupational therapy services*. Bethesda, MD: American Occupational Therapy Association.

American Occupational Therapy Association. (2004). Guidelines for supervision, roles, and responsibilities during the delivery of occupational therapy services. American Occupational Therapy Association Web site. Available at *http://www.aota.org*

American Physical Therapy Association. (2004). Levels of supervision. American Physical Therapy Association Web site. Available at *http://www.apta.org/governance/HOD/policies/HoDPolicies/Section_I/TERMINOLOGY/HOD_06001526*

Bernard, J. M., & Goodyear, R. K. (1992). *Fundamentals of clinical supervision*. Boston: Allyn & Bacon.

Bliss, W. (2001). The business cost and impact of employee turnover. Bliss and Associates Web site. Available at *www.blissassociates.com/thml/articles/employee_turnover01.html*

Brollier, C. (1985). Managerial leadership and staff OTR job satisfaction. *Occupational Therapy Journal of Research, 5,* 170–184.

Brollier, C. (1986). A multivariate predictive study of staff OTR job satisfaction: Some results of importance to psychosocial occupational therapy. *Occupational Therapy in Mental Health, 5,* 13–27.

Case-Smith, J. (2003). Using the AOTA professional development tool (PDT). *OT Practice, 8,* 1–7.

Ewen, A. J. (1994). Multi-source assessment increases healthcare employee satisfaction. *Journal of Ahima, 65,* 56–58.

Gowda, N. M. (1997). Factors associated with burnout and turnover intention among case managers who work with older adults. *Dissertation Abstracts International. B: The Physical Sciences & Engineering, 57,* 4760.

Harvey, V. S., & Struzziero, J. (2000). *Effective supervision in school psychology*. Bethesda, MD: National Association of School Psychologists.

Irvine, D. M., & Evans, M. G. (1995). Job satisfaction and turnover among nurses: Integrating research findings across studies. *Nursing Research, 44,* 246–253.

Kadushin, A. (1992). *Supervision in social work* (3rd ed.). New York: Columbia University Press.

Keller, C. (2000, February). Calculating the high cost of turnover. *Case Management Advisor,* 12–16.

Kraeger, M. M., & Walker, K. F. (1993). Attrition, burnout, job dissatisfaction and occupational therapy managers. *Occupational Therapy in Health Care, 8,* 47–62.

Latham, G. P., & Wexley K.N. (1994). *Increasing productivity through performance appraisal*. Reading, PA: Addison-Wesley.

Lawler, E. E. I. (1994). *Motivation in work organizations*. San Francisco: Jossey-Bass.

Leddick, G. R. (2004). Models of clinical supervision. ERIC Digests. Available at *http://www.ericfacility.net/databases/ERIC_Digests/ed372340.html*

Liebler, J. G., Levine, R. E., & Rothman, J. (1992). *Management principles for health professionals*. Gaithersburg, MD: Aspen.

Maslow, A. E. (1970). *Motivation and personality*. New York: Harper & Row.

McNamara, C. (2003). Basics: Definitions (and misperceptions) about management. The Management Assistance Program for Nonprofits Web site. Available at *http://www.mapnp.org/library/mgmnt/defntion.htm#anchor662641*

Miller, J. J., & Kilpatrick, A. (1987). *Issues for managers: An international perspective*. Homewood, IL: Irwin Press.

Nicklin, P. (1995). Super supervision. *Nursing Management, 2,* 24–25.

Nosse, L. J., Friberg, D. G., & Kovacek, P. R. (1999). *Managerial and supervisory principles for physical therapists*. Baltimore: Lippincott Williams & Wilkins.

Patterson, C. H. (1986). *Theories of counseling and psychotherapy* (4th ed.). New York: Harper & Row.

Salancik, G. R., & Pfeffer, J. (2003). Expectancy models of job satisfaction, occupational preference, and effort: A theoretical, methodological and empirical appraisal. *Administrative Science Quarterly, 23,* 224–253.

Salomon, W. (1999). *The new supervisor's survival manual*. New York: American Management Association.

Smith, P., Schiller, M. R., Grant, K., & Sachs, L. (1995). Recruitment and retention strategies used by occupational therapy directors in acute care, rehabilitation, and long-term-care settings. *American Journal of Occupational Therapy, 49,* 412–419.

Stoltenberg, C. D., & Delworth, U. (1987). *Supervising counselors and therapists*. San Francisco: Jossey-Bass.

Toolpack Consulting LLC. (2002). Effective performance appraisals and evaluation. Toolpack Consulting Web site. Available at *http://www.toolpack.com/performance.html*

Vroom, V. H. (1964). *Work and motivation*. New York: John Wiley & Sons.

Whetten, D. A., & Cameron, K. S. (1998). *Developing managerial skills* (4th ed.). Boston: Addison-Wesley.

Will, J. B. (1995). An analysis of attitudes toward measures of job satisfaction related to identified factors of paramedic education. *Dissertation Abstracts International. B: The Physical Sciences & Engineering, 60,* 2050.

7

Brent Braveman, Ph.D., OTR/L, FAOTA

Competency and the Occupational Therapy Manager

Real-Life Management

Emily has worked as an occupational therapy assistant for more than 20 years in a number of different settings but has specialized in spinal cord injury rehabilitation for the last 8 years and has developed specialized skills in a number of areas. Recently, Emily and her spouse relocated, and she began working within a spinal cord injury program at a different rehabilitation facility. Most of the components of the program are very similar to the program in which she was working, and, in her interview, it seemed that her job tasks would be almost identical to those she had been completing. It seemed that she would need to learn relatively little new information to return to the independent style of working she had adopted.

Given her experience, she was surprised by the very formal and in-depth orientation program she was expected to complete before she began treating patients without "line of sight" supervision. Because the facility was accredited by the Joint Commission on Accreditation of Healthcare Organizations (JCAHO) and the Commission on Accreditation of Rehabilitation Facilities (CARF), she could understand having to review videotapes and take written exams on fire and electrical safety and even on hand washing (although she assumed everyone knew the importance of hand washing).

However, Emily did not understand why she had to spend time reviewing orientation information on aspects of intervention that she considered basic, such as techniques for safely transferring patients or completing "skin checks" to prevent pressure sores. She had to admit privately that she was somewhat insulted to be supervised so closely given the excellent references she had received from her prior supervisors. Moreover, she could not understand why her supervisors were being so slow to assign her patients when her new supervisor reported that the facility was short staffed and had several vacancies. Emily had offered to jump in and suggested that she could help by beginning to treat patients in their rooms for activities of daily living sessions or to complete portions of the assessment appropriate for the occupational therapy assistant. However, her supervisor had responded that they took the "assessment of competencies" for new employees very seriously and did not cut any corners.

Emily had been excited about beginning to work at the facility because the other occupational therapy assistants who worked there reported feeling highly valued and respected by all of the occupational therapists, but all of this attention to her level of "competency" made her wonder if she had made a mistake. She decided to confront her supervisor during their next meeting and express her dissatisfaction at the close level of scrutiny she was under. She decided to make a list of the competencies noted on her orientation checklist that she had been completing independently for more than 5 years and to ask that she be able to forgo the rest of the orientation period.

Key Issues

- Terminology related to assessment of competencies, competency, and continued competency is very specific, and care must be taken to utilize the appropriate terms in the correct situations.
- The process of conducting assessment of competencies is related to and can support nu-
- merous other management functions, including employee recruitment, orientation, performance planning, and accreditation reviews.
- Evidence suggests that the skills necessary to demonstrate competencies in an area are often the very same skills necessary to evaluate competence in that
- area, and hence individuals are often poor judges of their own level of competence.
- Occupational therapy managers play a role in the assessment of competencies, continued competency, and the development of specialized and advanced skills recognized through processes such as certification.

During the 1980s and 1990s, the need to determine the initial competence of health professionals, to assess competencies in regard to a specific job as professionals are hired and begin to work, and to promote professionals' continuing competence began to be addressed with increasing urgency and concern by numerous professions. The level of concern has continued to grow, and competency and the assessment of competencies continue to be a focus today (Barney, Long, McCall, Watts, & Cash, 2000; Braveman, Gentile, Stafford, Berthelette, & Learnard, 2004; Grossman, 1998; Lenburg, 1999b; Redman, Lenburg, & Hinton-Walker, 1999). Concerns regarding competency-related issues span the period of time from which a health professional is initially judged to be competent to practice (e.g., National Board for Certification in Occupational Therapy, Inc. [NBCOT] certification), through the process of hiring and orienting staff, to fostering continued competence of health professionals across entire careers.

Occupational therapy managers often play critical roles in determining whether an individual has met the initial competency standards to practice within a setting through a review of an applicant's credentials. Upon hiring a new employee, the manager must assess the individual's ability to perform specific skills or recall specific information by assessing performance against a set of competencies, or specific statements of action representing competency in a skill or procedure. The manager also can facilitate the continued competency of staff through a variety of professional development activities.

Increased attention to issues related to the competence of occupational therapy practitioners and other health professionals has come about because of a variety of factors. The increased sophistication of health care consumers has led to increased scrutiny of the initial competence of health care professionals as well as a call for more severe penalties and consequences for lapses in competence. As a result, the process of *certifying* the initial competence of practitioners has also become more sophisticated. The rapid rate of technology change has had a dramatic impact on the rate at which new knowledge is developed and communicated. The workforce has become more mobile and, with personnel shortages in fields such as occupational therapy, physical therapy, and nursing, recruitment of personnel has become more competitive. Economic influences have resulted in expectations for higher productivity and flexibility on the part of workers. These factors and others have contributed to increased need for the assessment of *competencies* as employees enter a job or need to demonstrate various skills as well as the assessment of *continued competence* as employees.

This chapter will overview the key organizations involved in the assessment of competency and the promotion of continued competence, examine the reasons why these processes are important to any health profession, and introduce you to the components and tools of basic systems for assessing competencies and promoting continued competency of occupational therapy personnel. Advanced certification and specialty certification as methods of indicating competency in particular areas of practice will also be introduced.

Why Do We Need to Worry About Competency?

The answer to the question, "Why worry about assessing the competency of occupational therapy personnel?" might seem simple, and in fact there are some readily identifiable reasons. These reasons include the following:

- We want to promote the provision of the best possible quality of intervention for our patients and clients.
- We want to avoid litigation that comes with allegations of malpractice and "incompetence."
- Lifelong learning, practice based upon evidence, and keeping pace with the introduction of new knowledge and changing technology are commonly recognized values of the profession.

However, there are additional reasons for developing an ongoing and integrated system for the assessment of competencies and the promotion of continued competency. First, a fully integrated system will relate strategies and efforts to assess competencies to strategies and efforts for hiring, orienting, supervising, and evaluating staff. A system for assessing competencies can help you recruit and hire the right person with the right skills or identify the skills you need to develop in current staff. Second, evidence suggests you cannot rely on staff members to accurately assess their own skills or to accurately identify their own learning needs for the present or for the future (Jansen, Grol, Rethans, & Vleuten, 1998; Kruger & Dunning, 1999). Moreover, there is not always a high level of agreement between the self-assessment of level of competence and the assessment of managers of the level of competence of the same subordinate (Meretoja & Leino-Kilpi, 2003). In fact, staff members may underestimate their level of competence as often as they overestimate it. In either case, inaccurate assessment of level of competence may lead to poor utilization of resources, rework, lowered levels of staff satisfaction, and decreased quality of care.

Finally, occupational therapy managers play an important role in retaining staff once hired. In times of personnel shortage, competition for available personnel increases, and retaining staff and avoiding the costs of recruiting and orienting new staff becomes even more important. One key strategy for staff retention is continuing education and staff development, and evidence suggests that occupational therapy managers utilize this strategy often and view it as one of the most effective retention strategies (P. Smith, Schiller, Grant, & Sachs, 1995). Initiating planned efforts to help staff members develop specialized and advanced competencies (sometimes leading to formal certification) is one method of implementing this strategy.

Key Terms, Concepts, and Players

Multiple organizations related to health care delivery are concerned with developing and maintaining the "competency" of staff, and, as noted, competency-related issues arise at various points in the entrée of a professional to a profession. The American Occupational Therapy Association (AOTA), the NBCOT, the JCAHO, the CARF, and many state professional regulatory boards, among other organizations, have programs, policies, or efforts underway related to competency issues (AOTA, 2004; Braveman et al., 2004; NBCOT, 2004b). Because of the many organizations and bodies involved, and because of the range of points in the careers of professionals at which competency issues arise, the terminology involved can be confusing. Focusing on the context in which terminology is used can be a useful way of keeping the terminology straight.

For example, the AOTA distinguishes between the terms *competence* (an individual's capacity to perform job responsibilities) and *continuing competency* (the development of capacity and competency characteristics needed for the future as a component of ongoing professional development or lifelong learning) (Braveman et al., 2004; Hinojosa et al., 2000). Box 7–1 includes the definitions of some key terms that will be used throughout this chapter.

Box 7-1: Glossary of Key Terms

- **Competent** (adjective): Successfully performing a behavior or task as measured according to a specific criterion (Hinojosa et al., 2000).
  - *Example:* "Based on the established criterion, I am competent to take range-of-motion measurements."
- **Competency** (noun): An individual's actual performance in a particular situation (McConnell, 2001). Competency implies a determination that one is competent.
  - *Example:* "During my orientation to my job, my supervisor observed me and determined that I demonstrated competency in taking range-of-motion measurements."
- **Competencies** (plural of competency): Explicit statements that define specific areas of expertise and are related to effective or superior performance in a job (Spencer & Spencer, 1993).
  - *Example:* "New employees are required to demonstrate a range of competencies before they are allowed to treat patients without direct supervision, such as taking range-of-motion measurements, transferring patients, and making basic splints. These competencies are listed on an orientation check sheet."
- **Competence** (noun): An individual's capacity to perform job responsibilities (McConnell, 2001).

- *Example:* "My performance appraisal indicates that I demonstrate competence in assessing range of motion."
- **Continued/Continuing Competence:** The development of competency for the future, and a component of ongoing professional development or lifelong learning.
  - *Example:* "Because I do not take range-of-motion measurements every day, I need to do periodic reviews to maintain my continued competence; as new information is developed related to strategies for managing joint contractures, I will need to develop and demonstrate new competencies."
- **Professional Development:** May include a program of continuing competence, but also includes a focus on one's career development in terms of achieving excellence or achieving independent practitioner and expert role status, and in terms of assuming new, more complex roles and responsibilities.
  - *Example:* "Because I hope to one day become a college instructor, I plan to begin supervising fieldwork students to learn more about the process of teaching others skills such as taking range-of-motion measurements."

From Burkhardt, A., Braveman, B., & Gentile, P. (2000). Evaluating and documenting staff competence for accreditation reviews and staff development. *AMSIS Quarterly, 18,* 4,1–6. Bethesda, MD: American Occupational Therapy Association, with permission.

The process of establishing that a professional meets requirements representing *initial competence* includes multiple steps that are overseen by a variety of types of organizations. Often the NBCOT is thought of as having primary responsibility for establishing that an individual meets standards related to initial competency through administration of the certification examination. The NBCOT is a not-for-profit credentialing agency that oversees certification for the occupational therapy profession. The NBCOT serves the public interest by developing, administering, and continually reviewing a certification process that reflects current standards of competent practice in occupational therapy.

In addition, the NBCOT collaborates with state regulatory authorities, providing information on credentials, disciplinary actions, and regulatory and certification renewal issues (NBCOT, 2003). The mission statement of the NBCOT is as follows:

"Above all else, the mission of the National Board for Certification in Occupational Therapy, Inc., is to serve the public interest. We provide a world class standard for certification of occupational therapy practitioners. The National Board for Certification in Occupational Therapy, Inc., will develop, administer, and continually review a certifica-

tion process based on current and valid standards that provide reliable indicators of competence for the practice of occupational therapy." (NBCOT, 2003)

Undoubtedly, the NBCOT does play a vital role in the process of establishing the initial competence of occupational therapists and occupational therapy assistants. However, it is important to recognize that there are multiple steps in determining initial competence that occur before an occupational therapist or occupational therapy assistant reaches the point of taking the NBCOT certification examination.

Before candidates may sit for the certification exam, they must graduate from an educational program accredited by the Accreditation Council on Occupational Therapy Education (ACOTE). To graduate from such a program, students must not only receive a passing grade in a large number of courses by demonstrating competencies in multiple domains of learning but also successfully complete mandated full-time clinical fieldwork. Graduating from an accredited occupational therapy program is in fact the first step toward certifying initial competence. The process that the NBCOT oversees is referred to as *certification*. Certification is the process by which a professional certification agency grants a person permission to use a certain title if that person has attained entry-level competence. Certification is intended to assure the public that a professional has completed an approved educational program and has passed an examination that assesses the knowledge, skills, and experience needed to provide quality care (DeLisa, 2000). Professional certification agencies

- Serve the credentialing needs of the profession regardless of membership status (meaning that membership in the profession's association is not required to become certified or to maintain certification)
- Develop professional standards and measure compliance
- Promote a vision to improve the overall performance of a profession through a quality certification system

The NBCOT develops a certification examination through a process that they call a *practice analysis* that is completed every 5 years. The practice analysis is a method for determining key components required for entry-level occupational therapy practice across three levels: (1) domains, (2) tasks, and (3) knowledge. Domains broadly define the major performance components of the profession (e.g., evaluation; intervention planning; implementing intervention; identifying and implementing performance needs of populations; and managing, organizing, and promoting occupational therapy services). Tasks describe activities that are performed in each domain (e.g., job duties performed by an entry-level therapist). Knowledge statements reflect the information required to perform each task (e.g., knowledge of sources for staying current in legislative changes influencing practice). These levels are used to develop an *examination blueprint* that guides the percentage of the certification examination related to each domain. For example, beginning in 2005, the examination blueprint calls for 7% of examination questions to relate the domain of "manage/organize/promote OT services" (NBCOT, 2004a).

State professional regulatory agencies are also involved in establishing initial competence of professionals through the process of licensure. Licensure is the process by which an agency of government grants permission to an individual to engage in a given occupation upon finding that the applicant has attained the minimal degree of competence required to ensure that the public health, safety, and welfare will be reasonably well protected. Professional regulatory agencies serve a number of purposes, including

- Serving the public by legally monitoring entrée to public practice
- Establishing minimum standards to protect the public in a particular jurisdiction
- Monitoring minimal standards of practice via a practice act and ongoing disciplinary process

In Chapter 2, you learned that it is common to refer to any type of state regulation of who may practice within a profession as "licensure," although there are actually a number of different types of regulation often grouped under that term. Occupational therapy is currently regulated in all 50 states, the District of Columbia, Puerto Rico, and Guam. Different states have various types of regulation that range from licensure, the strongest form of regulation, to title protection or trademark law, the weakest form of regulation. Certification laws simply regulate who may refer to themselves as occupational therapists or occupational therapy assistants and may or may not provide a definition of occupational therapy. In some cases persons may practice as long as they do not refer to themselves as occupational therapy practitioners. Similarly, registration laws prevent nonregistered persons from stating that they are providing occupational therapy services, and trademark laws simply limit who may refer to themselves as occupational therapists or occupational therapy assistants (AOTA, 1999a).

Generally, unlike certification, registration, and trademark laws, a licensure law defines a lawful scope of practice for practitioners. Defining a scope of practice legally articulates the domain of practice and provides guidance to facilities, providers, consumers, and major public and private health and education facilities on the appropriate use of services and practitioners. Defining practice can further ensure important patient protections by offering guidance on appropriate care, particularly in the investigation and resolution of consumer complaints involving fraudulent or negligent delivery of services.

Competency, Skill Acquisition, and Theory

David McClelland was a Harvard University psychologist and founder of the Hay-McBer company, and is credited with founding the competency movement in the United States (Kierstead, 1998; Manley & Garbett, 2000). McClelland set out to define competency variables that could be used in predicting job performance and that were not biased by race, gender, or socioeconomic factors. *Competency* was thought to be a broader term than *skill* because it related to performance on the job that required integration of a number of skills. McClelland's colleague, Richard Boyatzis, furthered this work. He focused on identifying competencies that could differentiate superior performance from average or poor performance by focusing on a person who does the job well and the characteristics and qualities that enable a person to do a superior job, rather than focusing on the job itself (Boyatzis, 1982; Manley & Garbett, 2000). During the 1980s and 1990s, refinement of assessment of competencies continued in the human resources field and began to gain acceptance in other fields, including health care.

One commonly cited model related to the development of competence and competencies in health care is the Dreyfus and Dreyfus Skill Acquisition Model, which was originally based on the study of U.S. Air Force pilots (Dreyfus, 1981). In the 1980s, Patricia Benner adapted the Dreyfus and Dreyfus model to nursing and published an often-cited book, *From Novice to Expert* (Benner, 1984). This model frames skill acquisition as moving through various stages (Driscoll, 2002; Leach, 2002):

- *Novice:* learners focus on learning the rules of a particular skill.
- *Advanced Beginner:* learners focus on applying the rules of a skill in specific situations that become increasingly dependent on the particular context of the situation.
- *Competency:* learners see actions in terms of long-range goals or plans and are consciously aware of their skills.
- *Proficiency:* learners perceive situations as "wholes" rather than "aspects," and their performance is guided by intuitive behavior.
- *Expert:* learners integrate mastered skills with their own personal styles.

Applications of the Benner model have been widely reported within the nursing literature and to some extent within the literature of other health professions, often in relation to clinical decision making, education, and development of training programs or career ladders (Crook, 2001; Hargreaves & Lane, 2001; Manley & Garbett, 2000; Nichol, Fox-Hiley, Bavin, & Sheng, 1996; Nuccio et al., 1996; Winchcombe, 2000).

Interestingly, little discussion appears in the literature on competency and assessment of competencies regarding exactly *how* one comes to acquire a particular competency. Some reference is made to learning theories, and the assumption seems to be that managers should rely on bodies of knowledge related to education and skill development to guide training or education efforts aimed to help staff develop competencies. Discussion widely seems to focus on the roles of the individual, the manager, the organization, and the profession in facilitating the development of competence through processes such as self-assessment or professional development strategies (e.g., continuing education, portfolio development and use, or specialty or advanced certification) (Hinojosa et al., 2000; Tillema, 2001; Weinstein, 2000).

Limited empirical investigation is found in regard to any single approach to the development and assessment of competencies. For example, although the work of Dreyfus and Dreyfus and of Benner is perhaps among the most often cited as the basis for the creation of programs to foster the development of competencies, limited empirical evidence exists. To answer the question, "What evidence is there of the effectiveness of using the Dreyfus and Dreyfus and the Benner models for the development of competencies?", a search conducted in the PsycINFO, CINAHL, and OVID databases using the key phrase "professional competence" and a separate search using the key phrase "skill acquisition" revealed only a handful of articles that included a research focus. These studies are described in Table 7–1. A number of references included descriptions of applications of the Dreyfus and Dreyfus and the Benner models, such as through the development of career ladder systems, although these citations are not included in Table 7–1.

Assessment of Competencies and Other Functions of the Occupational Therapy Manager

Occupational therapy managers complete a range of functions that relate to the assessment of specific competencies. As described earlier, competency issues span the period from entrée to the profession to working with staff to try to assure that they maintain continued competence as they accept new responsibilities and as the profession's knowledge base rapidly grows and changes. Skilled managers will look across the various discrete management functions they perform and create bridges from one management function to another to establish a system that ties the assessment of competencies to other management tasks. This section will briefly overview some of the most important management functions to which the assessment of competencies is related.

Creating Job Descriptions

A job description is described in Chapter 10 as "the core personnel document that serves to codify best practice." It does this by establishing the essential functions that a particular employee or class of employees performs (e.g., occupational therapists versus occupational therapy assistants). In Chapter 10, you will be introduced to the components of job descriptions and strategies for developing job descriptions. Briefly, these components include the requirements for the job (e.g., eligibility for state licensure), the relationship of the employee to others in the organization, and the essential functions of the position or the fundamental job duties that the employee must be able to complete independently with or without a reasonable accommodation.

The essential functions performed by each employee should be reflected in specific competencies developed in relation to each function. The process of developing competencies may also help you reexamine the job descriptions of personnel to assure that they are accurate and complete. For example, including "Assists clients to develop positive support mechanisms to prevent relapse" in a job description might indicate the need for development of competencies related to understanding addiction to substances and the recovery process. In turn, knowing that a staff member often intervenes to help clients develop leisure activities and social supports that foster sobriety might indicate the need to add related tasks as essential functions within the individual's job description.

Recruitment of New Employees

Well-written job descriptions that accurately and completely identify the essential functions of a position and the related set of competencies can make the process of recruiting and hiring new employees easier and can increase the likelihood of recruiting an employee who is a good match for the position. Assessment of specific competencies may be useful in determining the skills, training, and education required for persons being hired to fill a specific vacancy, and can therefore guide the manager or supervisor in writing recruitment materials and screening and interviewing applicants (Braveman et al., 2004). Additionally, job offers can be made contingent upon the ability to demonstrate competency in the essential job functions as identified in the job description. Job descriptions and statements of competencies should be reviewed each time a vacancy occurs, because the knowledge re-

Table 7-1　Selected Evidence on Benner's Novice-to-Expert Model

Author	Design	Purpose of Study	n (Sample Size)	Level of Evidence	Results or Findings
Spalding (2000)	Case study	To gain an understanding of the professional development of two occupational therapists using the Dreyfus and Dreyfus model.	2 occupational therapists	Weak	The progressive nature of learning resembled the Dreyfus and Dreyfus model. Both therapists progressed to proficiency in a short time, suggesting that the amount of exposure to clinical experience was not as influential on skill acquisition as the reflective nature of the subjects.
Winchcombe (2000)	Questionnaire	To determine perceptions of various levels of competence in infection control professionals	464 infection control professionals	Strong	Findings highlighted the need for a framework to be developed to measure progression through the Benner levels.
Nuccio et al. (1996)	Qualitative, exploratory design	To understand nurses' perceptions of experiences with the implementation of a clinical practice development model	25 staff nurses	Weak	Nurses' perspectives ranged from negative to positive and were most influenced by the timing of transition events, communication about the transition process, and the organizational culture present.
Benner, Tanner, & Chesla (1992)	Qualitative, group narrative interviews	To further explicate the Dreyfus model of skill development	105 practicing nurses	Good	Two interrelated aspects were found to distinguish four levels of practice from advanced beginner through expert. Practitioners at different levels of skill respond to different directives for action, and a sense of agency is determined by one's clinical world and shows up as an expression of responsibility for what happens with the patient.
Maynard (1991)	Randomly selected cross-sectional design	To study the socialization process and subsequent development of professional nursing competen	121 nursing graduates	Good	Critical thinking had no relationship to competence or stage of skill acquisition.

quired for successful performance can change, sometimes over relatively short periods of time.

Initial Assessment of Competencies

The initial assessment of competencies is often associated with settings that undergo organizational accreditation by bodies such as the JCAHO. Such bodies often do require documentation of a comprehensive orientation of new employees, and initial assessment of competencies for essential job functions is an important part of a comprehensive employee orientation. However, documentation of initial assessment of competencies is not important only in settings subject to an accreditation process. In addition, managers should consider initial assessment of competencies in any setting in which they wish to assure provision of quality care and to safeguard to whatever extent possible against malpractice litigation (Braveman et al., 2004).

Initial assessment of competencies related to essential job functions, high-risk job tasks (e.g., transferring patients, working with a patient with cardiac precautions), and job functions requiring performance of specialized competencies (e.g., use of physical agent modalities) or advanced competencies (e.g., comprehensive cognitive evaluation of patients with neurologic conditions) should occur before the employee independently completes these job tasks (Braveman et al., 2004). Determination that an employee cannot demonstrate competence in an essential job function as part of the orientation process allows the manager or supervisor to safeguard consumers by taking steps to assist the staff member to develop competence in essential job function before the end of the orientation period.

It is often assumed that, if a therapist has obtained initial certification, he or she will indeed be able to adequately perform the functions expected of an entry-level therapist. Although this is typically the case, there are exceptions. At times a manager may hire a therapist, or may encounter staff members hired by previous managers, who in fact are not able to demonstrate all of the required competencies for adequate performance. If comprehensive job descriptions and statements of initial competencies exist, they can guide assessment of the staff member's level of competency. Hopefully the therapist will be able to develop the skills,

knowledge, and attitude required to demonstrate the necessary competencies. In worst-case situations, staff members who cannot demonstrate competencies at the end of an orientation period or in some cases later in their employment may have to be terminated. Situations such as this are rare, but they highlight the seriousness of managerial tasks and the importance of having structures and tools such as job descriptions and statements of competencies in place.

Annual Assessment of Competencies

In addition to the initial assessment of competencies conducted when a new employee begins work, there are some competencies that should or must be assessed on an annual basis. Competencies such as those required by the Occupational Safety and Health Administration (OSHA) can be documented as part of the process of conducting an annual performance appraisal. Often managers think that assessment of competencies differs vastly from performance appraisal. In fact, assessment of competencies is simply part of a performance appraisal based on defined skills and performance criteria. To reflect this single process and reduce paperwork, some organizations have re-engineered their job descriptions and performance appraisal systems. By basing the job description on the specific skills that are required, forms that previously did "double duty" as performance evaluations can serve also as the assessment of competencies documentation tool (LaDuke, 2001).

Examples of competencies assessed on an annual basis would include those related to fire safety and electrical safety or to blood-borne pathogen precautions, such as knowledge of effective hand washing and infection control techniques. Competency statements included in an annual assessment of competence might also include competencies related to a specific employee's job tasks or skills (e.g., competencies related to specialized practice skills such as conducting an evaluation for driver safety or the provision of low vision services) or to general skills such as customer service (Krozek & Scroggins, 1999a). Competencies included in annual assessments may build on established knowledge, skills, and capacities reflecting the ever-changing nature of some jobs in light of an organization's mission and goals. Braveman et al.

(2004) noted that these competencies might reflect new, changing, high-risk, or problem-prone aspects of the job as it evolves over time. Examples of when the need for such competencies might come about include the following:

- Competencies based on new initiatives, procedures, technologies, policies, or practices are identified.
- Competencies based on changes in procedures, technologies, policies, or practices occur.
- Competencies related to high-risk job functions are identified or added to a job description.
- Competencies related to problematic job functions are identified through continuous quality improvement (CQI) efforts, consumer or staff surveys, incident reports, or any other formal or informal evaluation processes.

Professional Development and Portfolios

As a result of implementing a comprehensive system for assessment of competencies, a manager may become aware of acute or long-term professional development needs of staff. Through the process of assessing competencies, you may identify learning needs that can be met through your department's in-service education program or through continuing education or training. Tying the development goals of staff to needs identified during the initial or annual assessment of competencies as well as the annual performance appraisal creates a synergy of effort that can save you time and help you to identify the most effective strategies for using limited continuing education resources.

One approach to professional development that relates to continued competency is the development and use of *portfolios*. Portfolios have become popular as assessment instruments and as learning tools for the development of competence because they provide opportunities to monitor and appraise changes in performance (K. Smith & Tillema, 1998). Portfolios contribute to the process of assessing competency (note that the more general term *competency* is used here rather than *competencies*) by compiling evidence about performance and relevant feedback about individual practices (Tillema, 2001). A portfolio may also be a useful tool in gathering and organizing information about involvement in professional development activities

to satisfy the requirements for professional development for NBCOT recertification or for maintaining state licensure (Alsop, 2001).

Three general types of portfolios have been identified (K. Smith & Tillema, 2001): (1) performance dossier portfolios, (2) course-related learning portfolios, and (3) reflective learning portfolios. Performance dossier portfolios are often suggested as tools for documenting work performance in relation to external evaluation requirements (such as requirements for experience of a certain type and duration required to obtain some specialty certifications). In using this type of portfolio, you focus on marking achievements that may be evaluated according to specified external standards. Evidence of performance is collected in fixed formats as a key feature of this type of portfolio (K. Smith & Tillema, 2001). Portfolios for course-related learning help learners to inform others and track or redirect competence developed through formal programs. These types of portfolios place high value on the recognition, interpretation, and utilization of relevant learning experiences according to the standards as laid out in a formal course or educational or training program. Collecting specific and predetermined types of information fosters meaningful decision making for further development (Winsor, Butt, & Reeves, 1999). Reflective learning portfolios document and highlight the cyclical process of professional growth in understanding work experiences through continued monitoring over an extended period of time. The process resembles a biography, and this type of portfolio is used as a document alongside professional practice to integrate evolving thoughts and actions as directed by personal goals and learning needs (K. Smith & Tillema, 2001).

Regardless of the type used, advantages of developing and using portfolios include (Tillema, 2001)

- Assistance in identifying strengths and weaknesses in performance
- Fostering development of awareness of competence
- Resolving discrepancies between external standards and achieved performance
- Capturing achievements under realistic circumstances and recording them using authentic evidence and tangible products

Staffing Plans, Including Per Diem or Registry Staff

According to a study by the National Association for Health Care Recruitment, the vacancy rate for occupational therapists in this decade has been at crisis levels, or more than 11% (Green, 2004). With continued high vacancy rates, many organizations have pursued a variety of strategies to respond to the shortage. One strategy is to purchase personnel services (referred to as contract staff) from an outside agency or vendor or maintain their own registry of per diem staff. In this situation, the organization must obtain information from that outside vendor to assure that the contracted staff members have the proper credentials (e.g., licensure as required by a state practice act).

Contract or per diem staff members are typically held to the same standards for demonstrating both initial and annual competencies as permanent staff. For example, the JCAHO has stated that, "Organizations must manage contracted services and personnel just as they must manage services and personnel who are provided by direct employees. They can either define in the contract or in policy criteria for performance of the contracted service; or, review and adopt the contract organization's policies and practices" (JCAHO, 2004). Assessing competencies for these staff members can be costly. Often the human resources department will verify basic credentials such as licensure, but typically the occupational therapy manager is responsible for verifying that the contract or per diem staff can demonstrate competencies related to essential job functions. To minimize expense, documentation of some competencies prior to beginning work (e.g., cardiopulmonary resuscitation [CPR] certification, blood-borne pathogen training) might be written into contracts with agencies or may be made the responsibility of per diem staff to be completed during nonpaid time (Braveman et al., 2004). Additionally, by making adjustments in how caseloads are assigned and assigning agency staff only patients within a specified age range and with a limited variety of conditions, you may be able to limit the scope of competencies that must be assessed initially.

A system for the assessment of competencies is a key component in the development of an overall staffing plan for a department. In settings accredited by the JCAHO, these plans are required, but such plans can help you identify the number of staff necessary and the competencies they must be able to demonstrate to meet the care needs of any setting. For example, identifying the needs that your department has for providing specialized types of intervention based on competencies would alert you that, because of staff turnover, you employ only a single staff member who has documented competencies related to treating patients with wound care needs. Competency-based staffing plans can help you identify that additional training must be provided to other staff to assure adequate coverage when employees who have demonstrated competency are not working. Accrediting bodies may require that the same level of care be provided regardless of the day of the week patients are admitted to your facility.

Agency Accreditation and Licensure

Both accrediting bodies and state regulatory agencies have increased their focus on the assessment of competencies and on continuing competency. Increasingly, state regulatory agencies are including requirements for continuing education as part of an effort to promote continued competence (AOTA, 2004). Managers working in accredited and licensed facilities and programs must ensure that their programs for assessment of competencies meet all accrediting and licensing standards. You should be aware that standards related to competency may vary from one accrediting body to another and may change over time, so you must be vigilant in monitoring these changes.

Licensure laws often include what are referred to as "sunset" provisions, meaning that a provision of the law is automatically repealed on a specific date, unless the appropriate legislative body re-enacts the law. This means that state licensure regulations often have to be re-enacted on a regular cycle. State professional associations often see sunset provisions as an opportunity to change provisions or add new provisions to the regulation, and updated versions of the regulation may have an impact on what competencies should be assessed or how, or the requirements for documenting efforts to maintain continued competency.

The most common accrediting bodies occupational therapy managers may be involved with are the JCAHO and the CARF. Standards related to the assessment of competencies for both JCAHO Leadership and CARF Business Practices are primarily found in the human resources section of their manuals. Managers should carefully review these standards when developing competency programs for their staff (Braveman et al., 2004).

Quality Control and Continuous Quality Improvement Efforts

Chapter 11 provides an in-depth discussion of quality control and CQI. Assessment of competencies and efforts to promote continued competency are natural fits with CQI initiatives. For example, the use of quality control measures such as "check sheets" to determine the level of conformance to pre-established standards for interventions such as splint fabrication, use of modalities, or documentation can flag the need for education or training of staff. Similarly, CQI efforts focusing on process improvement may indicate the need to establish new competencies or revisit established measures of competency by providing targeted training for staff.

As a result of a CQI effort, processes may be changed or new processes may be implemented. Introducing a changed or new process and assuring that it becomes "institutionalized" so all staff members are aware of the process and complete it in the same manner is a key final step in any CQI effort. Identifying the key competencies and developing assessment methods can help measure the extent of compliance to new procedures.

Outcomes Evaluation and Management

Many factors influence the outcomes of occupational therapy intervention, and the assessment of competencies will not automatically assure desired outcomes. Other factors related to patients or clients, their support, their medical condition, and the length and type of intervention provided might all impact the outcome of occupational therapy intervention. You must be aware that evaluating outcomes of interventions with individual clients calls for very different procedures than evaluating outcomes of occupational therapy intervention at the program level. Systems to assess competencies related to essential job functions can help to prevent

unusual cases or "outliers" from influencing the overall variability found in outcome measures (Braveman et al., 2004). It is important to recognize that not all outliers in a process are negative events. Sometimes we should attend to an outlier because it signifies that someone has found a more effective way of doing something or might be our most skilled employee, and we would benefit from others adopting that employee's procedures. Again, the process of developing statements of competencies can help guide the institutionalization of new and improved procedures.

Domains of Knowledge, Competency, and Assessment of Competencies

Traditionally, three domains of performance have been identified to guide programming related to education, training, and the development of competency. These three domains are the cognitive domain (knowing), the affective domain (appreciating and valuing), and the psychomotor domain (physical performance) (Gronlund & Linn, 1990; Redman et al., 1999). In addition, two other domains of performance for occupational therapists have been identified: ethical reasoning and critical reasoning. These domains were identified as related to competency by the AOTA's Commission on Continuing Competency in the "Standards for Continuing Competence," which are intended to "assist occupational therapy practitioners to assess, maintain, and document competence in all the roles they assume" (AOTA, 1999b). The standards address the following five domains: (1) knowledge, (2) critical reasoning, (3) interpersonal attitudes, (4) performance skills, and (5) ethical reasoning. Table 7–2 includes examples of competency statements related to the cognitive, critical reasoning, affective, psychomotor, and ethical reasoning domains for an occupational therapist involved in work-related occupational therapy practice.

Examples of Types of Competencies

Competencies can be generic to clinical practice in any setting (basic), specific to a clinical specialty, or reflective of specialized knowledge or advanced

Table 7-2	Examples of Competency Statements from the Cognitive, Critical Reasoning, Affective, Psychomotor, and Ethical Reasoning Domains
Cognitive domain (knowing)	• The therapist will be able to identify various physical, cognitive, and environmental factors that can affect performance within the worker role. • The therapist will be able to identify resources available to assist workers and employers in accessing services in their community.
Critical reasoning domain	• The therapist will integrate knowledge from multiple sources to formulate a comprehensive description of prior work performance. • The therapist will reflect on prior practice and be able to identify strategies that have not been effective in the past.
Affective domain (appreciating and valuing)	• The therapist will document in a manner that reflects an appreciation for cultural influences on personal values related to worker identity. • The therapist demonstrates valuing the involvement of parents in the process of planning occupational therapy intervention by asking their opinions and using information-seeking behaviors.
Psychomotor domain (physical performance)	• The therapist will be able to attach and detach all basic attachments to a work simulator. • The therapist will be able to demonstrate proper lifting techniques to clients when lifting up to 50 pounds.
Ethical reasoning domain	• The therapist will be able to identify ethical principles and their relationship to reporting to Workers' Compensation payers, employers, and others. • The therapist will be able to identify limits in knowledge and understanding of ethical principles in order to know when to seek guidance from others.

practice (Gurvis & Grey, 1995). In most practice settings, a manager will have to identify a wide range of types of competencies related to the setting, the population seen, a variety of personnel and staffing processes, and specific interventions and types of equipment. This section provides a brief introduction to the most common types of competencies that must be assessed.

AGE-SPECIFIC COMPETENCIES

This category of competencies documents that employees have the knowledge and skills to work with a specific age group and that the special needs of age-specific populations are addressed when developing the job descriptions, orientation, performance appraisal tools, and competence assessment tools for the staff members who care for them

(Chai, 2003). For example, employees who work in a neonatal intensive care unit require one set of knowledge and skills specific to that age group, whereas employees who work with adolescents in an outpatient psychiatric program and those who work with older adults in a skilled nursing facility require different sets of knowledge and skills specific to those age groups. With the frequent shortages in occupational therapy personnel, it may be tempting to move experienced staff from one program to another to accommodate vacations, vacancies, or fluctuations in work volume. You must remember in those situations, however, that when staff is rotated to different units or programs and is asked to provide intervention to a different age group, staff members should be assessed on competencies for this new group before they intervene independently. Such age-specific competencies are a requirement of the JCAHO (Chai, 2003). The use of the following five-step method is recommended to help you meet this standard: (1) reflect age-specific competence when developing job descriptions, (2) reflect age-specific competence when developing performance appraisal tools, (3) develop age-specific competencies for specific job titles, (4) provide age-specific education and training, and (5) provide evidence of age-specific care. As suggested earlier, although you might most commonly implement a process such as that just described because of the regulations of an outside accrediting agency, assuring that staff members have the knowledge and can demonstrate competencies specifically related to the age group to which you assign them is a mark of ethical managerial practice in any setting.

EQUIPMENT-RELATED COMPETENCIES

Assessment of equipment-related competencies may overlap with other competencies and relates to performance of skills, knowledge, attitudes, or critical or ethical reasoning involved with the use of specific equipment. These competencies may be part of initial assessment of competencies in some settings (e.g., use of mobile arm supports on a spinal cord injury unit) or of assessment of specialized or advanced competencies in other settings (e.g., the use of a computerized work simulation unit or cognitive assessment of a person with a brain injury). When purchasing some types of equipment, especially if the cost is significant, vendors may be able to assist you with the development of competencies. Often training materials for the equipment may include tests or checklists that can be easily adapted.

SPECIALIZED PRACTICE COMPETENCIES AND ADVANCED PRACTICE COMPETENCIES

There is often confusion over the difference between *specialized practice competencies* and *advanced practice competencies*. Specialized competencies relate to abilities that are not expected to be reflected in the entry-level practice of all professionals but that do not require advanced clinical judgment, prior experience, or complex clinical reasoning in order to demonstrate competence. Specialized practice competencies require specific education and train-

ing but may not require the type of complex clinical reasoning only expected from an experienced practitioner. New graduates might be expected to demonstrate competencies related to specialized practice after appropriate training. An example of specialized practice might be the use of physical agent modalities such as ultrasound. Licensure laws and other forms of practice regulation vary from state to state as to whether the use of physical agent modalities is within the domain of occupational therapy practice. It is the position of the AOTA that "physical agent modalities may be used by an occupational therapist or occupational therapy assistant as an adjunct or preparation for intervention that ultimately enhances engagement in occupation" (AOTA, 2003). The AOTA further stipulates that "physical agent modalities may only be applied by occupational therapists and occupational therapy assistants who have documented evidence of possessing the theoretical background and technical skills for safe and competent integration of the modality into an occupational therapy intervention plan" (AOTA, 2003). Other examples of specialized practice competencies might relate to the provision of low vision services or wound care.

Advanced practice competencies are those that require complex critical reasoning based upon prior clinical experience not expected to be able to be demonstrated by entry-level practitioners. An example of advanced practice skills might be the application of advanced neurologic rehabilitation techniques that require the assessment and integration of complex knowledge and clinical judgments based on prior experience.

Employees who use specialized practice skills or advanced practice skills should be evaluated specifically for competencies in these skills. Documentation of assessment of these competencies should become a formal part of employee records. Because techniques and equipment change frequently, specialized or advanced practice competencies should be re-evaluated for appropriateness and be updated frequently.

COMPETENCIES RELATED TO SPECIFIC SKILLS OR PROCEDURES

In most settings, occupational therapists perform specific procedures related to the process of assessing and intervening with clients for which specific assessment of competencies might be appropriate. These differ from the specialized practice competencies just discussed in that it might be expected that any entry-level practitioner would be able to quickly learn to demonstrate these competencies without first undergoing extensive training or education. These competencies simply reflect the common types of interventions carried out in a specific setting. For example, in most pediatric settings, competencies related to the administration of standardized assessments to identify developmental milestones might be appropriate. In other settings, competencies related to procedures routinely performed, such as the fabrication of certain types of splints, serial casting, or procedures related to safety precautions (such as on a mental health unit), may be appropriate.

Reviews of job descriptions, documentation procedures, and common referrals are some simple ways to screen for common procedures for which you might develop competencies. Having experienced therapists keep simple time logs in which they note the primary activities in which they are involved and the common procedures that they complete is another way of identifying competencies for which assessments might be developed. You may also do a review in which you involve staff in identifying high-risk procedures or interventions that were not typically completed but are occurring more often to determine if any of these might be appropriate to incorporate in your system for assessment of competencies.

Documenting Assessment of Competencies

A critical part of any system for assessing competencies is to assure that the assessment results and any action taken if the results are not to full satisfaction are documented. You must realize that, as far as an accreditation reviewer or legal entity is concerned, assessments of competencies that are not documented in a permanent written format may as well not have occurred at all. Assessments of competencies should be documented by a formal and standardized method, and it is recommended that such documentation become a permanent part of each employee's personnel file (Braveman et al., 2004). Documentation of assessments of competencies may be completed in concert with or as part

of other elements of managerial documentation, including

- New employee orientation forms
- Annual performance appraisal forms
- Personnel development and in-service education plans and post-tests
- Staffing plans
- Quality control and improvement forms, including check sheets and audits

ELEMENTS OF EFFECTIVE DOCUMENTATION

Documentation of assessment of competencies should include the following elements:

- Written specific statements reflecting essential job functions that identify specific and measurable tasks or behaviors
- The method(s) to assess each competency
- The person(s) who assessed each competency
- The date(s) on which a competency was assessed
- An action plan for competencies for which the employee is deemed less than fully competent
- The date for the next assessment of the competency if it is to be repeated

One observation regarding establishing time frames for reassessment is that it is not uncommon for a therapist in a setting to go for long periods of time without completing a particular aspect of evaluation or intervention, and that skills can become rusty over time when not practiced. A potential mistake that can be made by a manager is assuming that, once a competency is demonstrated, it need not be repeated. That may be the case for skills that are used frequently, but may not hold true for other skills such as splinting, use of some types of equipment, or even transferring patients safely. Including some type of review of work assignments and the need for reassessment of competencies is highly recommended. A good time for such a review is at the annual employee performance appraisal.

Writing Assessment of Competencies Statements

The primary question you must be able to ask before beginning to write an effective assessment of competencies statements is "What is it that you expect a person to know or do in order to demonstrate the competency?" This question must be answered such that an assessment of competencies statement can be written in clear, concise, and unambiguous terms so both the person expected to demonstrate the competency and the person conducting the assessment interpret the competency statement in exactly the same way. There should be no doubt as to when performance is adequate and when continued practice or learning is required. Box 7–2 includes four criteria for evaluating assessment of competencies statements presented as part of the Competency Outcomes and Performance Assessment (COPA) model described in the nursing literature (Lenburg, 1999a).

Methods of Assessing Competencies

The methods of assessing various competencies must be matched to the domains of learning being evaluated (e.g., cognitive, affective, psychomotor, critical reasoning, and ethical reasoning). In most cases, the completion of a specific intervention may require competency in multiple domains, so the comprehensive assessment of competency may require that you develop multiple competency statements and consider assessing the competency using more than one strategy. The following information may guide you when choosing specific methods to assess competencies (Braveman et al., 2004).

Some competencies (e.g., CPR or responding to ethical dilemmas) may not easily be assessed in

"real-life" situations and may need to be assessed through case studies, role-playing, or drills that simulate situations that might be encountered. For example, you are likely familiar with fire drills or mock simulations of disasters to estimate the readiness of an organization or system to respond to an emergency. Similar exercises can be used as part of an assessment of competencies system.

Any assessment of competencies program should be based upon sound adult learning principles. Box 7–3 lists some of these principles.

A variety of methods can be used when assessing competencies, and each method has its advantages in terms of the resources needed for administration, such as the time it takes or whether you can assess one person or multiple persons at a time. These methods can be categorized into one of three types: (1) simulated tests, (2) objective tests, and (3) observational tests. Simulated tests usually involve a video presentation or a written scenario. The person being tested watches a videotape or reads the scenario and then answers questions. Objective tests can contain true-or-false, multiple choice, and matching questions. Observational tests require the person being tested to be observed by a skilled assessor in a natural setting, and these tests typically list observable, objective measures (Barney et al., 2000).

The method you choose for assessing competencies should match the domain of knowledge related to each competency. Whenever possible, you should use multiple methods to assure that you have adequately addressed each domain of performance. Table 7–3 lists a variety of methods for assessment of competencies and factors to consider in their use.

Table 7-3	Methods for Assessment of Competencies and Factors to Consider in Their Use
Post-tests (written tests, oral exams, or worksheets)	• Measure cognitive skills (an individual's comprehension of basic knowledge). • Ineffective to measure behavioral performance (psychomotor skills).
Return Demonstration (demonstrating a set of skills to another skilled assessor)	• Appropriate for measuring behavioral performance (psychomotor domain). • May occur in an artificial environment (skills lab) or in a real-world setting. • Must go beyond description—describing an action may reflect the cognitive domain (knowing), but performance is required to assess competencies in the psychomotor domain. • Most effective if a standard set of criteria for evaluation (competency checklist) is used. • The assessor must be familiar with the criteria for evaluation and have demonstrated the indicated competency to another trained assessor.
Observation of Daily Work	• Appropriate for measuring skills in the psychomotor and affective domains. • Both supervisors and peers can be used for these types of observation.
Case Studies (provide individuals with a situation and ask them to explain their responses or choices in that situation)	• Appropriate for assessing critical thinking skills. • Manager or supervisor must create a check sheet or other evaluation tool to document specific competencies that are based on predetermined criteria related to the case content. • Can be prepared in many different ways • Can be used with individuals or discussion groups to facilitate team building and group problem solving.
Exemplars (a story describing a situation you have experienced or describing a rationale you thought about and choices you made in a situation)	• Appropriate to measure critical thinking skills and interpersonal skills. • Captures actions NOT taken as well as those chosen. • Appropriate for use with a variety of personnel, including staff and leadership. • Very useful for personnel who must establish trust with a client, provide customer service, or deal with sensitive issues.
Peer Reviews	• Appropriate for assessment of interpersonal skills and critical thinking skills. • Staff should be prepared via a thorough orientation to the process, including suggestions for giving constructive feedback so that receiving feedback from peers is viewed as a positive experience. • May use a written format or verbal "face-to-face" format.
Self-assessment	• Appropriate for assessment of critical thinking skills. • Appropriate for assessment of values, beliefs, opinions, and attitudes because it engages the individual in a reflective exercise that allows him or her to put into words his or her conscious and unconscious thoughts. • Has limited utility for assessment of psychomotor skills, and an additional method should always be used for high-risk procedures or skills that could result in harm to patients or clients.

Synthesizing Assessment of Competencies and Documentation

Developing an effective and comprehensive system for assessment of competencies requires that you identify categories of competencies, develop appropriate competency statements, match appropriate assessment methods to each competency, and select a method of documenting the results of the assessment and follow-up of actions taken if the result of the assessment of competencies is not satisfactory.

Table 7–4 includes examples to illustrate how a sample of categories of competencies, specific competency statements, methods of assessing competencies, and documenting assessment are combined. Sample forms for the documentation of the assessment of competencies are included as appendices at the end of this chapter.

Managerial Competencies

To this point, our discussion has focused primarily on competency and the assessment of competencies for those you might supervise. In addition, you may have asked the question "What about my competency as an occupational therapy manager?" Although the assessment of competencies for managers has not received the same attention by bodies such as accrediting agencies, competency development and the assessment of competencies

Table 7-4	Examples of Synthesis of Assessment and Documentation of Competencies		
Category of Competency	Example of Competency Standard	Example of Assessment Method(s)	Documentation Methodology
Initial evaluation of competence	Accurately reads a cardiac rehabilitation patient's blood pressure before engaging the patient in activities of daily living	• Observation by supervisor using a check sheet • Check of accuracy by supervisor, who also takes the patient's blood pressure	Checklist of initial competencies and observation form showing "competent" or need for intervention and action taken is dated and placed in file.
Annual evaluation of competence	Is able to state the steps taken if a fire occurs in a patient area with patients present	• Watch a videotape combined with a post-test • Mock drills twice yearly	Copy of post-test placed in personnel record signed by qualified reviewer. Results of drills reviewed at staff meeting.
Age-related competence	Identifies physical and cognitive changes experienced during puberty	• Written test based upon a filmed case • Verbal discussion after assessment of adolescent with peers using a check sheet	Test results and peer evaluation form signed by employee, observer, and supervisor, including any intervention plan placed in the personnel file.
Equipment-related competence	Completes monthly safety check of fluidotherapy machine	Self-review using checklist	Checklist turned into supervisor and placed in personnel record.
Physical agent modality competence	Identifies all contraindications for use of heat and cold	Post-test after training module	Copy of post-test placed in personnel record, signed by qualified reviewer.

for managers have been addressed by a number of professions and some empirical investigation of managerial competencies has been conducted. This information is useful in considering the major areas in which specific managerial competencies might be developed or for conducting self-assessment of managerial competencies as part of a professional development plan.

Some competencies might be considered "universal" for managers. One traditional method of identifying competencies is to use the commonly identified managerial functions (e.g., planning, organizing and staffing, directing, and controlling) as a guide. For example, Box 7–4 lists these traditional management functions and the related categories of competencies identified by Anderson and Pulich (2002). Other managerial competencies will be more dependent upon the nature of your job. Just as you would identify competencies specific to any clinical environment, some competencies for the occupational therapy manager will need to be developed with the specific organizational context in mind.

Competencies cannot be isolated from the institutional surroundings and must be defined by taking day-to-day "real-life" behavior into account (Noordegraaf, 2000). They should reflect the nature of what you do in the course of everyday work, including some of the activities that might be taken for granted. For example, most managers would agree that they spend a tremendous amount of their time in meetings. Running effective meetings, recognizing the power dynamics of meetings, preparing adequately and differently depending on the type and agenda of a meeting, or even organizing a room or seating to affect interactions in a meeting are all examples of competencies that you might identify for yourself as a manager.

Another way of considering competencies for managers is to distinguish between what have been referred to as *threshold competencies* and *high-performance competencies*. This approach draws on the work of McClelland and Boyatzis described earlier. A threshold competency is a cluster of related behaviors that is used by managers but that has not been empirically associated with superior job performance. A high-performance managerial competency is a cluster of related behaviors that has been found empirically to distinguish high-performing from average-performing managers (Cockerill,

---

Box 7–4: Traditional Management Functions and Managerial Competencies

Planning
- Use of goal setting
- Understanding the changing health care environment
- Making effective decisions

Organizing and Staffing
- Understanding team structure and flexible work design
- Using cooperation techniques
- Applying coordination techniques

Directing
- Interpersonal competencies
  - Communication skills
  - Communicating with the boss
  - Communicating with peers and others
  - Communicating with employees
  - Being politically astute
  - Managing conflict
  - Managing diversity
- Role model competencies
  - Demonstrating professionalism in conduct and demeanor
  - Enhancing technical competence

Controlling
- Using employee empowerment
- Applying continuous quality improvement efforts

Adapted from Anderson, P., & Pulich, M. (2002). Managerial competencies necessary in today's dynamic health care environment. *The Health Care Manager*, *21*, 1–11.

Hunt, & Schroder, 1995). An example of a threshold competency might be "concern with close relationships," or spending time with subordinates, whereas an example of a high-performance competency would be "concept formation," or building frameworks and models or ideas on the basis of information to become aware of patterns and cause-and-effect relationships. Table 7–5 lists 11 sets of

Table 7-5	High–Performance Managerial Competencies
Information search	Gathers many different kinds of information and uses a wide variety of sources to build a rich informational environment in preparation for decision making in the organization.
Concept formation	Builds frameworks or models or forms concepts, hypotheses, or ideas on the basis of information; becomes aware of patterns, trends, and cause-and-effect relations by linking disparate information.
Conceptual flexibility	Identifies feasible alternatives or multiple options in planning and decision making; holds different options in focus simultaneously and evaluates their pros and cons.
Interpersonal search	Uses open and probing questions, summaries, paraphrasing, etc. to understand the ideas, concepts, and feeling of another; can comprehend events, issues, problems, and opportunities from the viewpoint of others.
Managing interaction	Involves others and is able to build cooperative teams in which group members feel valued and empowered and have shared goals.
Developmental orientation	Creates a positive climate in which staff members increase the accuracy of their own awareness of their own strengths and limitations; provides coaching, training, and developmental resources to improve performance.
Impact	Uses a variety of methods (e.g., persuasive arguments, modeling behavior, inventing symbols, forming alliances, and appealing to the interest of others) to gain support for ideas and strategies and values.
Self-confidence	States own "stand" or position on issues; unhesitatingly makes decisions when required and commits self and others accordingly; expresses confidence in the future success of the actions to be taken.
Presentation	Presents ideas clearly, with ease and interest, so that the other person (or audience) understands what is being communicated; uses technical, symbolic, nonverbal, and visual aids effectively.
Proactive orientation	Structures the task for the team; implements plans and ideas; takes responsibility for all aspects of the situation even beyond ordinary boundaries—and for the success and failure of the group.
Achievement orientation	Possesses high internal work standards and sets ambitious, risky, and yet attainable goals; wants to do things better, to improve, to be more effective and efficient; measures progress against targets.

From Cockerill, T., Hunt, J., & Schroder, H. (1995). Managerial competencies: Fact or fiction? *Business Strategy Review, 6,* 1–12, with permission.

competencies identified by Cockerill et al. (1995) that have been empirically shown to correlate with high-performance management. Although high-performance management and average-performance management have been distinguished based on empirical evidence in the business literature, not all managerial behaviors have been empirically investigated, especially as they relate to health care settings. Using the underlying schema on your own to identify behaviors that separate high-performing managers from average performers in your organization may be useful as part of a self-assessment process to identify competencies that you desire to achieve.

Specialty and Advanced (Board) Certifications

Another form of indicating competency is obtaining specialty or advanced certifications. As described earlier, specialty practice relates to practice that requires specific training or education that is not expected to be part of all entry-level education, whereas advanced practice requires reliance on experience or advanced clinical or critical reasoning that would not be expected of any new graduate. Such certifications may be offered within a discipline such that only members of a specific profession are eligible for the certification.

For example, the AOTA is pursuing development of both specialty certifications and advanced (board) certifications for occupational therapists. The specialty certifications are relevant to the scope of occupational therapy practice and reflect a defined set of skills, techniques, and interventions. Areas appropriate for specialty certification include, among others, cognitive intervention, community mobility and driving, early intervention, feeding and swallowing, and low vision intervention. Advanced or board certifications reflect a major domain of practice with an established knowledge base in occupational therapy and reflect the scope of occupational therapy. Areas appropriate for advanced certification include, among others, pediatrics, gerontology, rehabilitation, and mental health (AOTA Specialties Board, 2004; Glantz, 2003).

Other certifications serve the same purpose but are open to persons from more than one professional discipline as long as they meet the criteria for the certification. For example, the American Society of Hand Therapists (ASHT) is a professional organization composed of licensed occupational and physical therapists, some of whom have earned the advanced designation Certified Hand Therapist (CHT) and who specialize in the treatment and rehabilitation of the upper extremity. The mission of the ASHT is "to advance the specialty of hand therapy through communication, education, research, and the establishment of clinical standards" (ASHT, 2003).

The ASHT certification process includes the following requirements:

- Documentation of 5 years of practice as an occupational therapist or physical therapist

- A copy of a current professional credential to practice in the United States, Canada, Great Britain, Australia, or New Zealand
- Documentation of 4000 hours of Direct Practice Experience in Hand Therapy, verified by a supervisor or employer
- A passing score on the certification examination

Although specialty and advanced certifications have become more common and are indeed indicators that practitioners have completed learning or practice experiences, they should not automatically be accepted as the sole indicator of competency. Credentials such as specialty or advanced certification are indicators of what an individual *should* be able to do and not what that individual *can* or *will* do (Redd & Alexander, 1997). Assessment of competencies should not automatically be waived simply because an individual has a certification.

Chapter Summary

This chapter introduced you to the concepts of competency, assessment of competencies, and continued competence and the critical role that the occupational therapy manager plays in the process of assessing and documenting competencies. You learned that numerous regulatory, certification, and professional bodies and organizations play a role in protecting the public by requiring assessment of competency using a variety of strategies. These strategies include initial certification of entry-level practitioners by the NBCOT, requirements for professional development to promote continued competency by the NBCOT and state regulatory boards, standards related to assessment of competencies by accrediting bodies including the JCAHO and the CARF, and specialty or advanced certification through professional associations such as the AOTA or the ASHT.

At the beginning of the chapter, you were introduced to Emily, who was an occupational therapy assistant with more than 20 years of experience who had just started a new job. Emily was surprised at the formal orientation she was expected to undergo, especially the amount of time she was asked to spend reviewing basic aspects of care such as hand washing and conducting skin checks for patients with spinal cord injury. Emily had decided to

Real-Life Solutions

Emily met with her supervisor as planned for their weekly supervision session. During the session she expressed her concern over the length of time and the amount of energy that were being spent in assessment of competencies as part of her orientation. Emily explained that she had been working for more than 20 years and had worked in close collaboration with the occupational therapists in her last job. She had established service competency with her supervisor and had been independently completing standard parts of patient evaluations and was certainly prepared to do the same in this facility. She also admitted to her supervisor that she was somewhat offended that her skills were not being better utilized given the high caseloads in the facility and that the department had several vacancies.

Emily's supervisor, Joan, began by thanking Emily for her concern over helping to meet the department's patient care needs. She shared that she, too, was very worried over how the department was going to handle its work given the vacancies on the staff. Joan also assured Emily that she had no concerns over Emily's skill level or whether or not she was a competent occupational therapy as-

sistant. She told Emily that she and the other occupational therapists on the spinal cord injury staff were confident in Emily's skills but that prior experience and even glowing reports from other occupational therapists could not be substituted for formal assessment of competencies. In addition to legal, licensure, and accreditation concerns, Joan saw the assessment of competencies system as an important indication of the level of professionalism and concern for quality care shared by the organization's leadership.

Joan provided Emily some readings on competency, assessment of competencies, and continued competency to help her become more familiar with how the concepts were related to each other and to other management functions. As Joan and Emily discussed Emily's concerns and experiences, they realized that all of the staff could benefit from additional information, and Joan enlisted Emily's help to develop an in-service presentation for the staff. After their discussions, although Emily remained concerned about increasing her contributions to the team as quickly as possible, she felt more comfortable that the time being taken to assess her level of competence should not be taken personally.

express her dissatisfaction at the level of scrutiny that she was under and the amount of attention that was being paid to her competency.

Resources for Learning More About Assessment of Competencies and Continued Competency

Journals That Often Address Assessment of Competencies and Continued Competence

NURSING MANAGEMENT

Nursing Management is a monthly journal that focuses on applied strategies and educational information for nursing managers. Topics included in the publication include legal and ethical aspects of nursing leadership to personnel management, recruitment and retention, budget issues, product selection, and quality control. While focused on

management in nursing, many articles address issues and topics of concern to managers in any area of health care including staff development, health care policy and the like.

JOURNAL FOR HEALTHCARE QUALITY

The *Journal for Healthcare Quality* targets health care quality professionals who are responsible for promoting and monitoring quality, safe, evidence-based, cost-effective health care as its audience. Published articles focus on a variety of management related topics including accreditation issues and successes, administration/ management, behavioral health care quality, compliance, confidentiality, evidence-based practice, government affairs and policy making, information systems and management, health care innovations, knowledge management, performance measurement and improvement, and health care quality research. Additional monthly columns provide reviews and announcements of Internet sites, reports on conferences and other resources. The journal provides coverage of state-of-the-art technology, quality management techniques, practical applications of quality improvement systems, and new and emerging trends and innovations.

Organizations and Associations Concerned with Assessment of Competencies and Continued Competence

JOINT COMMISSION ON ACCREDITATION OF HEALTHCARE ORGANIZATIONS

http://www.jcaho.org/
The mission of the JCAHO is to continuously improve the safety and quality of care provided to the public through the provision of health care accreditation and related services that support performance improvement in health care organizations. The JCAHO publishes standards related to competency in numerous health care settings and publishes resources on promoting competency and quality care.

COMMISSION ON ACCREDITATION OF REHABILITATION FACILITIES

http://www.carf.org/
The mission of the CARF is to promote the quality, value, and optimal outcomes of services through a consultative accreditation process that centers on enhancing the lives of the persons served. The CARF publishes standards related to competency in a variety of rehabilitation settings.

NATIONAL BOARD FOR CERTIFICATION IN OCCUPATIONAL THERAPY, INC.

http://www.nbcot.org
The NBCOT is a not-for-profit credentialing agency responsible for certification for the occupational therapy profession. The NBCOT develops, administers, and continually reviews a certification process that reflects current standards of entry-level practice in occupational therapy. It also works with state regulatory authorities, providing information on credentials, disciplinary actions, and regulatory and certification renewal issues. The NBCOT is responsible for establishing initial competency through its certification examination and has requirements for maintaining certification related to continuing education to promote continued competency.

AMERICAN SOCIETY FOR TRAINING AND DEVELOPMENT

http://www.astd.org/astd/
The ASTD is an association for human resources professionals and other fields related to training and development of employees. ASTD members represent multinational corporations, medium-sized and small businesses, government, academia, consulting firms, and product and service suppliers. Assessment of competency is a concern of human resources professionals in various fields. The ASTD publishes *T + D Magazine* and includes issues related to assessment of competency and a wide range of other topics relevant to managers.

Reference List

Alsop, A. (2001). Competence unfurled: Developing portfolio practice. *Occupational Therapy International, 8,* 126–131.

American Occupational Therapy Association. (1999a). Definitions of types of regulation for occupational therapy. AOTA State Policy Department, AOTA Web site. Available at *http://www.aota.org/*

American Occupational Therapy Association. (1999b). Standards for continuing competence. *American Journal of Occupational Therapy, 53,* 599–600.

American Occupational Therapy Association. (2003). Physical agent modalities: A position paper. American Occupational Therapy Association Web site. Available at *http://www.aota.org/*

American Occupational Therapy Association. (2004). State occupational therapy statutes and regulations. American Occupational Therapy Association Web site. Available at *http://www.aota.org/members/area4/links/link12.asp?PLACE=/members/area4/links/LINK12.asp*

American Occupational Therapy Association Specialties Board. (2004). *Panel reports on areas for certification.* Bethesda, MD: American Occupational Therapy Association.

American Society of Hand Therapists. (2003). About ASHT. American Society of Hand Therapists Web site. Available at *http://www.asht.org/geninfo.html*

Anderson, P., & Pulich, M. (2002). Managerial competencies necessary in today's dynamic health care environment. *The Health Care Manager, 21,* 1–11.

Barney, J. D., Long, K. G., McCall, E., Watts, J. H., & Cash, S. H. (2000). National call to test for competence: Strategies for clinical managers. *Administrative and Management Special Interest Section Quarterly, 16,* 1–3.

Benner, P. (1984). *From novice to expert.* Menlo Park, CA: Addison-Wesley.

Benner, P., Tanner, C., & Chesla, C. (1992). From beginner to expert: gaining a differentiated clinical world in critical care nursing. *Advances in Nursing Science, 14,* 13–28.

Boyatzis, R. E. (1982). *The competent manager: A model for effective performance.* New York: John Wiley & Sons.

Braveman, B., Gentile, P. A., Stafford, J., Berthelette, M., & Learnard, L. (2004). A guide for managers and supervisors to develop a system for assessment of competencies. The American Occupational Therapy Association Web site. Available at *http://www.aota.org/*

Burkhardt, A., Braveman, B., & Gentile, P. (2000). Evaluating and documenting staff competence for accreditation reviews and staff development. *AMSIS Quarterly,* 18, 4, 1–6. Bethesda, MD: AOTA.

Chai, K. (2003). *Age-specific competence...amended to comply with 2003 JCAHO standards.* Glendale, CA: CINAHL Information Systems.

Cockerill, T., Hunt, J., & Schroder, H. (1995). Managerial competencies: Fact or fiction? *Business Strategy Review,* 6, 1–12.

Crook, J. A. (2001). How do expert mental health nurses make on-the-spot clinical decisions? A review of the literature. *Journal of Psychiatric and Mental Health Nursing,* 8, 1–5.

DeLisa, J. A. (2000). Certifying and measuring competency in the United States. *Archives of Physical Medicine and Rehabilitation,* 81, 1236–1241.

Dreyfus, S. E. (1981). *Four models v. human situational understanding: Inherent limitations on the modeling of business expertise* (Air Force Office of Scientific Research, USAF Contract F49620-79-C-0063). Unpublished manuscript, University of California, Berkeley.

Driscoll, J. W. (2002). Paradigms for assessment: Women's knowledge and skill attainment. *The American Journal of Maternal/Child Nursing,* 27, 288–293.

Glantz, C. (2003). Update on AOTA certification initiatives. OT Practice Online, American Occupational Therapy Association Web site. Available at *http://www.aota.org/featured/area2/links/link16hf.asp?PLACE=/featured/area2/links/link16hf.asp*

Green, N. (2004, February 9). Demand and recruitment. *OT Practice,* 49.

Gronlund, N. E., & Linn, R. L. (1990). *Measurement and evaluation in teaching* (6th ed.). New York: Macmillan.

Grossman, J. (1998). Continuing competence in the health professions. *American Journal of Occupational Therapy,* 52, 709–715.

Gurvis, J. P., & Grey, M. T. (1995). The anatomy of a competency. *Journal of Nursing Staff Development,* 11, 247–252.

Hargreaves J., & Lane, D. (2001). Delya's story: From expert to novice, a critique of Benner's concept of context in the development of expert nursing practice. *International Journal of Nursing Studies,* 38, 389–394.

Hinojosa, J., Bowen, R., Case-Smith, J., Epstein, C., Moyers, P., & Schwope, C. (2000). Self-initiated continuing competence. The American Occupational Therapy Association Web site. Available at *http://www.aota.org/*

Jansen, J., Grol, R. C. H., Rethans, J., & Vleuten, C. (1998). Failure of feedback to enhance self-assessment skills of general practitioners. *Teaching and Learning in Medicine,* 10, 145–151.

Joint Commission on Accreditation of Healthcare Organizations. (2004). Human resource standards applicability to contracted and volunteer personnel. Joint Commission on Accreditation of Healthcare Organizations Web site. Available at *http://www.jcaho.org/accredited+organizations/hospitals/standards/hospital+faqs/manage+human+res/planning/human+resource+standards+applicability+to+contracted+and+volunteer+personnel.htm*

Kierstead, J. (1998). Competencies and KSAO's. Public Service Commission of Canada Web site. Available at *http://www.psc-cfp.gc.ca/research/personnel/comp_ksao_e.pdf*

Krozek, C., & Scroggins, A. (1999a). *Competencies for all positions—hospital wide.* Glendale, CA, CINAHL Information Systems.

Krozek, C., & Scroggins, A. (1999b). *Employee competency assessment tool.* Glendale, CA: CINAHL Information Systems.

Kruger, J., & Dunning, D. (1999). Unskilled and unaware of it: How difficulties in recognizing one's own incompetence lead to inflated self-assessments. *Journal of Personality and Social Psychology,* 77, 1121–1134.

LaDuke, S. D. (2001). The role of staff development in assuring competence. *Journal for Nurses in Staff Development,* 15, 221–225.

Leach, D. (2002). Building and assessing competence: The potential for evidence-based graduate medical education. *Quality Management in Health Care,* 11, 39–44.

Lenburg, C. B. (1999a). The framework, concepts and methods of the competency outcomes and performance assessment (COPA) model. *Online Journal of Issues in Nursing.* Available at *http://nursingworld.org/ojin/topic10/tcp10_2.htm*

Lenburg, C. B. (1999b). Redesigning expectations for initial and continuing competence for contemporary nursing practice. *Online Journal of Issues in Nursing.* Available at *http://nursingworld.org/ojin.topic10/tcp10_1.htm*

Manley, K., & Garbett, R. (2000). Paying Peter and Paul: Reconciling concepts of expertise with competency for a clinical career structure. *Journal of Clinical Nursing,* 9, 347–359.

Maynard, C. A. (1991). *The relationship of critical thinking ability, stage of skill acquisition, years of practice, and organizational context to professional nursing competence.* Unpublished manuscript, University of Minnesota, Minneapolis.

McConnell, E. A. (2001). Manager's fast track: Competence v. competency. *Nursing Management,* 32(5), 14.

Meretoja, R., & Leino-Kilpi, H. (2003). Comparison of competence assessments made by nurse managers and practicing nurses. *Journal of Nursing Management,* 11, 404–409.

National Board for Certification in Occupational Therapy, Inc. (2003). NBCOT principles and missions. National Board for Certification in Occupational Therapy, Inc. Web site. Available at *http://www.nbcot.org*

National Board for Certification in Occupational Therapy, Inc. (2004a, Spring). NBCOT 2003 practice analysis. *Report to the Profession,* pp. 4–5.

National Board for Certification in Occupational Therapy, Inc. (2004b). Professional development requirements. National Board for Certification in Occupational Therapy, Inc. Web site. Available at *http://www.nbcot.org/webarticles/anmviewer.asp?a=55&z=13*

Nichol, M. J., Fox-Hiley, A., Bavin, C. J., & Sheng, R. (1996). Assessment of clinical and communication skills: Operationalizing Benner's model. *Nurse Education Today,* 16, 175–179.

Noordegraaf, M. (2000). Professional sense-makers: Managerial competencies amidst ambiguity. *Journal of Public Sector Management,* 13, 319–332.

Nuccio, S. A., Lingen, D., Burke, L. J., Kramer, A., Ladewig, N., & Raaum, J. S. B. (1996). The clinical practice development model: The transition process. *Journal of Nursing Administration, 26,* 29–37.

Redd, M. L., & Alexander, J. W. (1997). Does certification mean better performance? *Nursing Management, 28,* 45–49.

Redman, R. W., Lenburg, C. B., & Hinton-Walker, P. (1999, September 30). Competency assessment: Methods for development and implementation in nursing education. *Online Journal of Issues in Nursing.* Available at *http://nursing-world.org/ojin.topic10/tcp10_3.htm*

Smith, K., & Tillema, H. H. (1998). Evaluating portfolio use as a learning tool for professionals. *Scandinavian Journal of Educational Research, 41,* 193–205.

Smith, K., & Tillema, H. H. (2001). Long-term influences of portfolios on professional development. *Scandinavian Journal of Educational Research, 45,* 183–203.

Smith, P., Schiller, M. R., Grant, K., & Sachs, L. (1995). Recruitment and retention strategies used by occupational therapy directors in acute care, rehabilitation, and long-term-care settings. *American Journal of Occupational Therapy, 49,* 412–419.

Spalding, N. (2000). The skill acquisition of two newly qualified occupational therapists. *British Journal of Occupational Therapy, 63,* 389–395.

Spencer, L. M., & Spencer, S. M. (1993). *Competence at work.* New York: John Wiley & Sons.

Tillema, H. H. (2001). Portfolios as developmental assessment tools. *International Journal of Training and Development, 5,* 126–135.

Weinstein, S. M. (2000). Certification and credentialing to define competency-based practice. *Journal of IV Nursing, 23,* 21–32.

Winchcombe, J. (2000). Competency standards in the context of infection control. *American Journal of Infection Control, 28,* 228–232.

Winsor, P., Butt, R. L., & Reeves, H. (1999). Portraying professional development in preservice teacher education. *Teachers and Teaching, 5,* 9–33.

Appendix 7–1: Sample Form for Assessment of Competency

Department of Occupational Therapy
Physical Agent Modality Assessment of Competency: Hot Packs

Name: _____   Date: _____

Reviewer: _____

Method of Assessment: Direct Observation by Skilled Reviewer

A.	SELECTION	YES	NO	N/A	COMMENTS
1.	Verbalizes clinical rationale for use of modality				
2.	Verbalizes contraindications for use of modality				
B.	**APPLICATION**	YES	NO	N/A	COMMENTS
1.	Conducts skin check and assesses patient sensation				
2.	Orients patient to use of hot pack, including process, impact, and complications				
3.	Matches size of pack to body part				
4.	Uses towels to wrap hot pack to sufficiently guard against burn				
5.	Positions patients for comfort and to assure that pack remains in place				
6.	Drapes hot pack correctly onto body part				
7.	Documents time of start of application and provides instruction to patient				
8.	Checks patient's skin within minutes of application				
9.	Adjusts hot pack if necessary when conducting skin check				
10.	Removes hot pack in timely manner				
11.	Checks skin within 2 minutes of removing hot pack and informs patient of outcomes				
12.	Checks impact of treatment on patient				
C.	**DOCUMENTATION**	YES	NO	N/A	COMMENTS
1.	Documents use of modality in medical record				
2.	Documentation includes reference to preparation for participation in occupational behavior				
3.	Documentation includes start time, end time, and length of treatment				
4.	Documentation includes reference to patient response and impact of treatment				

COMPETENCY MET: ☐ yes ☐ no

If no, document action plan on reverse of form and instruct staff member not to use modality unsupervised until competency is met.

Reviewer's Signature: _____

Staff Signature: _____

Appendix 7–2: Sample Form for Annual Assessment of Competencies

Department of Occupational Therapy

Competency	High Risk	High Volume	Problem Prone	Link to Quality Plan	Professional Standard	Assessment Method
Mandatory All Employees						
Patient Confidentiality (HIPAA)	X					
Fire Safety	X					
Electrical Safety	X					
Hazard Communication	X					
Infection Control	X					
Emergency Management	X					
Mandatory Patient Contact						
CPR						
Age-Specific Care						
TB Test						
Signs of Abuse						
Restraints						
Blood-Borne Pathogens						
Job Specific Annual Competencies						

Annual Assessment of Competencies
(To be completed and filed as part of Annual Employee Performance Appraisal)

Assessment Method Key:

1. Return Demonstration
2. Cognitive Test
3. Observation

4. Peer Review
5. Chart Review/Audit
6. Other

Employee Signature: _____

Supervisor Signature: _____

Appendix 7–3: Sample Form for Documentation of Assessment of Competencies

Organization Employee Competency Assessment

_____ (UNIT)

NAME: _____   JOB POSITION: _____   HIRE DATE: _____

COMPETENCY	SELF-ASSESSMENT			ACTION PLAN			VALIDATION			
Standard of Care, Practice, Procedure, Equipment, or Skill	0 = Never Done 1 = Need Review 2 = Can Perform Without Review			Minimal Level of Planned Activity LEARN P&P = Review Policies and Procedures C = Attend Class V = Video/Self Learning Packet		VALIDATE 1 = Once Only A = Annually	This is to certify that the above individual is competent (able to perform task safely and correctly) as demonstrated in a simulated or practice setting. VALIDATOR = Enter Date and Signature			
	0	1	2	LEARN/PRACTICE	VALIDATE	TARGET DATE	FIRST VALIDATION	RENEWAL	RENEWAL	RENEWAL
A.										
B.										
C.										
D.										
E.										

From Krozek, C., & Scoggins, A. (1999). _Employee competency assessment tool._ Glendale, CA: CINAHL Information Systems.

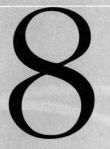

CHAPTER

8

Brent Braveman, Ph.D., OTR/L, FAOTA

Managing Change and Solving Problems

Real-Life Management

As an occupational therapy manager with 3 years of management and supervisory experience, I accepted the job of Director of Clinical Services for Occupational Therapy for a large academic medical center. The occupational therapy staff at the center had been through tremendous changes in the years just before I arrived. Two years earlier, a decision had been made to merge the medical center with another hospital and to close the facility in which the staff members were located; then, after many of the staff had resigned and taken jobs elsewhere, the decision was reversed and it was decided to keep the facility open. In addition, I was the third Director of Clinical Services hired in a period of a few years.

As a new director entering a department in turmoil, I had numerous concerns about policies, procedures, and expectations of staff that I felt needed to be addressed right away. I was excited about the opportunity to work with the staff mem-

bers and the organization to rebuild the department and came armed with many ideas about how to begin the process. Although my enthusiasm and optimism were appreciated by the staff members, my plans to introduce additional changes to the department were not!

As I began to introduce new policies, procedures, and increased performance expectations for staff, I encountered varying levels of resistance. I found it very confusing that the staff had many complaints about the current state of the department but resisted the efforts I was making to respond to those concerns. I had been introduced to theories and models of "change management" in graduate school but had not made any explicit use of the information. I decided to review the information and to explore and learn more about strategies that I could use to foster change and decrease the resistance that I was experiencing.

Key Issues

- Managers are concerned with creating, fostering, and managing change within individuals, groups, departments, and entire organizations.
- Solving problems includes *problem setting*, or naming the prob-

lem to be solved as specifically as possible, and then choosing different strategies to help with different parts of the problem-solving process.
- Managers are often under pressure to solve problems quickly,

but effective problem solving requires gathering data, information, and other forms of evidence to guide decision making.

Undoubtedly you have heard someone say, "Change is the only constant." In health care, this often seems to be the case. Occupational therapy personnel and other health care practitioners face almost constant changes within the organizations in which they work. Change also frequently occurs within the local, state, and national environments in terms of legislative and reimbursement policy, and within the many health care professions as views on practice shift. Sometimes it seems difficult to keep up with the rate of change. For example, in occupational therapy, the requirement for entry-level education for occupational therapists has changed so that all educational programs must be at the post-baccalaureate level by the year 2007. Yet, even before many educational programs made that change, much discussion and focus on education within the profession shifted to discussion of clinical doctoral programs and whether that should be the mandated entry-level education for occupational therapists. Clinical doctoral programs, or "OTD" programs, are indeed being introduced at universities all over the country.

As an occupational therapy manager, you will be responsible not only for responding to change within your department and your organization, and the range of external influences that affect your organization, but also for facilitating and creating change. The term *change management* has often been used to describe this function. Literature on change addresses four principle aspects of change management: (1) theoretical models and frameworks that reveal and guide organization members' and researchers' thinking about organizational change, (2) approaches and tools for creating and managing change, (3) factors important to successful change management, and (4) the outcomes and consequences of the process of change management (Branch, 2002). In addition, literature and empirical research on change have addressed change in terms of the individual both at the level of the work group or team, and at the level of the organization.

Scholarship related to change has included the development of a number of models for explaining how change occurs in individuals, groups, and organizations and models for creating change. Major areas of empirical investigation related to change have included change within organizations, promoting change or acting as a change agent, and resistance to change. Solving problems is often involved in creating and managing change, and scholarship on this topic has included investigation of effective negotiation strategies and clinical and procedural reasoning in the health professions as well as in business and economics literature.

The idea that managers should "make decisions based upon data and information" is commonly discussed; almost to the point of being taken for granted. However, many managers might admit to feeling pressured to make decisions and solve problems quickly regardless of the amount or accuracy of the data or information they have to guide these processes. Unfortunately, making decisions quickly rather than making quality decisions is what is taken as the sign of a skilled manager and rewarded all too often. The skills related to finding and evaluating evidence are critical for effectively managing change and solving problems. This chapter will focus on knowledge and strategies related specifically to fostering and managing change and on strategies to help solve problems.

Layers of Change

When you consider the topic of change and management, you should recognize that change can occur within multiple layers of the environments in which we interact. Consider the figure first shown in Chapter 3 representing organizations as open systems (shown again in Figure 8–1). Figures similar to this have been used to represent individuals in society as well as larger organizational systems themselves. If we view an individual as an open system, then we must recognize that the input, throughput, and output relate to change within that person just as they relate to change within organizations.

Occupational therapists and occupational therapy assistants are typically concerned with facilitating some type of change for, and within, the individuals with whom we work. Occupational therapy managers are concerned with change both within individuals (i.e., staff development) and within larger organizational units such as a therapy department.

A number of models have been presented within the public health literature that address change within individuals as it relates to *health behaviors*

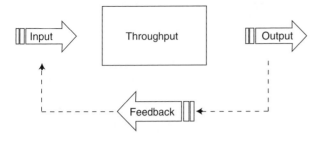

- Input for the individual may be information, experiences, or observations

- Throughput involves the processing of information and experiences, including health-related information

- Output may include health behaviors such as starting, stopping, or continuing a behavior that may improve or negatively affect health status

Figure 8–1 Individual as an open system.

(e.g., starting, stopping, or continuing to perform some health-related act). Health behaviors are many of the behaviors that we choose to perform or avoid in the course of our daily lives that have a positive or negative effect on our health. For example, each of the following would be considered a health behavior:

- Starting to exercise
- Stopping smoking
- Continuing to eat a well-balanced diet

These models are reviewed in Chapter 9 because they are often used when developing occupational therapy programming. The most relevant of these models to change management is the *transtheoretical model of change*, in which change behavior is considered through a series of stages (Prochaska & DiClemente, 1993). This model has most often been applied to understanding how change occurs in discrete health behaviors but can be useful in providing a general framework for considering how other change processes occur in people's behavior. The five stages are presented in Box 8–1.

In this chapter, as we consider change, we will focus on change theory and models as they relate to accepting or adopting new behaviors, practices, or systems within the work environment whether in regard to an individual, a department, or a work unit such as an interdisciplinary team, or an entire organization.

Bennis, Benne, and Chin (1985) identified three strategies for fostering individual change that are still commonly cited in the literature. These strategies are (1) educative/empirical-rational, (2) normative/persuasive, and (3) power-coercive. These strategies and examples of each are presented in Box 8–2 as applied to a common problem faced by occupational therapy managers in medical-model settings: convincing staff to adopt practices related to charging for services provided and to documenting those services.

Box 8–1: The Five Stages of Change

- **Precontemplation:** Individuals are unaware or underaware of a problem or the need to change.
- **Contemplation:** Individuals are aware of a problem and the need to change and considering taking action, but have made no commitment to any specific action.
- **Preparation:** Intention to begin change is combined with criteria for action that include a time frame to begin acting.
- **Action:** Individuals attempt to incorporate new behavior into their routine.
- **Maintenance:** New behaviors are successfully incorporated into daily routines so that the behaviors become habitual.

Adapted from Prochaska, J. O., & DiClemente, J. C. (1993). In search of how people change: Applications to addictive behavior. *American Psychologist, 47,* 1102–1114.

Box 8–2: Three Strategies for Fostering Individual Change

Educative/empirical-rational:

- If individuals are educated and guided by information, they will use logic and reason to make rational choices and behave accordingly.
  - *Example:* providing an in-service program on productivity and documentation stressing the negative impact on staffing and the ability to fill vacant positions if staff members do not charge and document according to policy.

Normative/persuasive:

- If knowledge about technology and systems is balanced with knowledge of noncognitive determinants of behavior, such as the processes of persuasion and collaboration, then individuals will be guided by internalized meanings, habits, and values and change behavior accordingly.
  - *Example:* creating a culture in which staff members support each other and remind each other to charge patients and document services, and establishing a norm in which staff members remind each other frequently to follow procedures related to charging for services and documenting.

Power-coercive:

- Individuals are exposed to strategies that emphasize political, economic, or regulatory sanctions. If they do not support change, then behavior will change accordingly.
  - *Example:* imposing penalties or removing rewards such as merit pay raises if staff does not follow policies and procedures related to charging for services and documenting.

Different situations may call for a different change strategy or for the use of more than one of these strategies in combination. The choice of strat-

egy or strategies for any given situation may be influenced by a number of factors (Nickols, 2004). These factors include

- *Degree of resistance:* strong resistance calls for use of more power and weaker resistance allows the use of rational strategies or education.
- *Target population:* larger populations may require a mix of strategies and smaller populations allow more limited choice of strategies.
- *The stakes:* when stakes are high, a mixture of strategies may lead to a greater likelihood of success.
- *The time frame:* shorter time frames call for increased reliance on power and longer time frames allow more rational or educative approaches to be used.
- *Expertise:* having considerable expertise available allows more mixing of strategies, whereas limited expertise may force reliance on power.
- *Dependency:* one party being dependent upon another affects the extent to which that party may rely on power versus other strategies.

A classic and simple model of change also related to both the individual and the organization was suggested by Kurt Lewin (1997). This model views change as occurring in three phases: (1) unfreeze, (2) change, and (3) refreeze (Figure 8–2). The largest contribution of this simple model may be that it suggests you may think about change as a staged process that can be broken down and analyzed, with different strategies being used at each of the phases. This simple approach is helpful for the new manager without extensive experience in creating and managing change processes. By focusing on each of the three stages, you can choose and plan strategies for introducing change, guiding staff through the change, and institutionalizing the new and desired state. Many of the continuous quality improvement (CQI) concepts, strategies, tools, and techniques discussed in Chapter 11 can be very helpful throughout the three stages.

The limitations of this model are that it does not consider that change often begins within an organization already in flux or unfrozen, or that organizations may need to remain unfrozen for extended periods of time (Nickols, 2004). In essence, the model may oversimplify how change really occurs in many situations; that is, often you find yourself dealing with processes or situations that were not

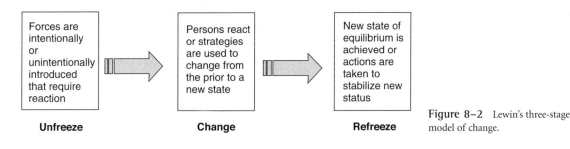

Forces are intentionally or unintentionally introduced that require reaction		Persons react or strategies are used to change from the prior to a new state		New state of equilibrium is achieved or actions are taken to stabilize new status
Unfreeze		**Change**		**Refreeze**

Figure 8-2   Lewin's three-stage model of change.

stable to begin with, and it may not be possible to completely stabilize the process or situation.

Lewin suggested that change could occur within organizations in one of three ways (Branch, 2002):

1. Change the individuals who work within the organization (skills, values, attitudes) and eventually behavior.
2. Change various organizational structures and systems such as rewards, reporting relationships, and work designs.
3. Change the organizational climate or interpersonal style (rate of interaction, conflict management, etc.).

These methods of change can be combined so that you facilitate change at both the individual and organizational levels. An example might be introducing a change to the process of completing seating assessments and recommending wheelchairs and seating systems on a rehabilitation unit. In the past, only one discipline has conducted the assessment, and you are changing the process so that occupational therapy and physical therapy will collaborate on the assessment and must come to agreement and present one recommendation. Such a recommendation might be met with resistance because of concerns over loss of control or power. Change might be fostered at the individual level by acting to change the knowledge, skills, and attitudes of staff. The knowledge of both disciplines could be addressed by providing factual information about the education and training of each discipline, the areas of overlap, and the areas of differences so that staff members could understand how, by collaborating, the knowledge brought to the assessment process would be greater than either discipline could possess alone. Skills could be addressed by developing competencies and a training program for seating assessments specific to both disciplines. Finally, attitudes might be addressed by a number

of strategies, including team-building activities to increase the personal comfort level of staff in interacting with each other, activities focusing on customer needs and what might not be adequately addressed if either discipline did not participate, and having leaders from each discipline model effective teaming. In addition to fostering change at the individual level, change could be fostered at the departmental and organizational levels by providing rewards and recognitions for staff members who effectively team together and by creating a climate in which open discussion of concerns is encouraged and welcomed. Other strategies for fostering this change process might include examining forms to require communication and to avoid separate processes being completed, and thinking about where assessments are conducted so that the power relationship between the two disciplines might be equalized.

Within organizations, two levels of *intentional change* have been identified and are discussed within the literature (Bridges, 1995; Burke & Trahant, 2000). Change related to organizational issues, such as mission, leadership, organizational culture or other "big picture" issues, has been referred to as *fundamental* or *transformational*. Change related to everyday "how to get things done" issues, such as management practices, overseeing employee satisfaction within a work unit, or job and task assignments, has been referred to as *transitional* or *transactional* change.

Large-scale organizational change is tremendously complicated, and there is a large and varied body of work presented in the organizational development, organizational behavior, and human resources literature, some of which is addressed in other chapters (see Chapter 3 regarding learning organizations and Chapter 11 regarding CQI). Occupational therapy managers will seldom be solely responsible for leading such a change, although the number of occupational therapists who own and operate their own business or engage in entrepreneurial ventures is increasing; those who become involved in higher levels of organizational administration or who do start their own business are encouraged to pursue a business education that will include strategies for organizational management and change. There are numerous examples of organizations that have been successful in changing in the face of economic and other challenges (Schermerhorn, Hunt, & Osborn, 1994). Unfortunately many others do not succeed. John Kotter (1996) identified eight common reasons that organizational change efforts fail in his book, *Leading Change*. These eight reasons are listed in Box 8–3.

Kotter argued that the biggest mistake people make when trying to change organizations is moving ahead without establishing a sense of urgency about what needs to be changed. In today's business environment, change happens quickly and organizations and managers must be prepared to react in kind. However, quick reaction does not mean acting without gathering sufficient information to make an informed (evidence-based!) decision. For Kotter, *complacency* means underestimating how difficult it is to move people out of their "comfort zones" and overestimating the amount of control they have over an organization. Throughout organizational change efforts, communication is key to success. Communication must be frequent and aimed at communicating not only what change is needed but also why, how, and when it is expected to occur. Most importantly, a vision of the future must be communicated in clear and sufficiently strong terms so that employees know where they are headed. Finally, it is the responsibility of the manager to identify and remove obstacles that will get in the way of achieving the vision or desired state.

The term *change agent* has been used to refer to those individuals, internal or external to the organization, who play a significant role in fostering and promoting change within organizations. The term is typically used to refer to those individuals who foster change with an organization's best interest in mind. Internal change agents may be formal or informal leaders. External change agents are typically paid consultants to an organization. Being an effective change agent requires that you (1) remain alert to situations that require change, (2) stay open to new ideas, and (3) become skilled in supporting the implementation of new ideas into actual practice (Schermerhorn et al., 1994).

In a review of the empirical literature on change agency, Caldwell (2003) identified four models of change agency that he advocated would encompass most of the existing literature. He emphasized that there is no *universal* or *single* model of change agency and provided a brief description of the four models of change agency as a heuristic tool. These four models are described in Box 8–4.

Box 8–3: **Eight Common Reasons Organizational Change Efforts Fail**

1. Allowing too much complacency
2. Failing to create a sufficiently powerful guiding coalition
3. Underestimating the power of vision
4. Under-communicating the vision
5. Permitting obstacles to block the vision
6. Failing to create short-term wins
7. Declaring victory too soon
8. Neglecting to anchor changes firmly in the new organizational culture

Adapted from Kotter, J. P. (1996). *Leading change.* Boston: Harvard Business School Press.

Skills for Creating and Managing Changing

Because change is created, is encountered, and needs to be managed within *open systems*, a wide variety of skill sets are required. Nickols (2004) identified what he believed were the most critical skills sets related to change management. These skill sets included (1) political skills, (2) analytical skills, (3) people skills, (4) system skills, and (5) business skills. Each of these skill sets and its relationship to creating and managing change will briefly be discussed.

Political skills involve understanding the real and imagined fears, desires, and consequences of action as perceived by others in the organization and environments in which you interact. Although the term

---

Box 8–4: Four Models of Change Agency

- **Leadership Models:** Change agents are identified as leaders or senior executives at the very top of the organization who envision, initiate, or sponsor strategic change of a far-reaching or transformational nature.
- **Management Models:** Change agents are conceived as middle-level managers and functional specialists who adapt, carry forward, or build support for strategic change within business units or key functions.
- **Consultancy Models:** Change agents are conceived as external or internal consultants who operate at a strategic, operational, task, or process level within an organization, providing advice, expertise, project management, change program coordination, or process skills in facilitating change.
- **Team Models:** Change agents are conceived as teams that may operate at a strategic, operational, task, or process level within an organization and may include managers, functional specialists, and employees at all levels, as well as internal and external consultants.

Adapted from Caldwell, R. (2003). Models of change agency: A fourfold classification. *British Academy of Management, 14,* 131–142.

- Learning to recognize the unwritten rules involved in organizational culture
- Understanding the importance of when to become more visible within meetings or projects and when to defer attention and/or credit to organizational leaders, your boss, and subordinates
- Understanding your assumptions and learning to recognize the assumptions of others about work, success, and change
- Becoming comfortable with talking to a wide variety of people in a wide variety of situations
- Becoming an effective communicator and skilled at giving feedback and delivering messages in nonconfrontational ways that maintain the dignity of others

Analytical skills include the skills that allow you to understand the whole of something by breaking it down into its component parts and in turn allow you to better understand the whole. One group of analytical skills includes those related to the evidence-based practice process of gathering and evaluating data and information. Nickols (2004) identified two important subsets of analytical skills: (1) workflow operations and (2) financial analysis. Workflow operations require that you be able to identify the start and finish of a process and the interim steps. Process analysis, including the use of *process flow diagrams*, is a central CQI strategy. Process flow diagrams are visual representations of work processes that identify the boundaries of a work process, the major stakeholders of the process, and the steps to complete the process. Process flow diagrams are very useful in identifying places where the process breaks down, where rework occurs, or where undesired variation may be introduced to a process. This and other workflow operation tools and techniques are discussed in depth in Chapter 11. Managers must also be able to identify the financial impact of changing a process or implementing a new process. For solutions to problems to be accepted and to be effective, they must also be affordable. Skilled managers will complete a financial analysis and recognize the financial impact of possible solutions before suggesting them.

People skills are those involved with motivating others in ways that show respect and recognize their efforts and contributions; these skills are mostly associated with communicating with others. People skills include both verbal and nonverbal communi-

office politics is often perceived as pejorative, it may also be thought to mean only that persons are acting in a shrewd and socially aware manner. None of us wants to feel bullied or embarrassed into taking action or changing, and developing more effective political skills means that you create and manage change in ways that show awareness that all employees want to be viewed favorably by their peers. Good politicians are leaders, effective communicators, facilitators, negotiators, marketers, advocates, motivators, visionaries, and, last but not least, "doers" (Gioia & Andersen, 2003). Political skills that will help you be effective in creating and managing change include

cation skills (see Chapter 12). Creating a positive culture and learning to develop and manage effective teams in addition to supervising individuals are also important subsets of people skills. As noted earlier, change can create a range of negative emotions, and learning to anticipate and recognize the emotional needs of employees in addition to other needs such as training will make the facilitation of change much easier. Managers face the difficult challenge of balancing *tasks* and *people*. During times of stress or when work processes are breaking down, attention to tasks often seems paramount. However, it is exactly those times when attending to people may be most important.

System skills include learning to develop, coordinate, and effectively use technical systems related to information management (e.g., charge systems, documentation systems, management of data for outcomes measurement) and general systems related to people and organizations (Nickols, 2004). *Medical informatics* is an emerging discipline that has been defined as the study, invention, and implementation of structures and algorithms to improve communication, understanding, and management of medical information (Zakaria, 2004). With the rapid changes and improvements in technology, management of information has become very sophisticated. In addition, medical informatics has become increasingly complex with the advent of laws such as the Health Insurance Portability and Accountability Act (HIPAA) of 1996, which includes regulations and proposes fines for mishandling of *protected health information* or information that could lead to the identification of patients. In larger organizations, the occupational therapy manager will need to become skilled in collaborating with an informatics specialist. In smaller organizations, such as a private practice, business owners are encouraged to examine closely and compare the advantages and costs of purchasing commercial systems or the time of a consultant with those of trying to manage information on their own. Similarly, most large organizations handle general systems, such as personnel, through the hiring of staff specialists to manage these functions. Managers or owners of businesses may have to develop a wide variety of skills, including general systems knowledge, that are handled by others in larger organizations; however, caution is recommended especially in areas such as human resources, where mistakes can be costly in terms of litigation and wasted resources.

Business skills include the various skill sets related to how business, and in particular a health-related business, works. Skills such as planning, human resources, marketing, and budgeting can all become part of solving a problem and identifying, evaluating, and implementing potential solutions. If it sounds to you like managers need to become skilled at a wide range of different types of activities, you are right. Much of the learning that occurs for many occupational therapy managers ends up being *on the job*; however, as the health care system and social systems in which we operate continue to become more complex, expectations for managers are increasing. As expectations for entry-level education also increase, graduates will be expected to have more advanced skill sets as they enter the profession. Still, most occupational therapy graduates will have had only one or two courses in administration and management that cover the full range of managerial tasks. Considering additional business-related graduate education or formal training in business-related skills is recommended for occupational therapy graduates who intend to focus on management as their area of practice or who plan to own and operate their own business.

Resistance to Change

Resistance to change refers to behaviors that discredit, delay, or prevent the implementation of a work change (Newstrom & Davis, 1997). Change can elicit a wide range of feelings in individuals, including fear, uncertainty, excitement, anger, or worry over loss, among others. Even when change is cognitively perceived as needed or beneficial, mixed feelings over experiencing the change process can cause individuals to resist. Curtis and White (2002) reviewed empirical literature from the fields of management and psychology and identified the most common reasons for resistance to change. These are summarized in Box 8–5.

Resistance to change has been the focus of much research and scholarship in the organizational development and management literature. Closely related research and scholarship has focused on ways

<table>
<tr><td>

Box 8–5: **Common Reasons for Resistance to Change**

</td></tr>
</table>

Box 8–5: **Common Reasons for Resistance to Change**

- *Increased stress:* Resistance can be not toward the change itself but toward the consequences of such change, such as loss of status or comfort, and the resulting feelings of stress that make it difficult for individuals to adjust.
- *Denial:* Denial of the need to change can be a natural reaction to perceived stress or other negative reactions to stress. Denial is recognized as a common defense mechanism used to deal with anxiety and is often thought of as a natural reaction that might be expected when individuals are initially confronted with change.
- *Self-interest:* Change often results in a shift in power or the addition of benefits to some members of an organization while other member's benefits remain the same or are decreased. Fear of personal loss has been identified as a major obstacle to change in organizations.
- *Lack of understanding, trust, and ownership:* People are less likely to accept and support change if they do not understand the purpose behind it or distrust those who are initiating change.
- *Uncertainty:* The lack of information about future events can increase feelings of lack of control and anxiety.
- *Motivation:* Motivation refers to the drive to meet our needs. When various types of needs (safety, security, belonging, or self-esteem) are threatened by the prospect of change, resistance may increase.
- *Different assessments or perceptions:* Resistance may increase when perceptions of a situation, the need for change, or the impact of change differ between persons at various levels of an organization.

Adapted from Curtis, E., & White, P. D. (2002). Resistance to change: Causes and solutions. *Nursing Management, 8,* 15–20.

of increasing *receptivity to change.* A noted example is work conducted by Pettigrew, Ferlie, and McKee (1992) examining receptivity to change in the British National Health Service. They identified eight factors associated with receptivity to change. These factors are summarized in Table 8–1.

It is also important to recognize that often individuals who are asked to change may experience conflicting feelings. Even while recognizing and valuing the advantages of adopting some change behavior, they may also recognize and fear negative effects. You may be able to tip the balance in favor of your desired change by (1) identifying the positive outcomes of change, (2) increasing the value of those outcomes, (3) making the path to achieving those outcomes easier, (4) identifying the negative outcomes of change, and (5) decreasing the perceived impact of negative outcomes and making them less likely to occur. One often-cited method of accomplishing this is *force-field analysis.* Force-field analysis is a management technique developed by Kurt Lewin that is useful when looking at the variables involved in determining the effectiveness of and when planning and implementing a change management strategy (Accel-Team, 2004).

Conducting a force-field analysis with your staff or a group of those who will be impacted by change is a great way of developing a sense of involvement. The first step in conducting a force-field analysis is to identify *driving forces* and *restraining forces.* Driving forces can be thought of as forces that are pushing in the direction of change. Examples of such forces might be changes in reimbursement, new competition, requests from customers, or demands for increased productivity from organizational leadership. Restraining forces can be thought of as forces that are working against change and work to maintain the status quo. When driving forces and restraining forces are equalized, a state of *equilibrium* is achieved and change is less likely to occur. However, when driving forces outweigh restraining forces, change may be inevitable. Another important concept is that of *valence,* or the capacity of a force to unite or join with other forces to cause action. In other words, not all driving forces or restraining forces are equal. Conducting a force-field analysis enables you to identify the smaller driving and restraining forces that might have otherwise gone unconsidered.

Table 8-1	Eight Factors Associated with Receptivity to Change	
Factor	**Definition**	
Coherent & effective policies and procedures	The extent to which policies and procedures are linked to each other and to the work that must be completed	
Continuity in key leadership positions	Maintaining consistency in the approaches and skills of those leading change efforts	
Environmental monitoring	Awareness of external factors in triggering change	
Supportive organizational culture	Values, beliefs, and behaviors that support the achievement of change goals	
Effective relationships between managers and clinicians	Managers and clinicians learning about each others' perspectives and making efforts to appreciate the challenges faced by others	
Effective relationships with key organizational collaborators	Productive relations with related organizations, such as social services and voluntary organizations	
Simplicity and clarity of goals	Establishing key priorities for the change agenda and articulating them to all in a clear and concise manner	
The fit between the change agenda and the locale	Awareness that particular features of the locality may inhibit or accelerate change	

Adapted from Pettigrew, A. M., Ferlie, E., & McKee, L. (1992). *Shaping strategic change: The case of the NHS.* London: Sage.

As an example, an organizational leader might ask your staff to implement new customer service procedures aimed at improving customer satisfaction. You might find one very strong driving force, such as the encouragement and support of a respected leader whom your staff does not want to disappoint. However, there may be several restraining forces that, when examined individually, do not seem strong enough to prevent change. For example, there may be minor staff resistance to taking time to learn new procedures, limited concern over the impact of new procedures on workload and productivity, and some discomfort regarding skill levels related to dealing with disgruntled customers. If you were presented with any one of these restraining forces separately, and paid attention to how strongly staff members felt and their level of concern over that single issue, it might be difficult to understand why staff members were resistant to change. However, through the process of conducting a force-field analysis and involving your staff, you might identify that there are several concerns (restraining forces) that, when combined, are suffi-

ciently strong to act against the staff's desire to change. Thus the value in conducting a force-field analysis is in both the process and the outcome (e.g., what you learn). This example is represented in Figure 8–3. The relative size of the arrows represents the valance of the individual force.

One set of behaviors that may be encountered during and after change efforts may be referred to as *victim behavior* (Balestracci, 2003). Victim behavior is likely to arise when individuals perceive that they have no influence over whether to change or how to change. They are likely to focus on what is happening "to" them as individuals and are unlikely to recognize what is happening in the environment around them or to other individuals. Victim behavior can be very frustrating to encounter as a manager, and what can be even more frustrating is that sometimes confronting it directly will only result in its increasing. Victim behavior may include complaining, lowered productivity, or missed workdays, or in worst cases can include behavior that works to sabotage the change efforts. At some point, such behavior must be dealt with

Driving Forces   **Restraining Forces**

Concern over time to learn new
procedures

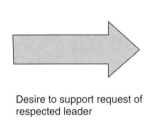

Concern over impact of new
procedures on workload

Desire to support request of
respected leader

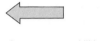

Concern over skill level in responding
to disgruntled customers

Figure 8–3   A force-field analysis of forces affecting adoption of new customer service procedures.

directly, but other less confrontational strategies that can be used to overcome victim behavior and facilitate change include the following:

- Admit openly that change is difficult and that you also have difficulty with change at times; be empathetic and show your human side.
- Model acceptance of change by being the first to follow new procedures, attending trainings required, or adopting new ways of working.
- Be flexible when you can. Stay true to the main purpose of the intended change but recognize when you can adapt to make staff see that you are listening to them.
- Ask the staff member's advice on how to proceed with the change; invite him or her to help you identify specific actions to take to increase the likelihood of the change being successfully implemented.
- Complete a force-field analysis and enlist the staff member by assigning him or her alone or with a small group the task of drafting a list of driving forces to present to you or a larger group.
- Try having a face-to-face conversation in which the focus is not on the staff member's behavior but instead you acknowledge that you are aware of his or her concerns and that you want to explain *why* change is needed. People may be open to change if they understand why it is needed,

and this may act to dispel irrational fears or inaccurate information.

Laframboise, Nelson, and Schmaltz (2003) suggested that resistance to change could be managed by envisioning change as a staged process similar to the commonly identified stages of grieving (i.e., denial, anger, bargaining, and acceptance). The four stages they suggested are (1) discovery, (2) denial, (3) resistance, and (4) acceptance. These four stages and strategies for each stage are briefly summarized in Table 8–2. As with many stage models, it is important to realize that not everyone will experience every stage, some may move forward and then fall back to an earlier stage, and not everyone will eventually get to the final stage of acceptance.

Top-Down and Bottom-Up Change

Conventionally, change management has been viewed as a function of management in which organizational leaders are responsible for identifying desired change and leading or forcing those whom they supervise to change. *Top-down* theories of change management assume that the focus of theory and research should be the creation of more effective models to support the traditional hierarchical system found in most organizations

Table 8-2	Four Stages of Change and Related Strategies

Stage of Change	Strategies
Discovery: when and how persons learn about the change	• Plan communication carefully so that all hear the same information at the same time. • For large-scale changes, develop a formal and written communication plan. • Put any facts, dates, or other concrete information that will help staff understand and be clear on what is to happen in writing.
Denial: when persons don't really believe that a change will occur or believe that, after a time, things will return to the way they were	• Continue wide communication in writing and in person. • Offer "town hall" meetings or allow time for questions and answers at a staff meeting. • Continue to express why the change is occurring and when. • Include persons in planning and implementing change so that they see that it will indeed occur.
Resistance: persons express frustration or anger and may avoid helping to implement change or work against it	• Continue to stress why change is occurring. • Allow opportunities to express concerns in writing and in person by using suggestion boxes or town hall meetings. • Make sure that communications includes details, and that persons are kept informed of steps as they happen. • Stress accomplishments.
Acceptance: persons understand what change will occur and agree to support it even if it is not how they would act if acting alone	• Celebrate accomplishments. • Recognize those instrumental in the change but thank all persons involved in the department or organization for their support. • Plan review of impact of change and to assure that the change is not temporary. • Review what went well and what did not go so well to help prepare for future changes.

(Lavasseur, 2001). More recent approaches to fostering and managing change within organizations have included *bottom-up* approaches, including those typically used within CQI process improvement efforts. Bottom-up change management approaches focus on tapping into the knowledge and expertise of those who are most familiar with work processes and may also be most familiar with the causes of rework, waste, and roadblocks within organizational processes.

Change as a Problem and Problem Solving

Often change is initiated because a problem arises that requires that new action be taken because existing procedures or circumstances are no longer satisfactory. If you view a problem as an opportunity for planning change, then you can apply frameworks for change discussed earlier, including seeing change as moving from one state to another, specifically from the *problem state* to the *solved state* (Nickols, 2004). Interestingly, although managers spend a considerable portion of time solving routine everyday problems as well as much more complex problems, problem solving itself is seldom taught.

A first step in problem solving is naming the problem, or *problem setting*. Problem setting is a critical first step because it only makes sense that, as you consider solutions and alternatives, you will pay attention to information that you identify as relating to the problem and ignore information that you feel is extraneous. For example, if you are at home and discover that you do not get a dial tone when you pick up a phone, there may be a number of different reasons why this could be the case. Initially you might consider that the problem is with the phone, but you might also consider that the problem is with the service outside of your home. When you pick up a second extension and discover that you still do not receive a dial tone, you likely stop attending to any information that does not relate to your outside service. Even if you have a third or fourth extension, you probably do not go to those extensions to see if you have a dial tone there because you assume that you will not learn any additional useful information by doing so. You attend only to information related to the problem you set.

In naming or setting the problem, it is helpful if you set the problem to be as specific as possible. The more specific the problem set, the easier it is to tell when the problem is solved. Setting a problem specifically also helps in ruling out unrelated causes. For example, knowing that a fuse blows in the occupational therapy kitchen every time the microwave and any other countertop appliance are in use at the same time is a more specific problem than simply knowing that a fuse occasionally blows. By identifying the key elements of a problem and setting it as narrowly as possible, you can avoid wasted efforts.

Problem setting is not an idea new to health care or to occupational therapy. Donald Schön introduced the idea in his investigations of *reflective practitioners* and the logic that practitioners used to solve problems (Schön, 1983). Schön described problem setting by saying, "Problem setting is a process in which, interactively, we *name* the things to which we will attend and *frame* the context in which we will attend to them. Tying the pieces all together, the practitioner then reframes the situation to fit her own previous experiences and tacit knowledge about that type of practical situation." These concepts were further developed in regard to the clinical reasoning and reflective practice of occupational therapists by Mattingly and Fleming (1994) in their book, *Clinical Reasoning: Forms of Inquiry in a Therapeutic Practice*. Often managers solve problems requiring a range of reasoning, but the works of Schön, Mattingly and Fleming, and others in regard to clinical reasoning are worth investigating to help managers with problems that involve human interaction.

Nickols (2004) suggested that the analysis of a change problem will focus on defining the outcomes of a change effort, on identifying the changes necessary to produce these outcomes, and on finding and implementing ways and means of making the required changes. Thus, a change problem may be broken into smaller problems that may be named "how problems," "what problems," and "why problems."

A second key element of problem solving, especially in regard to more complex problems related to human interactions, is to identify the assumptions you are making about a situation. Assumptions are necessary for three reasons (Harris, 2002). First, they set limits to the problem. Second, they may reflect desired but unstated values. Third, assumptions help to simplify the problem and make it more manageable by giving us fewer things to consider. However, at times we make assumptions about a situation, a process, or people that are inaccurate. By identifying the assumptions you hold in regard to any given problem, you can seek to validate the assumptions or let them go.

For example, a common problem that occupational therapy managers face in hospital settings is scheduling staff for weekend coverage. Often in facilities where daily coverage is needed, some type of rotation system is used so that staff members take turns working weekend days and in turn take a day off during the week before or following the weekend. In one facility where I had this responsibility, I struggled considerably with setting up a rotation system because there were several staff vacancies and I assumed that working weekends was not desirable to staff. It was quite accidental that I learned that one staff member liked working on the weekends because her fiancé typically had to work on the weekends and took days off during the week. Discovering that my assumptions about preferences for weekend scheduling might not be accurate prompted me to bring the problem back to the staff I supervised and look for more flexible solutions. As a result, staff members were not scheduled evenly for weekends. Rather, some staff members were scheduled more often and everyone ended up being happier. Harris (2002) provided a helpful checklist to identify some types of assumptions. The types of assumptions on his checklist are briefly presented in Box 8–6.

Another step that should be completed before jumping into problem solving is to identify criteria

Box 8-6: **A Checklist of Assumption Areas Related to Solving Problems**

- **Time:** You may have more time to solve a problem than you assume. Can you work with those who need to be involved to gain additional time to work on a satisfactory solution? If people are aware that you are working to solve a problem, they may be willing to wait for it to be solved, especially if allowing more time means a more effective solution.
- **Money:** Can you find more financial resources to invest in solving a problem *correctly* the first time? More importantly, do you need to spend *all* of the funds to which you have access? Sometimes simple solutions are the most effective and don't always cost a lot of money. You can win extra points for solving a problem *and* saving money.
- **Cooperation:** Have you made inaccurate assumptions about who will support you or your proposed solutions? Are there people whom you can recruit that you have not thought of? Do you need to confirm that

those whom you believe are with you really support you?
- **Law:** Have you assumed that you are limited by laws without consulting legal experts, or are there legal solutions you may not have considered?
- **Energy:** Is the benefit of solving the problem worth the time and energy you will need to invest to solve the problem at this time? Would it make more sense to have all involved recognize that you will live with the problem for the time being? Are you investing enough energy, or are you just putting a temporary "Band-Aid" on the problem? Does it make more sense to invest energy in fixing the problem correctly the first time than to come back to the problem again and again?
- **Information:** Do you have all the information you need to solve the problem? Do you need to begin by gathering more information, and is the information you have correct?

Adapted from Harris, R. (2002). Problem solving techniques. VirtualSalt.com Web site. Available at *http://www.virtualsalt.com/creebook4.htm*

for a successful and satisfactory solution. Too often, it is tempting to jump into problem solving by beginning to identify alternatives as solutions. In fact, *alternative swapping,* or a group of individuals who have a problem in common proposing first one solution, and then another and then another, is one of the most common roadblocks to successful problem solving. Rather than beginning by proposing solutions, groups should first focus on identifying the goals or objectives for a satisfactory solution. In other words, you should identify a set of criteria against which potential solutions can be evaluated. The perfect solution that makes all parties happy may not exist, but by identifying objective criteria to evaluate solutions first, you may not only identify the *best* solution, but may also prevent conflict among the problem solvers and limit individual agendas. One helpful tool to use that assists in comparing possible options to solve a problem by comparing them against a set of predetermined cri-

teria such as cost, feasibility of implementation, and anticipated effectiveness is a *proposed options matrix,* often used as part of a CQI effort. Further explanation and a sample matrix are included in Chapter 11.

A key concept in decision making and problem solving is that of *consensus.* Reaching consensus does not mean that there is full agreement among all parties involved in making a decision or in choosing a response to a problem. Consensus does indicate, however, that all parties have agreed to support the plan of action fully even if it is not how they would act if they were acting alone. This means that everyone commits to acting in ways that do not sabotage progress and that there is no saying "I told you so" if something goes wrong. A difficulty with reaching consensus is that it often takes time to reach real consensus, and managers are often under pressure to make decisions and solve problems quickly. However, as noted earlier, making the right decision the first time, even if it takes a little longer, often requires fewer resources than making the wrong decision multiple times!

Once you have set the problem as specifically as possible, have identified those assumptions that are accurate and that you want to maintain and use, and have established criteria against which to evaluate your possible solutions, you can decide upon the appropriate problem-solving strategies. Strategies should be chosen based upon the nature of the problem to be solved, and different strategies may be needed at different points in solving the problem. For example, John Malouff (2004), Senior Lecturer at the University of New England in Australia, has identified 50 different problem-solving strategies and categorized them into eight groups. These groups are listed in Box 8–7.

Dr. Malouff's Web site listing 50 different strategies for problem solving, and other resources like it, was found by conducting a simple Internet search using the key words "problem-solving theory" and then "problem-solving strategies." As discussed in Chapter 1, such sites should be evaluated to determine their level of validity and credibility, but many helpful sites are established and maintained by aca-

demicians and other credible sources. Inherent in this long list of strategies is that different strategies are appropriate at different stages of the problem-solving process. Some strategies will help you gather information to more specifically set the problem, some will help you identify root causes of the problem, others will aid you in gathering information to identify and evaluate potential solutions, and still others will help you decide how to implement solutions.

Chapter Summary

This chapter provided an introduction to change management and problem solving. A number of models and frameworks for conceptualizing change were presented, as were strategies for fostering change and dealing with resistance to change. Thinking about change as a process or problem that might be broken down into component parts was suggested as a way of recognizing that it is necessary to use different change or problem-solving strategies at different times. It was also recognized that managers must deal with change occurring within individuals, departments, organizations, and environments and that successfully managing change requires that we balance task needs with people needs.

It was suggested in this chapter that managing change and solving problems requires that a manager develop a broad range of skills, including political skills, analytical skills, people skills, system skills, and business skills. Many of these skill sets must be developed over time, and the knowledge underlying these skills typically is learned through on-the-job experience but may also be developed by pursuing graduate business education or taking advantage of the many formal training opportunities that are offered related to health care or business in general.

You were introduced to several tools and techniques that can be helpful in managing change and solving problems, including process flow diagrams, proposed options matrices, and force-field analysis. Several of the tools and techniques are discussed in more depth in other chapters of this book, but, in addition, you were encouraged to use the evidence-based practice strategies that you are learning to find current and more in-depth information spe-

---

Box 8–7: Types of Problem-Solving Strategies

- Strategies to help you understand the problem
- Strategies to help you simplify the task
- Strategies to help you determine the course of the problem
- Strategies involving the use of external aids to help identify possible solutions
- Strategies involving the use of logic to help you identify possible solutions
- Strategies using a possible solution as a starting point to help you solve a problem
- Strategies to help you determine which possible solution is best
- Strategies to help you function optimally while problem solving

Adapted from Malouff, J. (2004). Fifty problem solving strategies explained. University of New England, Australia, Department of Psychology Web site. Available at *http://www.unc.edu.au/psychology/staff/malouff/problem.htm*

cific to the situations you will encounter, because there are many helpful resources available on the Internet, in the professional literature, and from various professional and scholarly associations and organizations.

At the start of this chapter, I shared the experience I encountered when I accepted a job as the Director of Clinical Services at a large academic medical center that was in turmoil. The staff members that I supervised had been through tremendous change and, although motivated to rebuild the occupational therapy department, were also resistant to the additional changes that would be necessary to allow that to happen.

Real-Life Solutions

Initially, as I set about the various projects and activities that I envisioned would help to rebuild the occupational therapy department, I encountered considerable resistance to further change. I had been introduced to change management and strategies for creating change in my graduate program in Human Resources Development but had not yet made any formal use of that information. I began by returning to this literature and by enlisting the help of staff specialists within the human resources department and of managers in other departments who had lived through many of the changes themselves. Doing this helped me first and foremost to begin to understand the resistance that I was encountering and to recognize the fears, uncertainty, and concerns shared by many of the staff members. By doing this, I was able to see the various aspects of resistance as *problems to be solved* and, perhaps more importantly, I was able to frame the process of working with staff members to overcome their resistance as an *opportunity* rather than a problem.

I was encouraged by my mentors and peers to see the human side of what my staff was experiencing and to pay as much attention to staff members' emotional and psychological needs as I was to the procedural and technical task needs I had identified. By consciously using people skills to enlist the help of staff members as partners in the change process, I was slowly able to begin to use strategies and tools such as process flow diagrams. In doing so, staff members were able to recognize the "how, why, and what" of change problems we faced and were able to become active partners in identifying the needed changes and strategies for creating those changes.

One key strategy was to provide training and education to staff members related to change itself as well as some of the tools and techniques we would be using. Although I made tacit use of the transtheoretical model to plan strategies for increasing staff members' awareness for the need to change and to ready them for it, they found Lewin's simple three-stage model of change helpful to frame their experience. By recognizing that, as a result of the turmoil they had experienced, they had essentially become "frozen" in some nonproductive ways, they were able to ready themselves for additional and intentional change.

Over the next few years, many changes in policies, procedures, and philosophy were created, and at numerous points I found that I did not possess the skills or knowledge needed to be successful on my own. However, as I pursued doctoral study, I was able to take advantage of educational opportunities to gain new knowledge, and, by developing a network of peers both within and outside of the occupational therapy profession, I developed a ready bank of resources of which I took frequent advantage. I also set ambitious goals to increase my skills in business, information management, and general systems. Whenever possible, on the advice of my mentors, I volunteered for various organizational task forces and as a result received more advanced training in CQI and other change management skill sets.

I served as Director of Clinical Services in that occupational therapy department for a period of 8 years and saw the department grow to almost twice its size and become more stable. As the organization as a whole rebuilt itself, the rate of change decreased, but never stopped. In fact, as I left the position of director to assume other duties within the organization, my replacement came aboard with renewed energy and a vision of new changes. The case shared here is an example that change is indeed constant, but also that it can be productive and rewarding and that the knowledge, skills, and attitude to manage it successfully can be learned.

Resources for Learning More About Change and Solving Problems

Journals that Often Address Change or Solving Problems

JOURNAL OF ORGANIZATIONAL CHANGE MANAGEMENT

Articles published in *The Journal of Organizational Change Management* address theories, philosphies, and evidence related to managerial practices and strategies that create and foster successful organizational change. Topics often addressed in the journal include strategic planning, leadership research, CQI, and the psychology of change in the workplace.

THE LEARNING ORGANIZATION

The Learning Organization is one of the few sources of information to deal exclusively with the philosophy and practice of continual organizational improvement. The journal publishes articles related to understanding the learning organization and ways in which organizations can adopt learning strategies and apply theories of organizational learning.

Associations That Are Concerned with Change or Solving Problems

THE CHANGE MANAGEMENT ASSOCIATION

http://www.cmassociation.org/

The main goal of the Change Management Association is to provide a forum for discussion of Change management best practices. The association provides a forum for the exchange of ideas between members in order to promote identification of the most effective change management strategies for use within organizations. The Change Management Association is a global organization that includes members from varied professions who are affected by, or involved in, change management.

Other Resources

BUSINESS.COM "THE BUSINESS SEARCH ENGINE"

http://www.business.com

Business.com is a leading business search engine and business directory designed to help its users find the companies, products, services, and information they need to make business decisions. The site includes links to articles, business sites, and other resources on managing change.

CHANGE MANAGEMENT RESOURCE LIBRARY

http://www.change-management.org/

This site includes links to four areas related to change management that include articles, books, best practices and training. The site is sponsored by ProSci, a commercial process design and change management research company. The company Web site (*http://www.prosci.com/bpr_ph1.htm*) includes links to several management-related online learning centers.

Reference List

Accel-Team. (2004). Team building—force field analysis. Accel-team.com Web site. Available at *http://www.accel-team.com/*

Balestracci, D. (2003, November). Change management: Handling the human side of change. *Quality Progress*, pp. 38–45.

Bennis, W., Benne, K. D., & Chin, R. (1985). *The planning of change*. New York: Holt, Rinehart and Winston.

Branch, K. M. (2002). Change management. U.S. Department of Energy Web site. Available at *http://www.er.doc.gov/sc-5/benchmark/Ch%204%20Change%20Management%2006.10.02.pdf*

Bridges, W. (1995). Managing organizational transitions. In *Managing organizational change* (pp. 20–28). New York: American Management Association.

Burke, W. W., & Trahant, W. (2000). *Business climate shifts: Profiles of change makers*. Boston: Butterworth Heinemann.

Caldwell, R. (2003). Models of change agency: A fourfold classification. *British Academy of Management, 14*, 131–142.

Curtis, E., & White, P. D. (2002). Resistance to change: Causes and solutions. *Nursing Management, 8*, 15–20.

Gioia, E., & Andersen, A. (2003). Project managers need sharp political skills. Federaltimes.com Web site. Available at *http://www.portfoliomgt.org/read.asp?ItemID=1729*

Harris, R. (2002). Problem solving techniques. VirtualSalt.com Web site. Available at *http://www.virtualsalt.com/creebook4.htm*

Kotter, J. P. (1996). *Leading change*. Boston: Harvard Business School Press.

Laframboise, D., Nelson, R. L., & Schmaltz, J. (2003). Managing resistance to change in workplace accommodation. *Journals of Facilities Management, 1*, 306–321.

Lavasseur, R. E. (2001). People skills: Change management tools—Lewin's change model. *Interfaces, 31*, 71–73.

Lewin, K. (1997). *Resolving social conflict and field theory in social sciences*. Washington, DC: American Psychological Association.

Malouff, J. (2004). Fifty problem solving strategies explained. University of New England, Australia, Department of Psychology Web site. Available at *http://www.unc.edu.au/psychology/staff/malouff/problem.htm*

Mattingly, C., & Fleming, M. (1994). *Clinical reasoning: Forms of inquiry in a therapeutic practice.* Philadelphia: F. A. Davis.

Newstrom, J. W., & Davis, K. (1997). *Organizational behavior: Human behavior at work.* Boston: McGraw-Hill.

Nickols, F. (2004). Change management 101: A primer. Distance Consulting Web site. Available at *http://home.att.net/~nickols/change.htm*

Pettigrew, A. M., Ferlie, E., & McKee, L. (1992). *Shaping strategic change: The case of the NHS.* London: Sage.

Prochaska, J. O., & DiClemente, J. C. (1993). In search of how people change: Applications to addictive behavior. *American Psychologist, 47,* 1102–1114.

Schermerhorn, J. R., Hunt, J. G., & Osborn, R. N. (1994). *Managing organizational behavior* (5th ed.). New York: John Wiley & Sons.

Schön, D. (1983). *The reflective practitioner: How professionals think in action.* New York: Basic Books.

Zakaria, A. (2004). Medical informatics FAQ. www.faqs.org Web site. Available at *http://www.faqs.org/medical-informatics-faq/*

9

Brent Braveman, Ph.D., OTR/L, FAOTA
Gary Kielhofner, Dr.P.H., OTR/L FAOTA

Developing Evidence-Based Occupational Therapy Programming

Real-Life Management

David recently attended the annual American Occupational Therapy Association conference, where he sat in on a number of presentations on evidence-based practice. He has become convinced that he and the occupational therapy practitioners that he supervises need to integrate strategies for using evidence into their daily work.

Upon returning to the mental health agency where he works, David realizes that all of the presentations he attended focused on how practitioners could use evidence in making decisions about how to directly intervene with clients. Although those strategies are clear to him, he begins to wonder about how he can use evidence in *his* daily work. David's work often relates to making decisions at the program level as he plans, develops, implements, and evaluates occupational therapy services. For example, he has recently been asked to lead the development of a new day treatment program in conjunction with other clinical disciplines.

David and the occupational therapists and occupational therapy assistants he supervises have always been well respected by the physicians, social workers, nurses, and other professionals with whom they work for their use and application of theory. They have become skilled at combining both occupational therapy theory and conceptual practice models with theories and models developed by other disciplines.

As David begins to think about planning the new program, he identifies the following questions:

1. How can an occupational therapy manager use theory and evidence in planning, developing, implementing, and evaluating occupational therapy services?
2. What is the relationship between a program development model and a theory?
3. What kinds of theories or models are available to guide program development?
4. How are different theories and models combined as you proceed with program development using an evidence-based approach?

Key Issues

- Occupational therapy programming should be designed with consideration of available evidence, and it should clearly indicate the underlying mechanisms of action that are expected to promote the desired change in the target population.

- Occupational therapy conceptual practice models and related knowledge are often combined in order to address all mechanisms of action required for a comprehensive program.

- Occupational therapy theories, conceptual practice models, and frames of reference (and theories from related knowledge) have been developed to differ-

ent extents, and varying levels of evidence exist to validate their use.

- Use of a program development model will guide the occupational therapy manager through the process of applying appro-

priate theories while assessing the needs of the target population and the environments in which programming will be delivered.

Occupational therapy managers often find themselves with responsibility for developing, planning, implementing, and evaluating programming. Occupational therapy program development can be relatively simple, such as developing an intervention for individuals with a specific diagnosis in a familiar practice setting. An example of such program development would be formalizing a protocol for educating patients undergoing a total hip replacement as part of a critical pathway within an acute care hospital.

Conversely, program development can be complicated and challenging. It can require the assessment of how complex human and environmental factors impact totally new target populations in nontraditional practice contexts. An example of such an effort would be developing independent living and prevocational programming for persons living with human immunodeficiency virus/acquired immunodeficiency syndrome (HIV/AIDS) (a recently emerging disability group) in a transitional living residence that previously operated with a hospice focus. Such program development may call for the use of multiple theories and new approaches to organizing interventions.

Regardless of the complexity of a program, reliance on sound theory by evaluating and using available evidence is the best strategy for developing effective services with good outcomes. The value of evidence-based practice and strategies for finding and evaluating evidence has been presented in previous chapters. This chapter will focus on strategies for integrating theory and evidence with program planning. Before beginning this discussion, a review of a few key terms and concepts would be helpful.

What Are a Theory, a Paradigm, a Conceptual Practice Model, a Frame of Reference, and Related Knowledge?

In occupational therapy, different authors and scholars use different terms to describe the knowledge that managers might use to guide program development. For example, whereas Crepeau and Schell (2003) identified sensory integration as a "frame of reference" in Willard and Spackman's *Occupational Therapy* (10th edition), it was cited by Kielhofner (2004) as a "conceptual practice model" in *Conceptual Foundations of Occupational Therapy* (3rd edition). Terms such as *theory*, *model*, and *frame of reference* are sometimes used interchangeably in the field, although scholars often use these terms to refer to concepts that are quite different from each other. Moreover, the necessity of using bodies of knowledge from other disciplines (e.g., related knowledge) can lead to encounters with yet other terminology. This can readily cause confusion and frustration.

Although you should not become overly bogged down in the differences in terminology, it is useful to have some understanding of why different authors and scholars use different terminology. Having a clear understanding of the differences between terms used to describe the organization of knowledge can assist you in applying this knowledge to the process of planning, developing, implementing, and evaluating occupational therapy programming. Therefore, a brief discussion of some of these terms is presented in this section as a means of highlighting the key contributions that well-developed theories and models make to guiding program development. The terms that will be defined are *theory, paradigm, conceptual practice model, frame of reference*, and *related knowledge*.

A **theory** provides an explanation of how or why a particular phenomenon occurs and how that phenomenon might be influenced. Theories are often composed of both general concepts that refer to larger chunks of reality and specific concepts that refer to the elements of which they are organized. Thus the key element of a theory is explanation— that is, giving a plausible account for how something works (Kielhofner, 2004). Theory provides a way of understanding what is necessary for practice. For example, we might be interested in why people may choose to participate in specific occupations while choosing not to participate in other occupations, and how this process can be influenced or used when collaborating with persons with disabilities to re-establish a full compliment of roles. A theory that seeks to explain motivation and interests would be helpful in this case. It is unlikely, however, that a theory that seeks to explain motivation and interest would also seek to explain complex elements of neuromuscular function such as reflexes or motor planning. It is for this reason that occupational therapy managers need to draw from a wide range of theories in developing occupational therapy programming. Theory is found in the occupational therapy paradigm, in frames of reference, in conceptual practice models, and in related knowledge.

The occupational therapy **paradigm** is knowledge that specifically addresses the identity and perspective of the occupational therapy profession. It articulates a shared vision of members of the field that defines the nature and purpose of the discipline (Kielhofner, 2004). The paradigm addresses the following factors:

- What human need does the service address?
- What kinds of problems does it solve?
- How does it solve these problems (i.e., what is the nature of its service)?

Paradigms include theory to address these questions, but the theory in a paradigm is broad and focused on questions of what an occupational therapy program should focus on. It does not provide more concrete concepts and tools for practice.

A **conceptual practice model** generates theory and the methods (e.g., assessments and intervention strategies) that are used by therapists in their everyday work to apply that theory. These methods are sometimes referred to as *technology for application*. Each conceptual practice model addresses some phenomenon related to occupational functioning (e.g., motivation, perception, movement) and specifies theory and tools for application pertaining to particular kinds of problems in that area. Because each conceptual practice model focuses on specific phenomena or areas of function or capacity, you will likely need to rely on a combination of conceptual practice models to develop a comprehensive program that addresses the range of factors influencing your clients' occupational functioning. A conceptual practice model often builds upon theories from a variety of disciplines to create a new unique theory that explains the problems and challenges addressed by the model. For example, the Model of Human Occupation (MOHO) integrates theories related to motivation, habits, underlying human capacities, and the environment.

A **frame of reference** is a structure for guiding practice by delineating the beliefs, assumptions, definitions, and concepts within a specific area of practice. Frames of reference employ existing theory and focus on developing methods of applying that theory in occupational therapy. So, for example, a frame of reference may delineate a function-dysfunction continuum, evaluation processes, and intervention strategies that are consistent with a theory from outside occupational therapy (e.g., behavioral theory or object relations theory) (Crepeau & Schell, 2003).

Thus, the most important distinction between the use of the terms *conceptual practice model* and *frame of reference* is that conceptual practice models generate theory unique to occupational therapy, whereas frames of reference simply apply existing theory to practice (Kielhofner, 2004). A frame of reference may borrow a theory from another discipline and apply it to occupational therapy practice without formulating unique occupational therapy theory or giving consideration to how occupational therapists would use the knowledge differently from professionals in other disciplines. For example, sensory integration is a model of practice developed by occupational therapists. It includes theory that seeks to explain how the human nervous system perceives and processes information to guide performance. Although many of the concepts of sensory integration build on interdisciplinary theory, there is a unique theoretical explanation that is offered by this model and that guides occupational therapy intervention. An example of a frame of reference is object relations (Buckley, 1996). The underlying theory for this frame of reference comes from the psychoanalytic tradition of psychiatry and psychology. In occupational therapy, these concepts are applied to understanding how involvement in occupations and the relationship with the therapist can be used to achieve the kinds of personal change in occupational therapy patients that psychologists and psychiatrists seek to achieve in their psychotherapy patients.

Related knowledge comes from outside occupational therapy and thus has been developed and investigated primarily by members of another discipline. For example, a theory of motor learning may address redundancies in neurologic systems that allow individuals with a stroke or brain injury to relearn familiar tasks such as putting on a sock or opening a cabinet door. Although many occupational therapists may rely upon such knowledge to guide their interventions with these clients, occupational therapy scholars were not primarily responsible for developing this knowledge. Box 9–1 summarizes the key terms presented here and their definitions.

In developing most occupational therapy programs (regardless of level of complexity), managers will undoubtedly rely on a combination of the occupational therapy paradigm to guide thinking about what the service should be, and conceptual practice models and related knowledge to define more specifically what problems are addressed, what services are provided, what outcomes will be achieved, and how they will be achieved. An example of such a combination is presented at the end of this chapter in the case example on the Enabling Self-Determination for Persons Living with HIV/AIDS (ESD) Program. In this program, the developers used an occupational therapy conceptual practice model, the MOHO, as the overarching guide for program development. However, in developing discrete intervention elements of the program, reliance on multiple theories and models from related knowledge, including disability studies, so-

---

Box 9-1: **Definition of Key Terms**
• **Theory:** an explanation of how or why a particular phenomenon occurs and how that phenomenon might be influenced. Theories are often composed of both general concepts that refer to larger segments of reality and specific concepts that refer to the elements of which they are organized.
• **Frame of reference:** a structure for guiding practice by delineating the beliefs, assumptions, definitions, and concepts within a specific area of practice. Frames of reference employ existing theory and focus instead on developing methods of applying that theory in occupational therapy.
• **Conceptual practice model:** a model that generates theory and the methods (e.g., assessments and intervention strategies) that are used by therapists in their everyday work to apply that theory. Each model addresses some phenomenon related to occupational functioning (e.g., motivation, perception, movement) and specifies theory and tools for application pertaining to particular kinds of problems in that area.
• **Paradigm:** knowledge that specifically addresses the identity and perspective of the occupational therapy profession. The paradigm articulates a shared vision of members of the field that defines the nature and purpose of the discipline.
• **Related knowledge:** knowledge that comes from outside occupational therapy and thus has been developed and investigated primarily by members of another discipline.

---

cial cognitive theory, the Transtheoretical Model of Change, and the Health Belief Model, helped guide decision making (McLeroy, Bibeau, Steckler, & Glanz, 1988; Prochaska & DiClemente, 1993; Strecher, DeVillis, Becker, & Rosenstock, 1986).

Learning to become comfortable in thinking about ways in which to combine various theories and models represents an important skill set for occupational therapy managers. As with other skill sets, you will learn and develop your program development skills through application. Initially, heavy reliance on a program development model may be useful as a guide to decision making and sequencing of tasks for the new manager who is unsure of his or her skills. However, just as with assessment skills, documentation skills, or other skills sets, over time the program development process will become more fluid as you gain confidence and will likely take on a more "organic" nature.

Program Development Models

Numerous discussions of approaches to program development and case examples of programs can be found in the occupational therapy literature (Braveman, Goldbaum, Goldstein, Karlic, &

Kielhofner, 2001; Braveman, Kielhofner, Belanger, Llerena, & de las Heras, 2002; Braveman, Sen, & Kielhofner, 2001; Brownson, 2001; Grossman & Bortone, 1986; Scaffa, 2001). Parallel to the discussion earlier in this chapter of the different types of theories, this section presents a discussion of the focus of different types of program development models. Models for program development and evaluation may have different foci. Some program development models are more focused on systematic levels and are useful in guiding us in deciding where and with whom to intervene to address a particular challenge or health problem. Other models are more useful in guiding decision making once a setting and population for an intervention are known. For example, the Ecological Model of Health Promotion describes five societal levels at which intervention could be planned (Figure 9–1) (McLeroy et al., 1988):

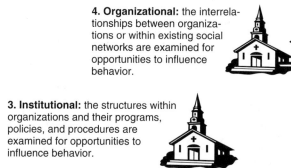

5. Public Policy: the policies, programs, and regulations of local, state, and federal bodies are examined for opportunities to influence or regulate behavior.

4. Organizational: the interrelationships between organizations or within existing social networks are examined for opportunities to influence behavior.

3. Institutional: the structures within organizations and their programs, policies, and procedures are examined for opportunities to influence behavior.

2. Interpersonal: relationships and interactions with persons such as friends, family, and peer groups are examined for opportunities to influence behavior.

1. Intrapersonal: individual factors and characteristics such as knowledge, beliefs, and values that may influence behavior.

Figure 9–1   The ecological model of health promotion.

- *Intrapersonal:* Individual factors and characteristics such as knowledge, beliefs, and values may influence behavior.
- *Interpersonal:* Relationships and interactions with persons such as friends, family, and peer groups are examined for opportunities to influence behavior.
- *Institutional:* The structures within organizations and their programs, policies, and procedures are examined for opportunities to influence behavior.
- *Organizational:* The interrelationships between organizations or within existing social networks are examined for opportunities to influence behavior.
- *Public Policy:* The policies, program, and regulations of local, state, and federal bodies are examined for opportunities to influence or regulate behavior.

Although the Ecological Model of Health Promotion is very helpful in deciding *where* one might intervene once a particular challenge or health problem is identified, it is not useful in deciding *how* to intervene. To make this decision, reliance on a more focused model to guide decision making regarding how to combine various theories (paradigmatic and related knowledge) and how to sequence program development actions is useful. Various models may emphasize different factors depending on the particular context in which the model is implemented, but most address the following four processes (Figure 9–2):

- *Needs Assessment:* the process of describing the target population, naming perceived and felt needs, and analyzing available resources and constraints both internal and external to the organization or context in which the program is being planned
- *Program Planning:* the process of identifying the steps and sequence of actions to be taken to plan for initiation of the program
- *Program Implementation:* the process of initiating intervention first in trial format and then in a more formal and sustained manner

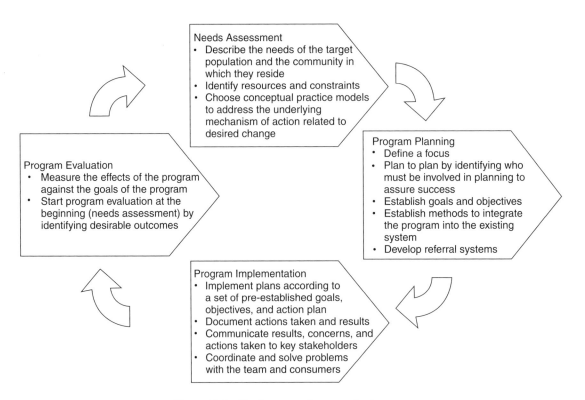

Figure 9–2 The four steps of program development.

- *Program Evaluation:* the ongoing process of assessing the impact and quality of program processes and outcomes and making continuous improvements in efficiency and effectiveness

What Are the Relationships Between Theory and a Program Development Model?

Theories or conceptual practice models and program development models are used in combination to guide decision making about where, how, and when to intervene given a chosen problem and/or target population. We seldom begin the process of developing occupational therapy programming without some critical variables, such as the context or organization in which the program will be delivered or the target population to whom it will be delivered, being predefined. For this reason, and because no single theory or practice model typically addresses all of the factors needed to plan intervention, it is recommend that you begin by identifying a program development model that will help guide the order of your managerial actions. In some cases, especially in emerging areas of practice, we may be familiar with the target population but not yet be aware of its needs, or we may be interested in addressing an area of occupational dysfunction and not be completely sure where to intervene or who might most benefit from the services. In such a case (as in the ESD Program case example later in this chapter), you might combine multiple program development models in the same way you might combine several conceptual practice models that seek to address different but complimentary phenomena.

To explain further, here is an example of how several models might be used in combination. Imagine that you wish to develop an intervention program for older adults living in high-rise apartment buildings in a large city who are becoming more isolated and having increased difficulty with daily activities such as getting groceries and maintaining social contacts. The Ecological Model of Health Promotion may be used to guide you to decide *where* to intervene, and you decide that you will do so at the intrapersonal, interpersonal,

organizational, and community levels. To plan the steps of developing your program, you use the four-step program development model presented in Figure 9–2. As you plan your program, you know that you need a model that helps you to understand motivation and why older adults may choose to become involved in various occupations, and you select the MOHO for this reason. As you develop specific intervention components, you find that you need to address physical aspects of function such as decreased strength, endurance, and other deficits due to normal aging or conditions such as arthritis. To address these problems, you rely on related knowledge such as the biomechanical model and neurologic model in combination with the MOHO.

Whether from the occupational therapy paradigm or from related knowledge, we should recognize that different theories and models have been developed to varying extents. In other words, different levels of evidence exist. Some theories and models are well investigated, have established assessments or other technologies for application, and have substantial and growing bodies of evidence to support their use. Other theories or models have been presented in the literature, but valid assessments or other technologies for application are limited and relatively little evidence exists to support their use. In some cases, a theory or model may receive initial attention but interest may wane because of the lack of strong evidence to warrant continued investigations. For example, Figures 9–3 and 9–4 illustrate the rates of publications on three conceptual practice models used by occupational therapy personnel (the MOHO, the Canadian Model of Occupational Performance [CMOP], and the Cognitive Disabilities Model). Figure 9–3 indicates the total number of publications on each model for the period from 1994 to 2004, and Figure 9–4 indicates the number of research-related publications for the same time period. Although the number of publications alone is not an indication of the quality of the evidence that exists, it does illustrate that different models utilized are often at different stages of development, and that fact should be part of our overall evaluation of the state of evidence in selecting models for use.

In the next section of this chapter, brief overviews of evidence will be provided on select related knowledge useful in the program develop-

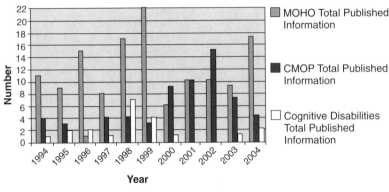

Figure 9–3 Total number of publications on three conceptual practice models for the years 1994–2004. CMOP, Canadian Model of Occupational Performance; MOHO, Model of Human Occupation.

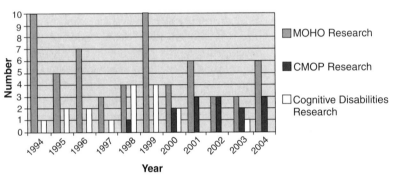

Figure 9–4 Total number of research publications on three conceptual practice models for the years 1994–2004. CMOP, Canadian Model of Occupational Performance; MOHO, Model of Human Occupation.

ment process. A full discussion of all related knowledge of use or concern to occupational therapy managers is beyond the scope of this or any other single book. However, the following are theories that may be of particular use in making program development decisions.

Overview of Evidence on Select Related Knowledge Relevant to Program Development

The Transtheoretical Model of Change

Much of occupational therapy programming is implemented with the expectation that, as a result of intervention, consumers will adopt some new behavior or change behavior in some way in order to better facilitate occupational performance. One model, the Transtheoretical Model of Change, suggests that change often occurs in a series of stages (Prochaska & DiClemente, 1993). This model has been well investigated in relation to behaviors such as smoking cessation, weight control, and exercise. It has not yet been studied in regard to adoption of behaviors that might be promoted by occupational therapists, such as adoption of joint protection techniques, wearing a splint, adhering to a physician-suggested medication regimen, or regularly completing skin checks to prevent pressure sores.

As with most staged models, it is important to remember that not everyone will experience each stage, and often individuals may cycle between stages, reverting to an earlier stage and progressing again to a later stage. Individuals may also skip a stage altogether. With behavior change, such as ceasing substance abuse, stopping smoking, or beginning to exercise, several failed attempts to start or stop a behavior may be made before finally incorporating the new behavior in a habitual pattern. We might expect this to be the case with adoption of new occupational behavior as well.

In the first stage, *precontemplation*, individuals are unaware or underaware of a problem or the benefits of adopting a new behavior pattern, so there is no intention to change behavior in the foreseeable future. In the second stage, *contemplation*, people are aware that a problem exists and are seriously thinking about overcoming it, but have yet to make a commitment to action. The third stage is *preparation*. In this stage intention is combined with behavioral criteria, so individuals are intending to take action in the next month or have unsuccessfully taken action in the recent past. In the fourth stage, *action*, individuals take action to modify their behavior or seek experiences to modify their environment in order to overcome their problems. In the final stage, *maintenance,* individuals work to prevent relapse and consolidate the gains that they attained during action. The five stages of the Transtheoretical Model are summarized in Box 9–2. Table 9–1 includes a selection of evidence on health behaviors in studies that used the Transtheoretical Model.

Although this model may appear relatively simple, the complexity of human behavior and the difficulty of altering behavior patterns must be

recognized. As noted by Kielhofner (2002), habits resist change because they are based on our most fundamental certainties about how the world is constructed. However, the construct of habits is one that is critical for us to consider in regard to health behavior because habits organize our underlying performance capacities so that we can perform within our environments. Occupational therapists and occupational therapy assistants can play a crucial role in helping individuals to habituate health behaviors by incorporating those behaviors into their daily routines. Understanding the process of change can assist the occupational therapy manager in developing a program by incorporating elements to assist individuals at any stage of change and to move toward maintenance. Table 9–2 provides an example of how each stage of the Transtheoretical Model can be incorporated into a program.

In the ESD Program case example presented later in this chapter, the health behavior addressed by the programming is the adoption of the strategy by a person living with HIV/AIDS of carrying a day's supply of medications in his briefcase so that he does not find himself without access to his medications. This strategy improves his adherence to his physician-recommended medication regimen, a behavior critical to preventing the development of drug resistance.

It should be mentioned here that the Transtheoretical Model explains the process of change in regard to a discreet behavior. In other words, the model must be applied to each behavior that you wish an individual to consider starting, stopping, or continuing, or to avoid ever beginning. So the model may be applied to many aspects of the program (i.e., each behavior you want to change). Although this may appear confusing at first, it can be highlighted by the following simple example. If you stand outside of any health club, you will soon notice people emerge who have just invested considerable time and energy taking part in one "healthy" behavior, that of exercising. Some of these same individuals will immediately take part in the "unhealthy" behavior of lighting up a cigarette. Application of the Transtheoretical Model to influence the health behavior of exercising will not automatically influence the health behavior of not smoking. Different interventions would need to be

---

Box 9–2: The Transtheoretical Model: Five Stages of Change

- *Precontemplation:* persons are unaware or underaware of a health problem or the benefit of performing a health behavior.
- *Contemplation:* persons are aware of a health problem and are considering taking action but have not committed to any specific action or to begin performing a health behavior.
- *Preparation:* intention to begin performance of a health behavior is combined with criteria for action that include a time frame to begin acting.
- *Action:* individuals attempt to incorporate health behaviors into their routine.
- *Maintenance:* health behaviors are successfully incorporated into daily routines so the behaviors become habitual.

Table 9-1	Summary of Selected Evidence Using the Transtheoretical Model of Change (TTM)			
Author	Study Type	N	Level of Evidence	Results
Riley, Toth, & Fava (2000)	Cross-sectional survey	9 women at risk and 10 HIV-infected women	Weak	The study supports use of the TTM to examine readiness to use stress management behavior in women regardless of their HIV serostatus.
Jammer, Wolitski, & Corby (1997)	Repeated cross-sectional sampling with matched intervention and comparison communities	3081 injection drug users	Strong	77% of injection drug users in the intervention area reported being exposed to an intervention to increase condom carrying. Rates of condom carrying increased from 10% to 27% ($p < .001$). There was also an increase from 2.32 to 3.11 in mean stage of change for using condoms with other partners, while stage of change decreased in the comparison area ($p < .01$).
Galavotti et al. (1995)	Cross-sectional questionnaire after intervention	296 women at high risk for HIV infection & transmission	Good	Results support the usefulness of the TTM for understanding and assessing contraceptive behavior among women at high risk for HIV infection and unintended pregnancy.
Glanz et al. (1995)	Cross-sectional survey after intervention	17,121 employees participating in the Working Well Study	Good	The TTM proved useful in an intervention to reduce fat intake and increase fiber and fruit and vegetable intake. Stage of change was associated with fat, fiber, and fruit and vegetables intake in a stepwise manner as predicted.
Prochaska & DiClemente (1993)	Randomized assignment to one of four intervention conditions	756 smokers	Strong	Results suggest that providing smokers with interactive feedback about their stages of change, decisional balance, processes of change, self-efficacy, and temptation levels in critical smoking situations can produce greater success than just providing the best self-help manuals currently available.
Marcus et al. (1992)	Correlational postintervention study	610 community members	Good	Most participants increased their stage of exercise adoption during a 6-week program designed using the TTM (62% of participants in contemplation became more active and 61% of participants in preparation became more active).

Table 9-2	Application of the Transtheoretical Model of Change Within a Program for Persons Living with HIV/AIDS
Stage of Change	**Elements of Occupational Therapy Programming**
Precontemplation	Health education groups are conducted that include information on the definition of satisfactory medication adherence and the negative impact of missing medications and health problems associated with resistance to medications.
Contemplation	Activities to identify current adherence rate with physician-recommended medication regimens and causes for missing scheduled medications are undertaken.
Preparation	Information on strategies to improve medication adherence (e.g., carrying a full day's dose of medications in one's briefcase, backpack, or purse) is included in multiple venues, including support and educational groups, handouts, and planning in individual occupational therapy sessions. Activities are undertaken to assist the individual in identifying reasons for missing medications doses and selecting strategies to resolve those problems.
Action	The individual attempts to implement selected strategies with the support of the occupational therapist, other program staff, and peers. The expectation that attempts often initially fail is freely shared, and positive reinforcement is provided for successful implementation of strategies. The individual is an active partner with the occupational therapist in identifying strategies that are not a good match for his or her routine, and dysfunctional strategies are dropped and alternatives are explored.
Maintenance	Occasional reassessment of adherence rates is included in group and individual occupational therapy sessions, positive reinforcement is provided often, and activities to help establish a positive view of a routine that includes the desired health behavior, such as having the individual mentor others, are incorporated.

included in any program intended to influence both behaviors. Choices about health behaviors are complicated. However, whereas some programs are targeted at improving health or quality of life by influencing multiple behaviors, you should recognize that often occupational therapy programming is targeted at incorporating discreet behaviors so that they become habits.

The Health Belief Model

The Health Belief Model was originally developed in the 1950s through an initiative by the U.S. Public Heath Service. The Health Belief Model describes the influence of individuals' beliefs in regard to a particular health behavior on whether the individuals are likely to adopt the behavior. The model posits that choices to behave or not behave in certain ways are influenced by four sets of *perceived beliefs*. These beliefs are perceived susceptibility, perceived seriousness, perceived benefits, and per-

ceived barriers. In addition, a *cue to action* is thought to trigger behavior (acting or not acting). Cues to action may be internal (such as pain or discomfort) or external (such as the presence of others involved in the behavior). An internal cue, such as fatigue or blurred vision, might cue a person with diabetes to check his or her blood sugar or take an insulin injection. An external cue such as seeing a traveling partner put on a seat belt might cue a person getting into a taxicab to put on his or her seat belt as well.

It is also helpful to distinguish between the constructs of *knowledge* and *belief*, because both may influence behavior, but different strategies may be required to change behavior depending upon the knowledge that an individual has, and what he or she believes. Knowledge is the condition of apprehending truth or fact. Knowledge entails the awareness that particular propositions or assertions are factual or true on the basis of some justification or evidence that sufficiently supports them. Beliefs are convictions or feelings that something is real or true. Belief systems rest at some point on a body of fundamental definitions or irreducible axiomatic principles whose truth is accepted a priori; they do not require, and may not be susceptible to, proof. Beliefs may be unassailable or closed propositions inaccessible to argument. *Belief* and *knowledge* are relative terms that are context dependent. It may be noted that we often have a tendency to claim our own worldview as knowledge and that of others as belief. For example, it might be reasonable to state that today most adults have the knowledge that a diet high in saturated fat and cholesterol may contribute to coronary artery disease. Such knowledge may be viewed as fact based on evidence presented through scientific trials. In contrast, some individuals believe that health status may be influenced by prayer. Although most would agree that, to date, such a belief has not been irrefutably proven by scientific inquiry, many hold a belief in a higher power that would make their belief in prayer impervious to argument.

It is worth noting that, in addition to using the Health Belief Model within a program to consider how to influence individual behaviors, it can also be used to consider how to improve compliance with a program. Because this model spells out the factors that influence a person's acceptance and maintenance of the necessary steps to achieve change, it is often helpful in organizing a program in a way that will enhance compliance or participation in the program itself.

Table 9–3 provides examples of each of the four sets of beliefs of the Health Belief Model and an example of cues to action as they might influence the health behavior of wearing a bicycle helmet. Table 9–4 provides examples of selected evidence on the Health Belief Model.

Social Cognitive Theory

Originally presented by Bandura in the 1970s as social learning theory, social cognitive theory holds that behavior is determined by expectancies and incentives. Expectancies can be divided into three types: (1) expectancies about environmental cues, which are called environmental expectancies; (2) expectancies about the consequences of one's own behavior, which are called outcome expectancies; and (3) expectancies about one's competence to perform a behavior necessary to achieve a particular outcome, which are called efficacy expectations. Incentives (or reinforcements) are the value that an individual places on particular outcomes. Examples of incentives that may influence the value of an outcome could include the praise or criticism of peers, improved perceived health, or financial impact (Rosenstock, Strecher, & Becker, 1988).

Expectancies and incentives influence behavior together. For example, a person who values the

Table 9-3	The Health Belief Model Applied to the Health Behavior of Wearing a Bicycle Helmet
Perceived susceptibility	The beliefs that you are susceptible to a head injury if you fall while riding a bike, and that a fall is possible or likely, will increase the chances of wearing a helmet.
Perceived seriousness	The belief that, if you fall and hit your head, the injury is likely to be serious will increase the chances of wearing a helmet.
Perceived barriers	The beliefs that you might look silly, that helmets are hot, and that friends may make fun of you will decrease the chances of wearing a helmet.
Perceived benefits	The beliefs that wearing a helmet will contribute to a sense of safety and well-being and set a good example for your children will increase the chances of wearing a helmet.
Cues to action	A sense of guilt for getting on a bicycle in front of your children without a helmet and seeing your spouse put on a helmet may cue you to wear a helmet.

Table 9-4	Summary of Selected Evidence on the Health Belief Model (HBM)				
Author	Study Type	N	Level of Evidence	Results	
Winfield & Whaley (2002)	Predictive	261 college students	Good	Perceived barriers were found to be a significant predictor of condom use.	
Ali (2002)	Predictive	178 women	Good	Perceived susceptibility and perceived seriousness predicted coronary heart disease preventive behaviors.	
Perkins (1999)	Predictive	144 adults	Strong	Patients who believe the risks of treatment outweigh the benefits are likely to discontinue their medication.	
Sapp & Jensen (1998)	Cross-sectional survey	1502 adults	Good	The HBM provided good prediction of perceived dietary quality and moderate prediction of actual dietary quality.	
Conrad, Cambell, Edington, & Faust (1996)	Quasi-experimental	310 smokers	Strong	Exposure to a worksite health-promoting environment as a cue to smoking reduction had significant effect on post-test smoking.	
Fischera & Frank (1995)	Descriptive	110 nurses	Weak	Found some support for the HBM, with noncompliers having significantly higher barrier scores.	

effects of beginning to exercise on a regular basis (incentives) will be more likely to attempt to exercise if he or she believes that (1) his or her current lack of exercise poses health threats (environmental cues); (2) exercising will decrease the threats and lead to improved health (outcome expectations); and (3) he or she is capable of adopting a new exercise regimen (efficacy expectations). Table 9–5 summarizes expectancies and incentives as they relate to adopting the health behavior of beginning to exercise.

Although all elements of social cognitive theory are important and helpful to the occupational therapy manager who is planning a health-related

Table 9-5	Social Cognitive Theory Applied to the Health Behavior of Beginning to Exercise
Environmental Expectancies: what leads to what	Belief that not exercising poses threats to health may act as cues to exercise.
Outcome Expectancies: how behavior is likely to influence outcomes	Belief that exercising improves health and decreases threat supports exercise.
Efficacy Expectations: confidence in the ability to perform a behavior	Belief that one is capable of incorporating exercise supports exercise.
Incentives: the value of an outcome	Valuing the praise of others for lost weight and lowered blood pressure supports exercise.

program, the concept of how to impact clients' perceived self-efficacy is of particular importance. *Self-efficacy* relates to beliefs about capabilities of performing *specific* behaviors in *particular situations*; it does not refer to a personality characteristic or a global trait that operates independently of contextual factors (Strecher et al., 1986).

In designing occupational therapy programming intended to foster changes in occupational behavior, it is important that we consider that efficacy expectations (the belief that one is capable of performing a certain behavior) are learned from primary sources; however, these sources are not of equal influence. These influences are described here and summarized in Box 9–3.

The first and most influential source refers to learning through experience or through *performance accomplishments*. Performance accomplishments are situations in which clients have the opportunity to achieve a sense of mastery through doing. An example of a performance accomplishment would be when we provide a client with an opportunity to use an assistive device such as a sock assist to don a sock, and the client discovers that he or she can be successful in using the equipment.

The second source of learning is through observation of others involved in the behavior in question, or through *vicarious experiences*. A typical example of this might be when we show a client a videotape of a model using assistive equipment but don't necessarily allow the client hands-on time to practice. When using vicarious experiences, it is im-

portant that we remember that the use of models has been shown to be more effective when the model is perceived to achieve mastery by overcoming difficulty rather than easily meeting the challenge presented. So if the model used in the videotape is a young occupational therapy fieldwork student who easily dons a sock using a sock assist, a client may perceive that the model is "not like me," and his or her sense of self-efficacy may not be impacted. The more closely the model resembles the client in age, level of function, and other characteristics, the more likely that the vicarious experience will affect perceived self-efficacy.

A third source of influence on perceived self-efficacy is that of *verbal persuasion*. Verbal persuasion is simply trying to convince a client to adopt a behavior. Trying to verbally convince a client who has undergone a total hip replacement to use a sock assist as part of his or her strategy to follow post-surgery precautions is a common example of verbal persuasion. Although this is a common method to try to convince occupational therapy clients to adopt new behavior, it is unfortunately much less effective than providing opportunities for performance accomplishment or to observe appropriate models.

Finally, a client's *physiologic state* can influence his or her readiness to experience an attempt to change behavior and can affect his or her perceived self-efficacy. Clients who are overly aroused because they are nervous, fearful of pain or failure, or under the influence of sedatives or highly fatigued may not be well prepared to attempt to learn a new behavior. Remembering this and providing multiple opportunities or returning to a client when he or she is more physiologically ready for intervention may increase the likelihood of successfully influencing occupational behavior.

In providing health education or in attempting to convince clients to adopt new occupational behavior that is health promoting, we must also consider the three following concepts in regard to perceived self-efficacy. Perceived self-efficacy may vary according to the *magnitude* or difficulty of the task. A client who has had hip replacement surgery may perceive that he or she can perform the simpler task of rising from a chair while following the recommendation not to flex the hip beyond 90 degrees but may not perceive that he or she can perform the more difficult task of getting in or out of a car while

---

> ### Box 9–3: Four Sources of Learning for Efficacy Expectations (Perceived Self-Efficacy)
>
> - *Performance accomplishments:* learning by doing; providing a hands-on opportunity for a master experience.
> - *Vicarious experience:* learning by observation; best if the "model" is perceived as being like the client and to achieve mastery through effort rather than ease.
> - *Verbal persuasion:* learning by listening.
> - *Physiologic state:* one's level of arousal can affect one's readiness to attempt new occupational behavior

following the same recommendation. Perceived self-efficacy may also vary according to the *strength* of level of confidence for completing a particular task in a particular situation. Strength and magnitude may be closely related, but the strength of a person's conviction that he or she can complete a behavior may be influenced by factors beyond the magnitude of difficulty of the task, such as prior experiences with similar tasks. Finally, we must consider the *generality*, or the degree to which expectations about a particular behavior in a particular situation will generalize to other situations. We often practice behaviors with clients only in medical settings, assuming that they will be able to generalize the behavior to the home or other settings in which they will need to perform a particular behavior.

Table 9–6 presents a summary of selected evidence on social cognitive theory.

Table 9-6	**Summary of Selected Evidence on Social Cognitive Theory**			
Author	Study Type	N	Level of Evidence	Results
Dilorio, Dudley, Soet, Watkins, & Maibach (2000)	Survey of a random sample of college students	1380 students, 18 to 25 and single, who reported initiation of sexual intercourse	Good	Self-efficacy, the central variable in the theory, was related both directly and indirectly to condom use behaviors. The findings lend support to a condom use model based on social cognitive theory and provide implications for HIV interventions.
Keller, Fleury, Gregor-Holt, & Thompson (1999)	Integrated literature review	Published research during the years 1990–1998 ($N = 27$ studies)	Weak	Descriptive studies found a statistically significant relationship between self-efficacy and exercise behavior. Intervention studies demonstrated that participation in an exercise program promoted self-efficacy, and programs designed to increase outcome expectations and self-efficacy significantly increased exercise behavior.
Langlois, Petosa, & Hallam (1999)	Nonequivalent comparison group design	Sixth-grade students: treatment group ($N = 81$); comparison group ($N = 80$)	Good	Students in the treatment group maintained a high level of confidence to refuse cigarette offers, whereas the confidence of the comparison group decreased significantly. They also increased their expectations for positive outcomes from refusing cigarette offers, whereas the expectations for positive outcomes of the comparison group decreased. The students' fear of negative outcomes is less impressionable and more stable. Behavioral capability to resist positive images of smoking was not affected by the program.

(continued)

Table 9-6	Summary of Selected Evidence on Social Cognitive Theory *(continued)*				

Author	Study Type	N	Level of Evidence	Results
Kalichan & Nachimson (1999)	Cross-sectional survey	Sexually active HIV-positive persons ($N = 266$)	Good	Men who had not disclosed to partners indicated lower rates of condom use and scored significantly lower on a measure of self-efficacy for condom use compared to individuals who had disclosed. Women who had not disclosed reported the lowest disclosure self-efficacy. Building self-efficacy for serostatus disclosure should therefore become a high priority in interventions designed for people living with HIV/AIDS.
Sheeshka, Woolcott, & MacKinnon (1994)	Survey	White-collar employees ($N = 490$)	Weak	This study demonstrates that elements of social cognitive theory may explain a substantial amount of the variance associated with intentions to adopt healthy eating practices.

Choosing Conceptual Practice Models and Related Knowledge for the Development of Occupational Therapy Programming

A key issue in selecting the theoretical underpinning of a program is to be able to identify the theoretical explanation for why a particular change occurs as a result of a specific intervention. A key portion of this explanation is often referred to as *mechanisms of action*. A mechanism of action specifies what changes, how change proceeds, the conditions under which an intervention achieves beneficial results, and why a change may occur for certain groups of consumers and not others (Box 9–4) (Gitlin et al., 2000). Because satisfactory occupational functioning is dependent upon a wide range of occupational behaviors and because different theories or conceptual practice models are intended to address a range of phenomena, developing programming most often requires managers to use more than one practice model in combina-

tion. For example, the MOHO is a model that seeks to explain the occupational nature of human beings and how we come to choose and participate in occupational forms. Although the MOHO recognizes that occupational performance is dependent upon underlying capacities such as the ability to move one's arm or to sequence a series of actions in the appropriate order to complete daily activities, it does not address how to remediate or compensate for a decreased active range of motion or impaired cognition. Thus, when designing programming for someone who is likely to have both motor and cognitive deficits, such as an individual with a head in-

---

Box 9–4: Mechanisms of Action

- Indicate how change proceeds
- Designate the conditions under which an intervention achieves beneficial results
- Suggest why change may occur for certain groups of consumers and not for others

jury, you must rely on multiple practice models to address all of the underlying mechanisms of action necessary to facilitate satisfactory occupational functioning.

Braveman et al. (2002) identified four questions that can guide the selection of model(s) for program planning (Box 9–5). These questions may be used to evaluate the appropriateness of models in regard to the phenomena that they address so that various models may be effectively combined within a program. They also guide a manager in considering the pragmatic issues that arise in trying to implement programs within varied contexts such as limitations in space, adequately trained personnel, or reimbursement. These questions will briefly be explained and applied to the development of the occupational therapy components of a cardiac rehabilitation program in this section of the chapter.

Question 1: Does the model specify the underlying mechanisms of action necessary to facilitate the desired type of change?

Box 9–5: Four Questions to Guide Selection of Conceptual Practice Models in Program Planning

1. Does the model specify the underlying mechanisms of action necessary to facilitate the desired type of change?
2. Is there sufficient evidence to support application of the model(s) to the consumer group and the type of change you wish to facilitate?
3. Do the model(s) fit with the social, organizational, cultural, political, professional, and financial contexts in which the program must be implemented?
4. Does implementation of the model have any special requirements for space, equipment, or personnel?

Adapted from Braveman, B., Kielhofner, G., Belanger, R., Llerena, V., & de las Heras, C. G. (2002). Program development. In G. Kielhofner (Ed.), *The Model of Human Occupation: Theory and application* (3rd ed., pp. 491–519). Baltimore: Williams & Wilkins.

Occupational therapists and occupational therapy assistants may be involved in a variety of types of interventions with a patient who is hospitalized after having a coronary artery bypass graft (CABG). These interventions may include activities of daily living, including self-care or home management; stress management, energy conservation, and work simplification techniques; environmental modification; and exploration of interests and hobbies that support a healthy lifestyle, such as exercise. The mechanisms of action that underlie return to satisfactory occupational performance in each of these areas are different, and no single conceptual practice model addresses all the necessary mechanisms. Table 9–7 gives examples of areas of intervention, hypothesized mechanisms of action, and a proposed conceptual practice model that would be used to facilitate improved occupational performance. The table highlights the need to combine conceptual practice models to encompass all the key mechanisms of action to be addressed by a single occupational therapy program.

Question 2: Is there sufficient evidence to support application of the model(s) to the consumer group and the type of change you wish to facilitate?

As introduced in Chapter 1, the process of evaluating evidence requires the development of specific clinical questions. Assuming that the most important clinical question, "Is there evidence to support that cardiac rehabilitation is effective?", has been answered to the satisfaction of the program developer, a next step would be to identify the key components of effective programs.

At this point the question that must be answered is whether there is a match between the underlying mechanisms of action thought to affect the desired occupational behavior, the key components of effective programming found in the literature (evidence), and the conceptual practice models chosen to guide program development. This matching process is an iterative one in which multiple comparisons and revisions to your thinking are likely to be made as you discover any type of mismatch between one component and another. Figure 9–5 represents the process of evaluating the fit between the suspected mechanisms of action, the components of effective programming supported by evidence, and the phenomena addressed by conceptual practice models.

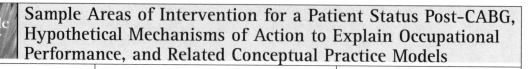

Table 9-7	Sample Areas of Intervention for a Patient Status Post-CABG, Hypothetical Mechanisms of Action to Explain Occupational Performance, and Related Conceptual Practice Models	
Area of Intervention	Mechanisms of Action	Related Conceptual Practice Model
Exploration of new leisure interests	Interests influence choice and participation in occupational forms, and indirectly health status, by lowering stress and improving cardiovascular fitness and conditioning. Exposure to new interests may encourage occupational exploration and involvement in new occupational forms.	Model of Human Occupation
Self-care activities, including bathing and dressing	Involvement in everyday occupational forms, such as bathing while standing, can improve strength and endurance of persons who have become deconditioned secondary to illness or hospitalization.	Biomechanical model
Environmental modifications and assistive and adaptive equipment to conserve energy and maximize safety	Adaptation of the environment can compensate for decreased performance capacity and increase independence.	Canadian Model of Occupational Performance

Question 3: Do the model(s) fit with the social, organizational, cultural, political, professional, and financial contexts in which the program must be implemented?

Many factors influence program development and implementation beyond just whether the program is theoretically sound and grounded in the most recent available evidence. Social, organizational, cultural, political, professional, and economic factors may also limit the capacity of an occupational therapy manager to develop and implement a program in exactly the manner that he or

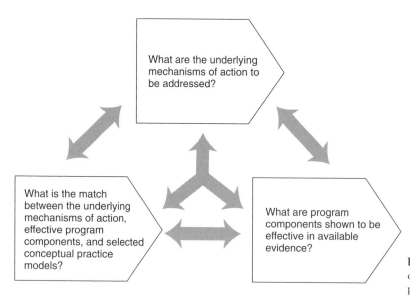

Figure 9-5 Matching mechanisms of action, evidence, and conceptual practice models.

she wishes. For example, theory drawn from an occupational therapy conceptual practice model might suggest that exploration of leisure pursuits and interests as a mechanism for managing and reducing work-related stress would be a valuable component of a cardiac rehabilitation program. However, the realities of staffing shortages, limits on the services that may be provided because of reimbursement mechanisms, or philosophical differences regarding the role of occupational therapy in an acute medical setting may force compromise or alterations in program design.

Considering the full range of factors that will influence how a conceptual practice model is used to guide program development can save valuable time by preventing investment of resources in program components that will be poorly received. It may also help the program developer consider ways in which the conceptual practice model (either in entirety or its primary tenets) might be introduced to key stakeholders in the organization or delivery context so that program elements will be more likely to be accepted. For example, an in-service education program might be provided to physicians, nurses, and physical therapists involved in the development of a cardiac rehabilitation program. The in-service might focus on the relationship between pursuit of leisure interests and decreased stress, as well as evidence to support addressing these issues in programming. Introduction to an occupational therapy conceptual practice model and possible interventions while acknowledging economic concerns could be included in such a presentation and be strengthened by linking the model to evidence on effective program components.

Question 4: Does implementation of the model have any special requirements for space, equipment, or personnel?

Although a theory supported by evidence might suggest a range of possible interventions, some interventions may require space, equipment, or personnel beyond the scope of the organization's resources. It is the responsibility of the program developer to plan for funding of staff salaries, training needs, new equipment, and space within available resources. Occupational therapists and occupational therapy assistants play different roles in different settings within the area of cardiac rehabilitation, ranging from involvement in only basic self-care intervention to much broader involvement in interventions, including stress management, energy conservation, and work simplification. In some settings, the occupational therapy practitioner may monitor physical activity. With the cardiac rehabilitation patient, involvement in any type of physical activity, from bathing to ambulation, typically requires monitoring of heart rate, blood pressure, and oxygen saturation, and monitoring these functions should require that occupational therapy personnel have undergone specific training and demonstrated specific competencies in these areas. The resource implications of involvement in such programming must be considered early in the process of program development.

In the section that follows, the information presented so far will be applied to an example of an occupational therapy program that was developed at the University of Illinois at Chicago by the authors of this chapter.

Case Example: Developing an Occupational Therapy Program Using Evidence—the Enabling Self-Determination for Persons Living with HIV/AIDS Program

The Enabling Self-Determination for Persons Living with HIV/AIDS (ESD) Program is an example of an occupational therapy program for which several program development models were utilized in conjunction with an occupational therapy conceptual practice model as well as a number of theories and models from related knowledge. The ESD program arose out

of a prior occupational therapy program (the Employment Options [EO] Program), also designed and implemented by the authors of this chapter. The EO Program was funded by a federal research and demonstration grant (Rehabilitation Services Administration Grant #H235A980170) and operated by the University of Illinois at Chicago Department of

(continued)

Case Example: Developing an Occupational Therapy Program Using Evidence—the Enabling Self-Determination for Persons Living with HIV/AIDS Program (Continued)

Occupational Therapy and the Howard Brown Health Center, a community-based health center serving Chicago's gay and lesbian population. The EO Program provided group educational services combined with vocationally focused occupational therapy to adults living with AIDS. The EO Program operated between 1998 and 2001 and enrolled 137 men and women living with AIDS in the Chicago area. At the completion of the project, 67% of participants had returned to work or were involved in a formal education effort (Braveman, Goldbaum, et al., 2001; Braveman, Sen, & Kielhofner, 2001; Braveman et al., 2002; Kielhofner et al., 2003).

At the completion of the project, we set about considering a subsequent project that would continue to meet the needs of people living with AIDS who wished to explore return to work and that would further develop knowledge about how occupational therapy personnel could effectively work with this population. In this case, the population (persons with HIV/AIDS) and the problems of concern (return to work and independent living in the community) were identified before beginning to develop the program.

The next step in the process of moving forward was to delineate more specifically where and how an intervention would occur. The EO Program had addressed primarily the intrapersonal level according to the Ecological Model of Health Promotion. It had done so by focusing on the knowledge, attitude, values, beliefs, and capacities of the participants. In the second project, we wished to have a more sustained impact on the community by building the capacities of organizations to deliver independent living and vocationally relevant services to persons with AIDS on an ongoing basis. In planning the ESD Program, the decision was made that, in addition to intervention at the intrapersonal level, the program would seek to impact services at the interpersonal, organizational, and community levels in order to have a wider and sustained impact on the target population. Table 9–8 provides examples of the focus of interventions at each level of the Ecological Model of Health Promotion addressed in the ESD Program.

Once the decision was made to focus on a program that would have a wider and more sustained impact than the EO Program, and it was evident that the

Table 9-8	Application of the Ecological Model of Health Promotion to the ESD Program
Level of the Ecological Model	**Focus of Interventions in the ESD Program**
Intrapersonal	Increase perceived self-efficacy in activities to support independent living in the community and return to work, such as budgeting, effective communication, and conflict management skills.
Interpersonal	Offer peer-led support groups or job clubs in which participants can discuss strategies, experiences, and frustrations related to returning to work or finding housing in the community.
Organizational	Work with facility leadership, peer educators, case managers, and transitional living staff to establish consistent expectations of behavior regarding involvement and attendance in programming.
Community	Work with nonprofit advocacy agencies, government-run "one-stop job centers," and transitional living facilities to develop effective and ongoing collaborative initiatives.

(continued)

program would include interventions aimed at multiple levels of the environment, steps to plan a specific program model could begin. In the remainder of this section, each of the four steps of program development shown in Figure 9–2 and described earlier will be illustrated as they were applied to the development of the ESD Program.

Needs Assessment

During the first step, needs assessment, a program planner must describe the needs of the target population and identify resources available to them as well as the constraints and challenges faced. In the case of the ESD Program, the process of needs assessment required us to examine both the needs of the residents of supportive living facilities and, because the program included the goal of building the capacity of the organizations to deliver services, the needs of the facility staff as well.

THE NEEDS OF THE TARGET POPULATION: RESIDENTS OF SUPPORTIVE LIVING FACILITIES FOR PERSONS WITH HIV/AIDS

Although the EO Program had been largely successful with clients who had stable housing, many of the clients who resided in supportive living settings had dropped out of the program. Their situation was examined more closely by conducting key informant interviews with facility staff and by surveying 58 residents in five supportive living facilities in Chicago. Data from the survey highlighted that the residents of supportive living facilities closely resembled the nationally emerging population of people with AIDS. They were 20% female, 59% African-American, and 15% Hispanic. More than 60% had a history of substance abuse and 50% had some form of mental illness. Most had lived chaotic lives characterized by unstable living situations or homelessness (68%), chronic unemployment (82%), hospitalization (84%), domestic violence (36%), and incarceration (41%). Half (50%) reported serious symptoms and/or medication side effects that complicated and interfered with performing daily tasks. Many had limited education (15% lacked a high school diploma).

Further, the survey revealed that these individuals were in a complex dilemma about their lives. Their lives had deteriorated such that they required support for daily living. Most had come to the facilities following a period of serious illness and/or chaotic personal circumstances. They were aware that they would eventually be required to move beyond supportive living and expressed sincere wishes to do so, but their confidence about living on their own was severely shaken.

As a result of their experiences, these residents had not developed strong confidence in their vocational skills, and this had affected their vocational interests and motivation. Most (95%) had recently relied on public assistance. Most (75%) desired to both live on their own and find employment, but they reported uncertainty over whether they could handle the challenges involved. They were concerned about the impact of their prolonged absence from the work force and how peers and supervisors would respond to their illness. They also worried about the impact that working would have on their social security and health benefits, especially given the cost of their life-sustaining medications. Consequently, they lacked a clear and hopeful vision about how to become self-determining.

Most residents had experienced a near-total breakdown of everyday habits of living and were just beginning to re-establish routines that supported health and well-being. Like other persons with chronic illness, they had lost their ordinary involvements and were consumed with the routines of managing their own illnesses. Many expressed concern about overcoming the inertia of habitual inactivity and the challenges of instituting a daily life routine to support community living and working.

In addition, residents' stories reinforced that individuals with AIDS face very real environmental pressures to move beyond their current circumstances. The institutions in which they lived could only provide temporary, transitional housing. They faced limited access to public or governmental benefits, such as Social Security Disability Insurance or Medicaid, because of improved health and function. Living and participating in the community not only required that residents develop skills that many lacked for managing a home, but, because of the escalating costs and limited availability of affordable housing, community living frequently required that residents gain employment to increase their incomes.

(continued)

Case Example: Developing an Occupational Therapy Program Using Evidence—the Enabling Self-Determination for Persons Living with HIV/AIDS Program (Continued)

However, the community and workplace presented attitudinal and other barriers to independence, integration, and work for a person with AIDS. For example, they legitimately worried over what would happen if they disclosed their HIV status to obtain services or request accommodations. By disclosing their status, they risked discrimination associated with AIDS. Alternatively, trying to "pass" in the workplace entailed difficulties (e.g., managing medication side effects such as fatigue and diarrhea without detection by others) that could, in turn, produce high levels of stress.

THE NEEDS OF TRANSITIONAL LIVING FACILITIES FOR PERSONS LIVING WITH HIV/AIDS

Nationally, programs previously accustomed to serving clients with a terminal prognosis were struggling to make the transition to rehabilitative models of service delivery. Supportive living facilities for people with AIDS had been organized to provide care to meet basic needs such as housing, nutrition, basic case management, and often hospice care. The staff of these facilities simply lacked the knowledge, skills, and organizational structures for offering services to support self-determination.

Importantly, we learned from the facilities that residents were not accessing existing services oriented to promoting independence in living or return to employment. This lack of utilization was because of several factors, including: (1) residents lacked the knowledge, skills, and habits to access services; (2) supportive living facilities' staff lacked the knowledge of agencies providing such services; and (3) agencies serving persons with disabilities did not actively target people with AIDS. For example, limited service utilization by people with AIDS was confirmed by the Illinois Office of Rehabilitation Services (Debra Russell, personal communication, 2001). During the year prior to development of the ESD Program, only 11 people with a diagnosis of AIDS received vocational rehabilitation services statewide, despite the large numbers living with AIDS in Illinois. Agencies such as the Jewish Vocational Service and the Chicago Industrial League (two of Chicago's largest private providers of vocational services) reported that few people with AIDS utilized their services. Consequently, it became evident that an effective model of service must link people with AIDS to existing, relevant services.

CHOOSING A CONCEPTUAL PRACTICE MODEL

Two guiding frameworks were used to design the ESD Program. The first framework was the Social Model of Disability, which views disability as the result of interaction of the person with the environment (Charlton, 1998; Hahn, 2003; Oliver, 1996). This framework underscores how problems at the community or societal level, such as lack of housing and societal stereotypes, can impose disability on the individual and how eliminating social and physical barriers and creating proactive policies can reduce disability.

Complimenting the Social Model of Disability, we used the MOHO, which also emphasizes person-environment interaction and had been successfully used for two decades to design rehabilitation programs focused on supporting success in community living and employment. These programs had addressed groups that shared characteristics with our target population (e.g., people experiencing AIDS, homelessness, mental illness, and imprisonment) (Braveman et al., 2002; Kielhofner & Brinson, 1989; Pizzi, 1989; Salz, 1983).

In planning the ESD Program, we relied on our 15 years of experience and success in using this dual conceptual approach to design comprehensive programs focused on supporting self-determination in everyday life. In addition, we based our decision to utilize the MOHO on the evolving evidence that supported the model. More than 80 studies have been published on the MOHO (Kielhofner & Iyenger, 2002). These studies include both basic research designed to test the theory and applied research that examines its utility in practice. Basic research on the model includes the following kinds of studies:

(continued)

- Construct validity studies that seek to verify concepts (e.g., Doble, 1991; Mallinson, Kielhofner, & Mattingly, 1996; Oakley, Kielhofner, Barris, & Reichler, 1986; Pan & Fisher, 1994)
- Correlative studies that examine the accuracy of relationships between constructs proposed in the theory (e.g., Barris, Dickie, & Baron, 1988; Duellman, Barris, & Kielhofner, 1986; Neville-Jan, 1994; Peterson et al., 1999)
- Studies comparing groups on concepts from the theory to test whether they explain group differences (e.g., Barris, Kielhofner, Burch, Gelinas, Klement, & Schultz, 1986; Davies Hallet, Zasler, Maurer, & Cash, 1994; Ebb, Coster, & Duncombe, 1989; Lederer, Kielhofner, & Watts, 1985)
- Prospective studies that examine the potential of the model's concepts and propositions to predict future behavior or states (e.g., Chen, Neufeld, Feely, & Skinner, 1999; Rust, Barris, & Hooper, 1987)
- Qualitative studies that explore the model's concepts and propositions in depth (e.g., Braveman, Helfrich, Kielhofner, & Albrecht, 2003; Jonsson, Josephsson, & Kielhofner, 2000, 2001; Jonsson, Kielhofner, & Borell, 1997)

Applied research based on this model falls into the following categories:

- Psychometric studies leading to development of assessments (e.g., Brollier, Watts, Bauer, & Schmidt, 1989; Forsyth, Lai, & Kielhofner, 1999; Fossey, 1996; Viik, Watts, Madigan, & Bauer, 1990)
- Studies of how the model's concepts influence therapeutic reasoning and practice (e.g., Muñoz, Lawlor, & Kielhofner, 1993; Oakley, Kielhofner, & Barris, 1985)
- Studies that examine what happens in therapy (e.g., Helfrich & Kielhofner, 1994; Kielhofner & Barrett, 1998)
- Studies examining the outcomes of services based on the model (e.g., Josephsson, Backman, Borell, & Nygård, 1995; Kielhofner & Brinson, 1989)

Over time, research on the MOHO has grown more sophisticated and rigorous. Many of the earlier and continuing studies have focused on validation of model of human occupation concepts and assessments. Studies that examine the therapy process and the outcomes of therapy are less well represented in

the body of research, though there is a growing emphasis on such studies related to this model.

Program Planning

In the second step, program planning, we defined a focus for the program, identified who must be involved in planning to assure success (e.g., who were key decision makers in the supportive living facilities who would have to approve the program), established goals and objectives, established methods to integrate the program into the existing systems, and developed referral mechanisms.

We carefully designed a corresponding four-phase continuum of services. At each phase, we focused on supporting the development of personal skills, habits, and confidence as guided by the conceptual practice model (the MOHO) upon which the program was based. Each program element was tied to the underlying mechanisms of action that we believed would facilitate change in behavior and personal capacity of the residents. Equally important was to address the environmental interventions and supports. People with disabilities in general face severe gaps in housing, education, transportation, jobs, and participation in many areas of life, along with discrimination and negative attitudinal barriers regarding disability. This was no less true for people with AIDS.

Ongoing research into factors that influence independence and employment success among persons with disabilities (including those with AIDS) indicated that self-determination involves transition through a process that can be conceptualized in four phases: (1) capacity for self-management, (2) identifying future goals and managing routines, (3) developing competence and vision, and (4) achieving success and satisfaction in everyday living and working (Barrett, Beer, & Kielhofner, 1999; Braveman & Helfrich, 2001; Kielhofner et al., 1999). The self-determination tasks expected to be accomplished in each phase are outlined in Table 9–9.

The vocational components of the ESD program also incorporated relevant elements from a "menu approach" and the Individual Placement and Support Model, two other areas of related knowledge for which we found sufficient evidence (Becker & Drake, 1994; Bond, 1998). These components included (1) early placement in actual work contexts,

(continued)

Case Example: Developing an Occupational Therapy Program Using Evidence—the Enabling Self-Determination for Persons Living with HIV/AIDS Program (Continued)

(2) integrated attention to vocational and mental health needs, (3) a consumer-focused "menu" of choices and paths, (4) continuous and comprehensive assessment, and (5) ongoing support as necessary for ultimate success.

We designed the program sequence to consider that a majority of the residents living in the transitional facilities with which we would be working would be managing recovery from substance abuse concurrently with their efforts to establish self-determination. Early phases of the program would focus on self-management and establishing routines and habits of self-management, including sobriety and medication

adherence. The first two phases were of a length sufficient to allow for resolution of cognitive problems often present early in the recovery process. These "time-dependent results of abstinence" include marked improvement in memory, concentration, and problem solving in the first months of abstinence, followed by gradual improvements over time (Goldman & Goodheim, 1988). Again, we relied on evidence found in the substance abuse literature that would impact change to guide our decision making about the program model. Emphasis on employment increased in phases 3 and 4 (the last 7 months of the program), consistent with the well-documented positive impact

Table 9-9	Tasks Involved in Four Phases of Achieving Self-Determination			
Capacity for Self-Maintenance	Developing Future Goals and Managing Routines	Developing Competence and Vision	Achieving Community Living and Work Success and Satisfaction
• Maintain positive health status (medication compliance, diet, and exercise). • Maintain sobriety/abstinence. • Manage fatigue and other symptoms while performing self-care and basic routines. • Explore alternatives for future independence and productivity. • Begin to identify and pursue short-term goals. • Build relationships with a peer group.	• Develop confidence and satisfaction in performance and plans for independence and productivity. • Identify goals related to independent self-manager, community participant, and & worker roles. • Develop skills and basic habits for independence and productivity. • Continue positive health status and sobriety/abstinence. • Identify and contribute to a peer group.	• Clarify a personal vision of desired life. • Identify and work as an active member within positive peer group(s). • Consistently work toward long-term goals. • Seek support to garner resources for goals attainment. • Enact values and interests, find satisfaction in daily life. • Take on roles (volunteer/training). • Sustain patterns of independence, productivity, health, and sobriety.	• Sustain work performance. • Find work satisfaction. • Balance worker and other life roles. • Maintain routine that consolidates self-maintenance, community living, and productivity. • Actively advocate for personal needs/rights. • Identify and establish connections with relevant group(s) in the community.

(continued)

Table 9-10	Overview of ESD Program Phases and Program Elements			
Phase 1: Capacity for Self–Maintenance (1 month)	**Phase 2: Developing Future Goals and Managing Routine (3 months)**	**Phase 3: Developing Competence and Vision (4 months)**	**Phase 4: Achieving Community Living and and Work Success Satisfaction (3 months)**
• Individual assessment and goal setting • Medication adherence • Nutrition and exercise program • Stress management • Orientation to local community • Development of positive support systems • Support groups led by peer mentors	• Home management/instrumental activities of daily living • Grooming and personal appearance • Interpersonal communication skills • Developing health interests and leisure pursuits • Household responsibilities • Facility-based jobs • Financial management skills • Support groups led by peer mentors	• Placement in volunteer positions or internships • Referral to the Office of Rehabilitation Services and one-stop job centers • Referrals to related training programs or schools • Job search preparation • Support groups led by peer mentors • Planning for transition to community living	• Job placement • Job coaching and peer mentoring • Managing benefits • Self-advocacy training • Obtaining community housing • Home visits and support in establishing and maintaining the home • Support groups led by peer mentors

of vocational rehabilitation and employment on successful substance abuse recovery and reduced rates of relapse (Platt, 1995). The program elements of the four phases of the ESD program are summarized in Table 9–10.

Program Implementation

During the third step, program implementation, we began to implement the ESD program according to our pre-established goals, objectives, and action plan. We documented actions taken and the results; communicated results, concerns, and actions taken to key stakeholders; and worked to coordinate and solve problems with facility staff and clients.

The plan of the program was developed as part of a grant submitted for funding to the National Institute for Disability and Rehabilitation Research (NIDRR Grant H133G020217). This project was funded for 3 years, and implementation began in January 2003. Following the design of the ESD Program, implementation required developing the specifics of the program, hiring and training appropriate staff, integrating

program services into the existing structures of the supportive living facilities that were participating in the program, and coordinating and documenting activities to facilitate program evaluation.

As the program was implemented, staff already familiar with the conceptual practice model upon which the program was planned (the MOHO) were hired and provided with additional training in the assessments and tools to be used within the program. The program coordinator, who had developed and directed the prior EO Program, provided hands-on supervision and guidance to new project staff. Key to success of the project was the presence of existing facility staff such as case managers and life skill counselors. Program staff had to work carefully to introduce facility staff to concepts and strategies based on the MOHO in lay terms. Continuous effort was made to include facility staff in day-to-day decision making and to develop program materials with an eye to their long-term use by staff members who likely would not be occupational therapists. As facility staff became more familiar with occupational therapy and

(continued)

Case Example: Developing an Occupational Therapy Program Using Evidence—the Enabling Self-Determination for Persons Living with HIV/AIDS Program (Continued)

with the MOHO, they were able to provide helpful observations and insights about individual clients' interests, habits, and values and the progress they were making toward re-establishing independent worker and self-management roles.

Program Evaluation and Outcome Measures

During the last step, program evaluation, we developed a plan to measure the effects of the program against the program goals. However, we started development of our program evaluation plan at the beginning of the program development process when we identified the desired outcomes for the program (the first step in program evaluation). Because this program, like the EO Program before it, had been funded to specifically identify and measure both process and outcomes of the program, an extensive program evaluation system was developed.

Our program evaluation system included both quantitative and qualitative strategies and was both formative (information was collected from all parties during program development to continuously improve the program) and summative (information was collected after implementation of the program on outcomes, effectiveness, and efficiency). Beginning in the earliest phase of the program, we collected qualitative information by conducting focus groups at each transitional living facility with both residents and staff. This approach was designed within a participatory action research (PAR) framework that calls for all persons involved in research, including the subjects being studied, to be partners in the research process and to help guide the research process itself in addition to any interventions (Balcazar, Keys, Kaplan, & Suarez-Balcazar, 1998; Selener, 1997). Although PAR approaches are most often described in the context of research, they can be extremely useful in the formative stages of program development.

Multiple strategies were used to provide for continuous quality improvement of the program. These included obtaining feedback from residents after group and individual sessions, including residents in choosing topics for future intervention sessions, and meeting frequently with facility staff to discuss how

program implementation could be improved. The program team met on a regular basis to discuss the challenges and successes they encountered during implementation of the program, and changes in strategies were made to accommodate the needs and cultures of the individual facilities.

Quantitative elements of the program evaluation system focused on determining the end impact of the program on residents. Therefore, two primary outcomes of the intervention were identified. The following outcome indicators were collected for all program participants 6 months after completing the program:

- The number of hours of paid employment per week
- The type of living situation that the resident was in (supported living or independent)

Program and outcome evaluation are ongoing in this program and will continue as the staff members hired for the ESD Program gradually remove themselves from the facilities and facility staff assumes responsibility for the program.

This case example highlights how several theories and models related to the occupational therapy paradigm and derived from related knowledge were combined to guide development and implementation of a new program. Full outcome statistics on the program are not yet available; however, facility staff report the following key changes:

- An increasing number of residents are accessing and utilizing state vocational rehabilitation services and services offered by nonprofit organizations related to educational and vocational preparedness.
- An increasing number of residents are seeking and finding paid employment.
- The percentage of residents who leave the facility in a planned manner on "good terms" and maintain contact with the facility is increasing, and the percentage who are asked to leave because of behavior problems is decreasing.
- The supportive living facility staff perceives dramatically increased levels of knowledge and skill to provide vocational readiness and independent living programming.

Chapter Summary

This chapter focused on the use of various types of theories and models to guide the development of occupational therapy programming. You were introduced to terminology including *theory, conceptual practice model, frame of reference, occupational therapy paradigm,* and *related knowledge.* The theme of using data, information, and other forms of evidence to guide practice was repeated, and this chapter demonstrated how an occupational therapy manager might use evidence to evaluate the applicability of various theories and models to guide development of a program.

You were introduced to the concept of a *mechanism of action* for change that specifies what changes, how change proceeds, the conditions under which an intervention achieves beneficial results, and why a change may occur for certain groups of consumers and not others. You were also provided four questions that can be used to help you in the process of choosing which theories and models address the underlying mechanisms of action for the type of change you hope to promote through a given type of programming.

A number of different examples were provided in this chapter to illustrate both how a model might be used to guide the steps of program development and how theories and conceptual practice models can be combined. The ESD Program was presented as a case example of occupational therapy programming developed by combining paradigmatic theory with related knowledge. This example also illustrated how existing evidence was used to guide the development of a new program.

At the start of the chapter, you were introduced to David, an occupational therapy manager who was considering how the principles and strategies of evidence-based practice could be applied to his daily work as a manager. Specifically, he wondered about the connections between evidence-based practice and program development.

Resources for Learning More About Developing Programs

Journals That Often Address Program Development

T & D Magazine

T & D Magazine is published by the American Society of Training and Development. The primary

---

Real-Life Solutions

As David moved forward on working with his colleagues to develop a new day treatment program, he gave more thought to how he could utilize the strategies that he had just learned on finding and evaluating data, information, and other forms of evidence in his managerial responsibility for program development. David shared his questions with his colleagues who were managers in the disciplines of psychology, nursing, and social work and with the psychiatrist with whom they worked. Each of these managers noted that their disciplines were also promoting the principles of evidence-based practice and the strategies associated with its implementation.

After consulting with peers who had experience in the area of program development and searching the literature for descriptions of program development and for examples of evidence-based programming, David decided to pursue the following activities:

- Read about and become familiar with key theories from related knowledge useful in program development, such as the Transtheoretical Model of Change, the Health Belief Model, social cognitive theory, and theories related to the mechanisms of action that would underlie the challenges faced by the target population for the day treatment program.
- Adopt the use of a simple program development model to act as a guide for decision making, to be supported by case examples using the model in occupational therapy or other professional literature.
- Become familiar with the primary occupational therapy conceptual practice models for which evidence exists so that he can make better informed decisions about choosing practice models in the future.

audience for the magazine are training and development professionals and line managers who range from new practitioners to seasoned executives in business, government, academia, and consulting. The magazine provides practical information, advice and strategies, reports on new technologies and their application and discussion of current and emerging best practices.

JOURNAL OF ORGANIZATIONAL BEHAVIOR

The *Journal of Organizational Behavior* is dedicated to the study of how organizations impact people and how people shape organizations. It publishes worldwide work-related issues, including leadership and leadership development. The editorial staff encourages both theoretical and empirical inquiry from a diversity of perspectives, methods, and national cultures.

Associations That Are Concerned with Program Development

THE AMERICAN SOCIETY OF TRAINING AND DEVELOPMENT

http://www.astd.org/

The membership of the American Society of Training and Development (ASTD) includes over 70,000 individuals from various fields related to workplace learning and performance from over 100 countries. The ASTD's mission is to provide leadership to individuals, organizations, and society to achieve work-related competence, performance, and fulfillment.

THE AMERICAN PUBLIC HEALTH ASSOCIATION

http://www.apha.org/

The American Public Health Association (APHA) is the oldest and largest organization of public health professionals in the world, representing more than 50,000 members from over 50 occupations of public health. The APHA is concerned with a broad set of issues affecting personal and environmental health, including federal and state funding for health programs, pollution control, programs and policies related to chronic and infectious diseases, a smoke-free society, and professional education in public health.

Useful Web Sites on Program Development

PROGRAM DEVELOPMENT AND EVALUATION UNIT, UNIVERSITY OF WISCONSIN

http://www.uwex.edu/ces/pdande/index.html

The Program Development and Evaluation Unit provides training and technical assistance that enables cooperative extension campus and community-based faculty and staff to plan, implement, and evaluate high-quality educational programs. This Web site includes a program development model, and numerous .pdf files on "quick tips" related to aspects of program development and evaluation.

UNITED CEREBRAL PALSY ASSOCIATION, GREATER UTICA (NEW YORK) AREA INTERNET RESOURCES FOR NONPROFITS

http://www.ucp-utica.org/uwlinks/ nonprofitlinks.htm

The United Cerebral Palsy Association of Greater Utica maintains a Web site with links to other Web sites on a wide range of topics related to developing and managing nonprofit organizations. The directory is organized by topic of interest and includes a section on outcome measurement and program evaluation that includes many topics of interest to those developing new programs. As with any Web site of this type, some of the links were not current, but this site has been well maintained and the majority of links are functional.

Reference List

Ali, N. S. (2002). Prediction of coronary heart disease preventive behaviors in women: A test of the Health Belief Model. *Women & Health, 35,* 83–96.

Balcazar, F. B., Keys, C. B., Kaplan, D. L., & Suarez-Balcazar, Y. (1998). Participatory action research and people with disabilities: Principles and challenges. *Canadian Journal of Rehabilitation, 12,* 105–112.

Barrett, L., Beer, D., & Kielhofner, G. (1999). The importance of volitional narrative in treatment: An ethnographic case study in a work program. *Work, 12,* 79–92.

Barris, R., Dickie, V., & Baron, K. (1988). A comparison of psychiatric patients and normal subjects based on the Model of Human Occupation. *Occupational Therapy Journal of Research, 8,* 3–37.

Barris, R., Kielhofner, G., Burch, R. M., Gelinas, I., Klement, M., & Schultz, B. (1986). Occupational function and dysfunction in three groups of adolescents. *Occupational Therapy Journal of Research, 6*, 301–317.

Becker, D. R., & Drake, R. E. (1994). Individual placement and support: A community mental health center approach to vocational rehabilitation. *Community Mental Health Journal, 34*, 71–82.

Bond, G. R. (1998). Principles of the Individual Placement and Support Model: Empirical support. *Psychiatric Rehabilitation Journal, 22*, 11–23.

Braveman, B., Goldbaum, L., Goldstein, K., Karlic, L., & Kielhofner, G. (2001). *Employment options: A program leading to the Employment of Persons Living with AIDS Program manual.* Chicago: Model of Human Occupation Clearinghouse.

Braveman, B., Helfrich, C., Kielhofner, G., & Albrecht, G. (2003). The narratives of 12 men living with AIDS. *Journal of Occupational Rehabilitation, 13*, 143–147.

Braveman, B., & Helfrich, C. A. (2001). Occupational identity: Exploring the narratives of three men living with AIDS. *Journal of Occupational Science, 8*, 35–31.

Braveman, B., Kielhofner, G., Belanger, R., Llerena, V., & de las Heras, C. G. (2002). Program development. In G. Kielhofner (Ed.), *The Model of Human Occupation: Theory and application* (3rd ed., pp. 491–519). Baltimore: Williams & Wilkins.

Braveman, B., Sen, S., & Kielhofner, G. (2001). Community-based vocational rehabilitation programs. In M. Scaffa (Ed.), *Occupational therapy in community-based practice settings* (pp. 139–161). Philadelphia: F. A. Davis.

Brollier, C., Watts, J. H., Bauer, D., & Schmidt, W. (1989). A content validity study of the Assessment of Occupational Functioning. *Occupational Therapy in Mental Health 8*(4), 29–47.

Brownson, C. (2001). Program development for community health: Planning, implementation and evaluation strategies. In M. Scaffa (Ed.), *Occupational therapy in community-based practice settings* (pp. 95–116). Philadelphia: F. A. Davis.

Buckley, P. (1996). *Essential papers on object relations.* New York: New York University Press.

Charlton, J. (1998). *Nothing about us without us.* Berkeley: University of California Press.

Chen, C., Neufeld, P. S., Feely, C. A., & Skinner, C. S. (1999). Factors influencing compliance with home exercise programs among patients with upper-extremity impairment. *American Journal of Occupational Therapy, 53*, 171–180.

Conrad, K. M., Cambell, R. T., Edington, D. W., & Faust, H. S. (1996). The worksite environment as a cue to smoking reduction. *Research in Nursing & Health, 19*, 21–31.

Crepeau, E. B., & Schell, B. A. B. (2003). Theory and practice in occupational therapy. In E.B. Crepeau, E. S. Cohn, & B. A. B. Schell (Eds.), *Willard and Spackman's occupational therapy* (10th ed., pp. 203–207). Philadelphia: Lippincott, Williams & Wilkins.

Davies Hallet, J., Zasler, N., Maurer, P., & Cash, S. (1994). Role change after traumatic brain injury in adults. *American Journal of Occupational Therapy, 48*, 241–246.

Dilorio, C., Dudley, W. N., Soet, J., Watkins, J., & Maibach, E. (2000). A social cognitive-based model for condom use among college students. *Nursing Research, 49*, 208–214.

Doble, S. E. (1991). Test-retest and inter-rater reliability of a process skills assessment. *Occupational Therapy Journal of Research, 11*, 8–23.

Duellman, M. K., Barris, R., & Kielhofner, G. (1986). Organized activity and the adaptive status of nursing home residents. *American Journal of Occupational Therapy, 40*, 618–622.

Ebb, E. W., Coster, W., & Duncombe, L. (1989). Comparison of normal and psychosocially dysfunctional male adolescents. *Occupational Therapy in Mental Health, 9*(2), 53–74.

Fischera, S. D., & Frank, D. I. (1995). The Health Belief Model as a predictor of mammography screening. *Health Values, 18*, 3–9.

Forsyth, K., Lai, J., & Kielhofner, G. (1999). The Assessment of Communication and Interaction Skills (ACIS): Measurement properties. *British Journal of Occupational Therapy, 62*, 69–74.

Fossey, E. (1996). Using the Occupational Performance History Interview (OPHI): Therapists' reflections. *British Journal of Occupational Therapy, 59*, 223–228.

Galavotti, C., Cabral, R. J., Lansky, A., Grimley, D. M., Riley, G. E., & Prochaska, J. O. (1995). Validation of measures of condom and other contraceptive use among women at high risk for HIV infection and unintended pregnancy. *Health Psychology, 14*, 570–578.

Gitlin, L. N., Corcoran, M., Martindale-Adams, J., Malone, C., Stevens, A., & Winter, L. (2000). Identifying mechanisms of action: Why and how does intervention work? In R. Schulz (Ed.), *Handbook of dementia caregiving: Evidence-based interventions for family caregivers* (pp. 225–248). Philadelphia: Springer.

Glanz, K., Patterson, R. E., Kristal, A. R., DiClemente, C., Heimendinger, J., Linnan, L., et al. (1995). Stages of change in adopting healthy diets: Fat, fiber, and correlates of nutrient intake. *Health Education Quarterly, 21*(4), 499–519.

Goldman, R. S., & Goodheim, L. (1988). Experience-dependent cognitive recovery in alcoholics: A task component strategy. *Journal of Studies in Alcohol, 2*, 142–148.

Grossman, J., & Bortone, J. (1986). Program development. In S. C. Robertson (Ed.), *SCOPE: Strategies, concepts, and opportunities for program development and evaluation* (pp. 91–99). Bethesda, MD: American Occupational Therapy Association.

Hahn, H. (2003). Disability policy and the problem of discrimination. *Behavioral Scientist, 28*, 293–318.

Helfrich, C., & Kielhofner, G. (1994). Volitional narratives and the meaning of occupational therapy. *American Journal of Occupational Therapy, 48*, 319–326.

Jammer, M. S., Wolitski, R. J., & Corby, N. H. (1997). Impact of a longitudinal community HIV intervention targeting injecting drug users' stage of change for condom and bleach use. *American Journal of Health Promotion, 12*(1), 15–24.

Jonsson, H., Josephsson, S., & Kielhofner, G. (2000). Evolving narratives in the course of retirement: A longitudinal study. *American Journal of Occupational Therapy, 54*, 463–470.

Jonsson, H., Josephsson, S., & Kielhofner, G. (2001). Narrative and experience in an occupational transition: A longitudinal study of the retirement process. *American Journal of Occupational Therapy, 55*, 424–432.

Jonsson, H., Kielhofner, G., & Borell, B. (1997). Anticipating retirement: The formation of narratives concerning an occupational transition. *American Journal of Occupational Therapy, 51*, 49–56.

Josephsson, S., Backman, L., Borell, B., & Nygård, L. (1995). Effectiveness of an intervention to improve occupational performance in dementia. *Occupational Therapy Journal of Research, 15,* 36–49.

Kalichan, S. C., & Nachimson, D. (1999). Self-efficacy and disclosure of HIV-positive serostatus to sex partners. *Health Psychology, 18,* 281–287.

Keller, C., Fleury, J., Gregor-Holt, N., & Thompson, T. (1999). Predictive ability of social cognitive theory in exercise research: An integrated literature review. *Journal of Knowledge Synthesis in Nursing, 5*(January), 6–8.

Kielhofner, G. (2002). *The Model of Human Occupation: Theory and application* (3rd ed.). Baltimore: Williams & Wilkins.

Kielhofner, G. (2004). *Conceptual foundations of occupational therapy* (3rd ed.). Philadelphia: F. A. Davis.

Kielhofner, G., Baron, K., Braveman, B., Fisher, G. S., Hammel, J., & Littleton, M. (1999). The Model of Human Occupation: Understanding the worker who is ill or injured. *Work, 12,* 3–12.

Kielhofner, G., & Barrett, L. (1998). Meaning and misunderstanding in occupational forms: A study of therapeutic goal setting. *American Journal of Occupational Therapy, 52,* 345–353.

Kielhofner, G., Braveman, B., Finlayson, M., Paul-Ward, A., Goldbaum, L., & Goldstein, K. (2003). Outcomes of a vocational rehabilitation program for people with AIDS. *American Journal of Occupational Therapy, 51,* 64–72.

Kielhofner, G., & Brinson, M. (1989). Development and evaluation of an aftercare program for young and chronic psychiatrically disabled adults. *Occupational Therapy in Mental Health, 9,* 53–74.

Kielhofner, G., & Iyenger, A. (2002). Research: Investigating MOHO. In *A Model of Human Occupation: Theory and Application* (3rd ed., pp. 520–545). Baltimore: Williams & Wilkins.

Langlois, M. A., Petosa, R., & Hallam, J. S. (1999). Why do effective smoking prevention programs work? Student changes in social cognitive theory constructs. *Journal of School Health, 69,* 326–331.

Lederer, J., Kielhofner, G., & Watts, J. (1985). Values, personal causation and skills of delinquents and non delinquents. *Occupational Therapy in Mental Health, 5*(2), 59–77.

Marcus, B. H., Banspach, S. W., Lefebvre, C. R., Rossi, J. S., Carleton, R. A., & Abrams, D. B. (1992). Using the stages of change model to increase the adoption of physical activity among community participants. *American Journal of Health Promotion, 6,* 424–429.

Mallinson, T., Kielhofner, G., & Mattingly, C. (1996). Metaphor and meaning in a clinical interview. *American Journal of Occupational Therapy, 50,* 338–346.

McLeroy, K. R., Bibeau, D., Steckler, A., & Glanz, K. (1988). An ecological perspective on health promotion programs. *Health Education Quarterly, 25,* 351–377.

Muñoz, J. P., Lawlor, M., & Kielhofner, G. (1993). Use of the Model of Human Occupation: A survey of therapists in psychiatric practice. *Occupational Therapy Journal of Research, 13,* 117–139.

Neville-Jan, A. (1994). The relationship of volition to adaptive occupational behavior among individuals with varying degrees of depression. *Occupational Therapy in Mental Health, 12*(4), 1–18.

Oakley, F., Kielhofner, G., & Barris, R. (1985). An occupational therapy approach to assessing psychiatric patients' adaptive functioning. *American Journal of Occupational Therapy, 39,* 147–154.

Oakley, F., Kielhofner, G., Barris, R., & Reichler, R. K. (1986). The Role Checklist: Development and empirical assessment of reliability. *Occupational Therapy Journal of Research, 6,* 157–170.

Oliver, M. (1996). *Understanding disability from theory to practice.* New York: St. Martin's Press.

Pan, A. W., & Fisher, A. G. (1994). The assessment of motor and process skills of persons with psychiatric disorders. *American Journal of Occupational Therapy, 48,* 775–780.

Perkins, D. O. (1999). Adherence to antipsychotic medications. *Journal of Clinical Psychiatry, 60,* 25–30.

Peterson, E., Howland, J., Kielhofner, G., Lachman, M. E., Assmann, S., Cote, J., et al. (1999). Falls self-efficacy and occupational adaptation among elders. *Physical and Occupational Therapy in Geriatrics, 16*(1/2), 1–16.

Pizzi, M. A. (1989). The model of human occupation and adults with HIV infection and AIDS. *American Journal of Occupational Therapy, 44,* 257–264.

Platt, J. J. (1995). Vocational rehabilitation of drug abusers. *Psychological Bulletin, 117,* 416–433.

Prochaska, J. O., & DiClemente, J. C. (1993). In search of how people change: Applications to addictive behavior. *American Psychologist, 47,* 1102–1114.

Riley, T. A., Toth, J. M., & Fava, J. L. (2000). The Transtheoretical Model and stress management practices in women at risk for, or infected with HIV. *Journal of the Association of Nurses in AIDS Care, 11*(1), 67–77.

Rosenstock, I. M., Strecher, V. J., & Becker, M. H. (1988). Social learning theory and the Health Belief Model. *Health Education Quarterly, 15,* 175–183.

Rust, K., Barris, R., & Hooper, F. (1987). Use of the Model of Human Occupation to predict women's exercise behavior. *Occupational Therapy Journal of Research, 7,* 23–35.

Salz, C. (1983). A theoretical approach to the treatment of work difficulties in borderline personalities. *Occupational Therapy in Mental Health, 3,* 33–46.

Sapp, S. G., & Jensen, H. H. (1998). An evaluation of the Health Belief Model for predicting perceived and actual dietary quality. *Journal of Applied Social Psychology, 28,* 235–248.

Scaffa, M. E. (2001). *Occupational therapy in community-based practice settings.* Philadelphia: F. A. Davis.

Selener, D. (1997). *Participatory action research and social change.* Ithaca, NY: Cornell Participatory Action Research Network.

Sheeshka, J. D., Woolcott, D. M., & MacKinnon, N. J. (1994). An evaluation of a theory-based demonstration worksite nutrition promotion program. *American Journal of Health Promotion, 8,* 263–264.

Strecher, V. J., DeVillis, B. M., Becker, M. H., & Rosenstock, I. M. (1986). The role of self-efficacy in achieving health behavior change. *Health Education Quarterly, 13,* 73–91.

Viik, M. K., Watts, J. H., Madigan, M. J., & Bauer, D. (1990). Preliminary validation of the Assessment of Occupational Functioning with an alcoholic population. *Occupational Therapy in Mental Health, 10*(2), 19–33.

Winfield, E. B., & Whaley, A. L. (2002). A comprehensive test of the Health Belief Model in the prediction of condom use among African American college students. *Journal of Black Psychology, 28,* 330–346.

10

Barbara Schell, Ph.D., OTR/L, FAOTA
Brent Braveman, Ph.D., OTR/L, FAOTA

Turning Theory into Practice: Managerial Strategies

Real-Life Management

At one point in her career, Barbara accepted a position at a large rehabilitation facility. As the Director of Occupational Therapy, Barbara was responsible for overall management of about 40 individuals, most of whom were occupational therapists and occupational therapy assistants. As is common in facilities such as this, staff members were assigned to teams, and these teams focused on programmatic areas, such as dealing with people with head injuries, strokes, spinal cord injuries, and the like. Barbara's major challenge as the new director was to develop more current and cohesive occupational therapy approaches, which in turn would improve patient outcomes, as well as strengthen the recognition of what occupational therapy services had to offer.

Although there were many positive points about the staff and programs, there were also several challenges, starting with the fact that the physical therapy department was very strong, and had provided the major rehabilitation leadership in the facility. They had led the way in facilitating consistency in service delivery, most notably by encouraging occupational therapists, nurses, speech-language pathologists, and others to use neurodevelopmental techniques for positioning, tone management, and facilitation of movement. Occupational therapy had a somewhat fragmented program approach, with most self-care training provided by occupational therapy assistants and licensed practical nurses, and the homemaking

training provided by rehabilitation home economists. This approach had evolved as a result of the tremendous shortage of occupational therapy personnel in the region. Much of the intervention by occupational therapists was clinic-based and involved a lot of mat work and contrived tabletop activities with a goal of improving upper extremity function. Not surprisingly, the occupational therapy staff members were a bit insecure about the recognition of their contributions, as well as their relative status as compared with physical therapy. On top of all this, there still was significant turnover, primarily because the job market was so volatile as a result of the shortage of occupational therapy personnel. There were four occupational therapy supervisors who worked under Barbara's direction, and who in turn both carried caseloads and supervised the occupational therapy staff assigned to the various teams. Each interdisciplinary program team also had a program manager, so there was a significant need to coordinate occupational therapy practices with each particular program.

As Barbara began her new job, the key questions she had included the following:

- How do I start to gain the trust of the staff, which will be necessary to build better practice?
- How should we decide what constitutes "good practice"?

Real-Life Management (*continued*)

- Once an understanding of good practice is negotiated, how can we get (and keep) everyone "on the same page"?
- What are the implications for staff roles, productivity, and billing of any changes made?

- How can we communicate the nature and value of our services?
- How will we know if all this is working for the patients as well as for the staff?

Key Issues

- Effective management and supervision require an integration of departmental policy and personnel management strategies in light of the theories and practice models chosen to guide practice.
- The tangible tools and resources used to conduct and document occupational therapy services must be designed in light of the theories and related evidence guiding practice.
- The personnel practices within the department, including staff selection, orientation, development, and performance appraisal, must support and reward practices that are consistent with the espoused theories.
- Managers can play a critical role in *leading* occupation-based and evidence-based practice in their settings.

It is one thing to understand theory, research, and evidence, and to use them for program planning. In Chapter 9, you read an in-depth discussion of this process. It is another thing to bring those programs to life, and to create systems that support the people responsible for implementing the programs. The previous real-life management scenario describes the experiences of one of the authors of this chapter. Moreover, it portrays the challenges inherent in managing evidence-based practice that are faced by occupational therapy managers. As we reflected on the experiences and the actions that Barbara took in response, we realized that Barbara's actions in that setting, and in additional programs developed by both of us, were designed to cultivate a *community of practice*. A community of practice can be defined as follows (Wenger, McDermott, & Snyder, 2002):

> "*Communities of practice are groups of people who share a concern, a set of problems, or a passion about a topic, and who deepen their knowledge and expertise in this area by interacting on an ongoing basis.*"

At first glance, it might seem odd to think about a *community* of practice. However, the concept and definition of what has been considered a community has varied widely in social science literature. Towns and cities have been called communities, but

so have prisons and religious groups. Even corporations, factories, and trade unions have been referred to as communities (Minar & Greer, 1969). Fellin (1993) described the useful concept that the persons we encounter may also have membership in nonplace, "identificational communities." In this way, we might think about a group of occupational therapy practitioners who work in the same setting and share the same concerns as a community. The nature of the community may vary in size, in how homogeneous the members are, and in how long the community lasts. Table 10–1 provides examples of occupational therapy communities of practice, their focus, the participants, and the nature of their relationships. By seeking to understand the management task of building and maintaining a community of practice, managers can be sensitized to sociologic as well as psychological issues that must be addressed.

Many communities of practice are not tied to a specific management unit, and are composed of individuals from different disciplines with different knowledge bases. In private industry, organization consultants are advocating the support of such "knowledge communities" as a method of responding to globalization of companies, and the rapidly changing configurations of teams and organizational units (see Wenger et al., 2002, for examples). Skilled occupational therapy managers and super-

Table 10-1	Communities of Practice in Occupational Therapy (OT)			
Example	**Focus**	**Participants**	**Nature of Relationships**	
OT department	Delivery of effective service	Staff, supervisors, manager	Formal organizational hierarchy	
OT Discipline Group within a Program Management System	Mutual development and effective service	Staff assigned to programs	Informal or matrix relationships	
Local Pediatric Special Interest Group–Interdisciplinary	Advancement of knowledge and networking to improve service delivery across settings	Variety of therapists (i.e., OT, PT, SLP) from varied settings	Informal, voluntary	
AOTA Administrative & Management Special Interest Group	Sharing of knowledge and skills related to managing occupational therapy services	Members of AOTA who elect to join, generally people who are or want to become managers, supervisors, and/or administrators	Voluntary subset of professional society	
International researchers looking at occupation & habits	Examination of cross-cultural aspects of human occupation and the implications for health	Faculty members & scholars in many countries interested in occupational science & occupational behavior	A mix of informal voluntary to formalized research relationships, some mentoring relationships	

PT, physical therapist; SLP, speech-language pathologist.

visors can facilitate the creation and support of a community (or communities) of practice with the staff members in their assigned area. In this chapter, we will explore the specific management strategies that can be used to develop and support a community of practice.

 ## Communities of Practice Structures

Wenger et al. suggested that there are three common aspects to the structure of communities of practice, and that the combination of these structures is in part what makes each community of practice unique. These common aspects are as follows (the definitions in quotes are all from Wenger et al., 2002):

- The "*domain* of knowledge, which defines a set of issues." For instance, for Barbara and her staff, there were some significant issues regarding the appropriate domain of knowledge for occupational therapy. By virtue of the way the department was organized, knowledge and skill related to improving self-care and some instrumental activities of daily living had been relegated to occupational therapy assistants, licensed practical nurses, and rehabilitation home economists. The occupational therapists were most focused on neuromotor function, positioning to prevent or minimize abnormal tone, and task training devoted to improving coordination. This focus varied according to the program in which each staff member worked. For instance, on the spinal cord injury unit, there was great attention to muscle testing and use of adaptive technology, whereas, on the chronic pain unit, key knowledge included the behavioral management aspects of treating people with chronic pain. Curiously, from the managerial perspective (and from that of others viewing occupational therapy services), there was little that carried over from unit to unit, so that it was difficult to see the common core of occupational therapy services.

- The "*community* of people who care about this domain," which in this case included most of the individuals in the department: the occupational therapists, occupational therapy assistants, licensed practical nurses, and rehabilitation home economists. This community was nested within the larger community of rehabilitation team members, which typically included one or more physical therapists, speech-language pathologists, recreation therapists, psychologists, rehabilitation nurses, physiatrists, and internal medicine physicians. Similarly, the occupational therapists and occupational therapy assistants were part of the larger occupational therapy community within the city, and in some cases the state and nation.
- The "shared *practice* that they are developing to be effective in their domain." McCormack, Jaffe, and Frey (2003) suggested that shared practice includes *roles*, such as what aspect of rehabilitation each team member attends to, or who reports at team meetings; *rules*, such as how soon initial evaluations need to be done and how vacation coverage is arranged; and *tools*, such as the actual assessment tools available and the forms used to document results.

Many of the chapters in this book emphasize the *domain of knowledge*, particularly the use of theory and evidence to develop and implement programming. The *community* for purposes of this discussion is the unit or program for which the manager is responsible. Let's turn our discussion to the application of the roles, rules, and tools (many of which were introduced in Chapters 5 and 6) that must be addressed to support good practice.

Managing Practice: Roles, Rules, and Tools

What are the typical aspects of practice that must be addressed? McCormack (2003) noted that, in contrast to the classic descriptions of management functions as planning, organizing and staffing, coordinating, and controlling, most managers have little time to reflect, and are in fact "doers" whose "planning is done in real time as the job demands are being addressed." If that is the case, it is all the more important that managers have a guiding idea or mental framework to use as the basis for making the myriad daily decisions that range from where to spend limited continuing education money to what to purchase for departmental equipment and supplies. Let's return to the key questions posed in the real-life management scenario at the beginning of this chapter and examine the strategies that Barbara used as she sought to shape practice and to develop a community of practice by attending to the structures that support practice.

How Do I Start to Gain the Trust of the Staff, Which Will Be Necessary to Build Better Practice?

BUILD TRUST

You should start building trust immediately. Whether you are a newly hired manager or one promoted from within, you must understand what your staff members currently think and believe. One of the first things Barbara did as a new manager in the rehabilitation center was to meet with every person on her staff individually. This may sound overwhelming, but, by limiting the meetings to 20 to 30 minutes, she was able to connect personally with the entire staff in less than a month.

The most effective format for such interviews is a semistructured interview. Examples of good questions to ask are provided in Box 10–1. Once you have obtained the answers, you can summarize them and feed them back to the group as a whole. This is an efficient way to demonstrate to staff members that you listened to them. It is preferable to do this in person at a staff meeting, if at all possible, because then you can ask for validation or clarification if needed.

Box 10–1: Questions for Getting to Know Your Staff

- What do you like about working here?
- What things are problems for you in working here?
- What would you like to see done to improve patient care?
- What would you like to see done to improve your ability to do your job?
- What things would you like to help with?
- What do you see as the strengths of the department?
- What resources currently assist you most to effectively perform your job?

IDENTIFY A LEADERSHIP GROUP

From your interviews, as well as the structure of your unit, you should identify a core group to work with you on shaping the scope of practice. Barbara's strategy was to use the supervisory group within her department. Other strategies might be to use informal leaders or the more expert practitioners within a department. You can use this group as a sounding board, and encourage them to help you challenge current practices that may not be consistent with emerging evidence. It is important to find individuals who have sufficient expertise to handle the routine demands of the job. These individuals are more likely to have the capacity to challenge their own thinking, in light of evidence that newer practitioners are likely to be struggling to develop practice patterns (Schell, Crepeau, & Cohn, 2003).

DEVELOP OR REFRESH THE UNIT'S MISSION, VISION, AND GOALS

With the information you learn about your staff, the services provided, and your department's strengths and areas for growth, and with the assistance of a core group, you can complete a review of your department's mission, vision, and goals. You were introduced to the concept of mission and vision statements in Chapter 3. If your department does not have its own mission and vision statements, taking your staff members through the process of creating them is an effective strategy for identifying the key things that bring them together as a community of practitioners. In addition to identifying what you have in common, it also can identify differences in beliefs and understanding of which you may not be aware. Investigating these areas of differences can lead you to identify evidence-based questions to research as a group.

Barbara used the feedback from the staff interviews as the basis for a department-wide activity that generated possible solutions, which were prioritized by group members. Because she was dealing with close to 40 people, she clustered them into groups of 8, making a point of mixing staff and supervisors across various units. She then had a team leader in each group facilitate the generation of ideas by using the nominal group technique (described in Chapter 11). This, in addition to the strategic information provided by top management and the information from the individual interviews, formed the initial data on which the group based their departmental vision, as well as the operational objectives for the year.

How Should We Decide What Constitutes "Good Practice"?

By now you should have a good idea of the importance of keeping up with theory and emerging evidence as the cornerstone of shaping effective practice. The reality of keeping up with best practices is challenging for anyone, much less managers and supervisors who are often juggling multiple demands. Further, even if you and your staff do try to keep up with the advances, chances are that keeping up with a wide variety of issues may create the potential for a lack of consensus on the shared practice expectations and standards.

Focusing your efforts and those of your staff can help, starting with your responsibilities. One way of focusing efforts is to lead your staff through the process of identifying your strengths and weaknesses in terms of skills and knowledge. You must prioritize the learning needs of the department and organize to meet those needs first. There is no way around doing this. Incorporating theory and evidence into practice takes time to review and read the literature and to learn. Supporting each other in this process in an organized way, such as covering patients for an identified staff member who is conducting an evidence-based literature review related to a prioritized learning need, can make the process less daunting. You should focus your responsibilities in this process and show your team that you are willing to support their efforts and that you value the process.

RECOGNIZE THAT LEADING PRACTICE IS PART OF YOUR JOB

Perhaps the most important "strategy" is actually the recognition that you have a responsibility to shape practice as well as manage it. Managers sometimes choose to focus on the mechanics of management, such as budgeting or productivity, with the notion that they should let the staff take an "eclectic" approach. In fact, some managers seem to have developed the idea that there is something wrong with taking a role in *directing* the theoretical basis for practice in their setting. Although understandable, especially for new managers who are developing their managerial skills, this abdication of responsibility can result in very efficient therapists doing the wrong things well.

Leading practice may be particularly intimidating if you are accepting responsibility as a manager in an existing occupational therapy department, where the culture of the department, or "the way we do things around here," is well established. However, it is important to remember that changes in culture do not happen overnight and initial resistance to change is natural. One effective strategy would be to begin by introducing the principles of evidence-based practice to your staff so that, rather than being perceived as telling your staff that what they have been doing is wrong, you are questioning whether evidence supports a better approach. This strategy can result in both you and the staff learning something new because it forces you to examine your own assumptions while asking your staff to do the same.

You should make it your business to keep up with emerging theories, research, and evidence. This may require that you place an equal priority on attending advanced theory presentations and on continuing education related to management and supervision. In particular, you should look for advances that may have implications across various specialties, because these can often serve as unifying themes. You can be a role model by admitting that there are aspects of occupational therapy the-

ory, research, and practice with which you struggle, and that integrating these three is not always easy, even for you. Barbara used several resources that assisted her. Initially, she relied heavily on some key American Occupational Therapy Association (AOTA) documents, including those that defined the terminology most commonly used by occupational therapy personnel and sanctioned by AOTA to conceptualize the scope of the department's practice. Today, managers have a number of resources, including the AOTA Occupational Therapy Practice Framework (American Occupational Therapy Association, 2002) and *The Guide to Occupational Therapy Practice* (Moyers, 1999). Such documents generally reflect the current consensus on professional topics of interest. They have credibility both within and outside of the profession, because they represent a carefully generated and widely reviewed analysis.

Attempts to operationalize the concepts represented in these documents will necessitate discussions with your leadership group and the staff, which in turn sets the stage for a more reflective stance toward current practice. Throughout this book, membership in both the AOTA and your state occupational therapy association has been emphasized as an effective strategy for networking and obtaining resources. Not only do resources such as the AOTA Occupational Therapy Practice Framework represent the work of top occupational therapy scholars, but it and other official documents are frequently reviewed and updated so that they can assist you in staying current with changes in thinking and terminology as you gain experience.

In addition to AOTA documents, Barbara had been following the development of the Model of Human Occupation (MOHO), because it seemed to hold some promise to unify the various disparate practices she supervised in the different programs. However, early iterations of the model were difficult to comprehend, particularly because it seemed to be associated more with mental health practice. Nevertheless, because she had a sense that it held important potential, even though she was not sure exactly where it would lead or what it meant for their practice, Barbara continued to learn about the MOHO as the theory was further developed and to pursue options for increasing contact with others who were using the theory. This led Barbara to the next strategy.

Go to the Experts or Bring Them to you

One of the most critical functions a good leader and manager can perform is to support the development of clinical reasoning in his or her staff. Such development is supported by a blend of careful supervision combined with professional development activities. From a practical standpoint, managers need to think strategically about how they expend department travel and consulting funds, which are often limited if they exist at all. Rather than allowing staff members to go to any continuing education conference they suggest, you should make clear what the departmental priorities are, and fund them accordingly.

By tying continuing education experiences to established professional development plans (which are in turn tied to the department's strategic plan), you can gradually build a synergistic pool of knowledge within your practice community. Sometimes you can get more impact by bringing in a consultant to work with your staff directly with respect to specific practice approaches. After working for several years as the manager of the department described in the real-life management scenario, that is exactly what Barbara felt needed to happen. Although expensive in terms of both consultant costs and staff time, she felt that she and the staff needed to have a more sophisticated "department conversation" about what best practice should look like in their setting. That meant she had to find the money, which is when she started paying more attention to funding sources beyond her departmental budget. In this situation, Barbara focused on finding a consultant who could help her identify an occupational therapy theory or framework that could serve to unify the department and guide examination of practices. The MOHO turned out to be an effective resource, once it was more fully explained by the consultant she chose.

Work Within Your System to Obtain Special Monies or Grants

Barbara initially took the lead on raising conceptual issues, but, over time, she found she was having trouble keeping up with the literature and managing a complex department. A small grant from her institution's foundation allowed her to hire a consultant who had recently completed postprofessional graduate work within occupational therapy.

She took the role of identifying recent literature and critical concepts that she felt might help the staff reflect more deeply on their practices as a whole. Additionally, the grant paid for overtime hours, so that all staff could attend.

Although obtaining a grant or some type of other funding will certainly make your task of leading practice easier, there are many strategies that you may use that do not require extra funding. These strategies include (among others)

- "Brown bag" informal lunch discussions of clients, daily dilemmas, clinical problems, or reports from continuing education events attended by staff
- "Journal clubs" in which staff members rotate responsibility for reading a journal article and reporting to the other staff members using a predetermined format
- Co-treating patients with your staff or at least occasionally treating patients in front of your staff so that you may role-model the intervention approaches you are trying to promote
- Developing an active fieldwork education program and creating fieldwork assignments that foster evidence-based review of literature and sharing of new knowledge between staff and students
- Case discussions that not only allow the presentation of clinical problems but also allow discussion and exploration of new strategies by involving the entire staff

Use Your Leadership Skills to Address Practice

The consultant and Barbara designed a 6-month staff development project in which regular meetings were held with each group, organized by program units. Staff members were assigned some readings, and this provoked discussion on current practice. Then, supervisors took the lead in analyzing one of their current patients, using some of the parameters that emerged from the readings (Table 10–2 and Box 10–2 present a case study analysis guide). This case study approach, using real and current patients at the rehabilitation facility, provided a live laboratory with which to explore how new ideas might improve current practice. Supervisors took the lead by discussing a patient on their caseload. During this discussion, an attempt

Table 10-2 Case Analysis Guide—Model of Human Occupation

MOHO Elements	Clinical Reasoning Question
THROUGHPUT **Volition** Personal causation	• Does the person anticipate success? • Does the person feel in control or controlled by others?
Values	• What is important to the person? • What goals does the person have?
Interests	• What does the person like to do?
Narrative	• What is this person's story? • How does the person's life story guide his or her values, interests, and sense of control? • What meaning do the person's performance abilities and limitations have for that person?
Habituation Roles	• What are this person's major occupational roles? • To what degree does the person feel he or she is meeting those role demands? • What expectations does the person have regarding roles, and how flexible are these? • How well balanced are the person's role behaviors?
Habits	• What is this person's typical routine? • How has this been changed? • How well organized are the habit patterns?

Performance Capacity	• Does the person have the necessary performance capacities needed for required occupational skills?
	   • Musculoskeletal
	   • Neurologic
	   • Perceptual
	   • Cognitive
	 • Have there been developmental, traumatic, or environmental stresses that limit skill acquisition?

OUTPUT	• Does the person participate in activities that are personally and socially significant?
	 • Does the person use performance skills competently and consistently?
	   • Motor skills
	   • Process skills
	   • Communication/interaction skills
	 • Is the person satisfied with current occupational performance and identity?
	 • Is the person able to generate adaptive responses to challenges?

ENVIRONMENT	• What are the physical settings in which this person must perform? • What are the temporal expectations in the setting? • What are the social expectations for this person? • What cultural issues must be considered in the person's environment? • Overall, how would you characterize the importance of the person's occupational performance environments, relative to his or her opportunities, resources, demands, and constraints?

(continued)

MOHO Elements	Clinical Reasoning Question

FEEDBACK	• How does the physical environment support and limit desired occupational performance?
	  • Natural and built terrain
	  • Tools
	• How does the social environment support and limit desired occupational performance?
	  • Support systems
	  • Developmental expectations
	  • Cycle of illness or injury
	  • Role demands and flexibility
	• How do these factors impact the person's occupational identity, both now and in the future?

Data from Cubie, S. H., & Kaplan, K. (1982). A case analysis method for the Model of Human Occupation. *American Journal of Occupational Therapy, 36*, 646–648; and Kielhofner, G. (2002). *Model of human occupation* (3rd ed.). Baltimore: Lippincott, Williams & Wilkins.

was made to see what information was available about each of the clinical reasoning questions, whether this information was documented or communicated in any way, and, where information was lacking, what implications that had for practice. During this time, it became apparent that Barbara needed to attend all these sessions, because staff members were threatened by possible changes, and

Box 10–2: Reflective Questions for Case Analysis

Questions About the Case Itself:

• What information do we have about each of the clinical reasoning questions in the case analysis?
  • What is the quality of that information?
  • Is that information considered in intervention planning and implementation?
  • Is that information important to document?
  • Is that information communicated to team members who might find it helpful?
• What information is lacking?
  • Is there a practical way to obtain that information?
  • Does anyone else on the team already collect that information?
  • How might the information that is lacking influence intervention planning?

Questions About Departmental Practices That Arise from the Case Review

• Do we need to change our documentation forms or practices?

• Initial evaluations
• Progress reports
• Discharge summaries
• Patient/client education materials
• Do we need to change our verbal reporting practices?
  • Team meetings and rounds
  • Discharge planning
  • Patient/client education sessions
• Do we have the appropriate intervention resources?
  • Do we have the furniture, tools, and other items available in our clinical areas to provide occupationally centered intervention?
  • Do our policies support timely acquisition of resources needed to customize care?
• How can we gain better access to the person's natural environment?
  • Are site visits or home visits possible?
  • Can we obtain videotapes or photos?

needed her assurance that she would collaborate to identify changes, once the staff had a better idea of what needed to be changed. At the end of this process, the staff spent time reflecting on what specific changes were needed in policies, forms, and other "roles, rules, and tools" to incorporate the new knowledge. This then became the basis for shifting a departmental practice from being "stuck in component-land" (a phrase Barbara used to summarize the overemphasis on body structures and function) to a more client-centered, occupation-based, and evidence-based approach.

BE PREPARED FOR RESISTANCE TO CHANGE AND EVEN SOME STAFF TURNOVER

During the 6-month staff development project process, probably the greatest concern of staff members was that they would no longer be able to use the neurodevelopmental theories (NDTs) that were such a large part of the therapy community of practice. What Barbara hoped would happen is that therapy techniques, such as those exemplified by NDT approaches, would in fact be embedded within meaningful activities designed to help clients regain their desired life skills. Once again, the supervisors played a key role by actively trying out the new concepts and modeling the blending of these new practice approaches with older established approaches. For most staff members, ongoing personnel management strategies were effective in supporting them to make the desired changes. However, there was at least one staff member who decided that she did not like the direction the department was going, and she opted to change jobs and go to a center that was emphasizing NDT techniques as the primary method of intervention.

Once an Understanding of Good Practice Is Negotiated, How Can We Get (and Keep) Everyone "on the Same Page"?

Because service delivery in occupational therapy is a staff-intensive process, it should be no surprise that both the departmental policies and the personnel management structures within the department need to be shaped to support effective practice. Once you have a general vision of how you believe best practice should occur within your unit,

it is time to start operationalizing those concepts into structures that support staff functioning and development.

JOB DESCRIPTIONS

The job description is perhaps the core personnel document that serves to codify best practice. It helps shape employee roles within communities of practice, and serves to communicate valued employee activities. Key components of an effective job description are found in Box 10–3, and strategies for developing job descriptions are found in Box 10–4. A sample job description is provided at the end of this chapter (Appendix 10–1), as are resources for writing job descriptions.

Managers will find that they have varying levels of autonomy to create job descriptions in different organizations. If you are the owner of a private practice, then you may have complete control. Even so, you are cautioned to take the process of developing job descriptions very seriously. Job descriptions may be key documents in responding in a legal and responsible manner to situations such as the request by an employee for a reasonable accommodation under the Americans with Disabilities Act. They are also critical elements of the performance appraisal and disciplinary processes described in Chapters 5 and 6. If you are part of a large health care organization, community organization, or educational system, you may find that the job descriptions are standardized across the entire extended organization. If that is the case, you still may be able to develop addenda to these job descriptions to use within your own community to further define expectations.

In Barbara's situation, the job descriptions of all personnel were reviewed and revised to reflect the current understanding of good practice. For example, it became clear that staff needed to shift their attention from a primary focus on body functions, such as hand use and muscle tone, to a focus on occupational performance. They needed to identify a person's desired task performance, and then determine how actual performance was influenced by the person's body functions. In light of this shift, the job descriptions were modified to explicitly state that evaluation data must include assessment of clients' roles, interests, and performance concerns. Additionally, the descriptions were further

---

Box 10–3: Key Elements of Job Descriptions

Job Title: A brief two- to three-word phrase characterizing the job.
Example: Staff occupational therapist
Job Function: One or two sentences that capture the major purpose of the job.
Example: Provide comprehensive occupational therapy services, including assessment and evaluation; intervention planning and implementation in conjunction with assigned Certified Occupational Therapy Assistant; discharge planning; and documentation and administrative tasks associated with service delivery and assigned team roles.
Reporting Relationships: Indicate to whom the person in this job reports to as well as who he or she is responsible for supervising.
Example: Reports to Occupational Therapy Manager. Supervises assigned Occupational Therapy Assistants, aides, and fieldwork students.
Key Performance Expectations (Also Called Major Job Duties): A listing of frequent and important job tasks that the person in this job must perform in order to meet the organization's expectations. These typically represent baseline expectations, rather than all the possibilities within the job. These may be subdivided into frequency of expectation, as shown in the example.
Example:
- Routine duties:
  - Responds to requests for services within 24 hours by screening clients relative to occupational performance concerns.

- Educates client and client's significant others on how to use adaptive strategies to perform desired occupational tasks.
- Periodic (or occasional) duties:
  - Completes monthly analysis of assigned quality improvement indicators and notifies supervisor of any areas not meeting expectations.
  - Serves as interim team supervisor to cover for short-term vacancies or absences of team supervisor.

Qualifications: A listing of required and preferred education, experience, and credentials required for the job.
Example:
- Licensed or licensure-eligible as an Occupational Therapist, Registered, in the state of Georgia
- Minimum 3 years of experience working with adults with physical disabilities
- Excellent interpersonal skills

Essential Functions: Critical physical, cognitive, or emotional abilities that are required for job performance. Used to assist people with disabilities to identify whether they will require reasonable accommodation in order to perform job.
Example:
- High tolerance for stress
- Ability to lift 50 lbs. from knee to shoulder level
- Judgment to appropriately implement departmental criteria to prioritize referrals

---

modified to indicate that selected interventions addressed performance of occupations that were meaningful to the patient.

Carefully developed and accurate job descriptions then become the basis for supporting the community of practice. They become one of those core documents that the busy manager uses as a reference when implementing all of the managerial

functions, such as recruitment, orientation, and staff development.

STAFF DEVELOPMENT

Earlier in this chapter, we discussed the importance of strategically using staff development resources. This is important not only during times of change, but on an ongoing basis to assure that your man-

---

Box 10-4: Developing Job Descriptions

Find Out What the Job Consists Of

- Interview people currently in the job or who have similar jobs.
- If it is a totally new job, interview the people who will interact the most with employees in this position.
- Find out what tasks that must be done in a typical day.
- Find out what additional tasks are done in a typical week.
- Find out what tasks recur with little frequency, such as monthly, quarterly, or annually.

Explore What Qualifications Are Needed

- Are there specific credentials required by legal or accrediting agencies?
- Are there experiences that are likely to best prepare the person for this role, or is no experience required beyond basic credentials?
- Is special knowledge or a set of specific skills needed?
- Are there standard expectations for all employees in this setting (i.e., ability to speak Spanish, religious preferences in faith-based institutions)?

Draft the Job Description for Review

- Using the key elements shown in Box 10-3, draft the job description.
- Refer to official documents or guides to ensure that the job description is adequately comprehensive and consistent with regional and national standards.
- Obtain feedback from critical reviewers, such as your supervisor, the human resources department, or peers outside your organization who have experience with this type of job.

Finalize the Job Description

- Format according to institutional requirements.
- Put date completed and initials of author in footnote.
- Place in appropriate reference manual or computer file for ready accessibility.

---

agement unit as a whole is systematically gaining and sharing new knowledge relevant to your practice goals. You should keep in mind that staff development requires more than just attendance at educational seminars or courses. Therapists and assistants need time to reflect on the ideas gained from such experiences, and to discuss the possibilities for implementation. Many complex health care groups have interdisciplinary team activities, as well as discipline-specific time for staff development. These group times can be used as sounding boards for the potential implementation of new knowledge in that setting. These opportunities also provide support for each individual staff member as he or she seeks to meet professional obligations to maintain continuing competency (something else that can be explicitly stated in the job description).

Policies and Practices

As simple as it seems, some of the greatest barriers to implementing effective practice often have to do with routine policies and practices such as the purchase of necessary supplies and equipment (Schell, 1994). It is surprising how often occupational therapy managers will work to justify very sophisticated computerized equipment for assessing and intervening to improve performance capacity, while neglecting much more mundane, inexpensive, but critical resources such as a good supply of the tools used by their clients for work, leisure, and everyday life. Managers who want their staff members to exhibit evidence-based and occupation-based practices must take the time to make these practices convenient. This literally means taking a look at what supplies are available (and what are not).

In many occupational therapy departments, you can easily find colored cones, pegboards, or Velcro checkerboards, although seldom do you observe anyone actually playing checkers or using the items in any type of daily occupation. In other settings, there may be hours of unstructured time during which clients drop in to the occupational therapy department to paint ceramic bowls or chess pieces, even though they may not have made the bowls or may never have played chess. The products often go unfinished or are left in the department after the client is discharged and are never used for their intended purpose. Often these items and activities have existed in the department for many years and continue to be used out of imitation by new staff members who observed more experienced staff members making use of them without questioning whether there was underlying theory and evidence to support their use.

Alternatively, in some occupational therapy departments you might observe clients who have had a stroke ironing a shirt using a real iron and ironing board, opening a can of cat food and putting it into a bowl, or making a picture frame as a niece or nephew's birthday present. You might even find someone practicing hanging a shirt or pair of pants in a *real* closet! Using real-life *occupations* in therapy is dependent upon having or being able to obtain the appropriate objects, however.

Because as "occupational beings" we have such a great variety of interests and routines, supporting the type of intervention just described would require a careful look at purchasing policies, and availability of support staff to quickly obtain important items for assessment and intervention. Mounting theory, evidence, and expert opinions (Bodiam, 1999; Darragh, Sample, & Fisher, 1998; Mathiowetz & Bass-Haugen, 2002; Park, Fisher, & Velozo, 1994; Pedretti & Umphred, 1996; Poole & Whitney, 2001) suggest that the most effective assessments and interventions to improve performance capacity require that assessment and intervention occur in the context in which the performance occurs.

For example, consider assessment and intervention related to motor performance. Table 10–3

Table 10-3	Sample Evidence on Assessing and Intervening to Improve Performance Capacity in Context				
Author	**Design**	**Strategies Investigated**	**N (Sample Size)**	**Level of Evidence**	**Results or Findings**
Gilmore & Spaulding (2001)	Combined literature review	Treatment of individuals following stroke	N/A	Weak	Identified four factors contributing to motor learning (type of task, practice, feedback, and stages of learning).
Richardson (2000)	Randomized two-condition study	Compared application of motor learning principles in traditional clinic versus simulated (Easy Street) environment in older adults	80	Strong	Did not exclude benefits of contextually appropriate rehabilitation but found no benefit of expensive simulated environments over traditional settings.
Darragh et al. (1998)	Comparison study	Household task performance versus unfamiliar clinic performance of persons with brain injury	20	Good	Significant positive difference in household task performance in process ability but not in motor ability during administration of the Assessment of Motor and Process Skills.
Park et al. (1994)	Comparison study	Household performance versus clinic performance on IADL performance of older adults	20	Good	10 of 20 subjects performed significantly better in their homes, with process ability improving and motor ability remaining stable.
IADL, instrumental activities of daily living; N/A, not available.					

shows a sample of selected evidence related to assessment and intervention to improve motor performance. A search was conducted in the PsycINFO, CINAHL, and Cochrane databases using the key words "functional assessment" and "motor learning." The search was limited to citations published in English since 1990 and limited to references to adults. This evidence generally supports assessment and intervention to improve motor performance in a naturalistic context. Moreover, studies support that such contextually based assessment and intervention does not require expensive equipment or simulated settings. Gathering and evaluating evidence such as that provided in Table 10–3 with your staff and identifying strategies to begin integrating such evidence in your setting is an example of *leading* practice as a manager.

As a manager, you soon realize that is not always possible to visit or to exactly reproduce the context in which a client will perform an occupation. Even the best efforts to fill a clinic space with objects and furniture commonly found in homes or other settings will inherently fall short of perfectly duplicating the influences of a client's natural environment. However, whatever efforts you can take to make interventions more *naturalistic* may increase the likelihood that the occupational performance within interventions will hold increased meaning to your clients. You can do this by trying to have available those items that are common items among the clientele you serve, and also by asking clients to bring in objects they routinely use.

Anne Fisher, in her 1998 Eleanor Clark Slagle Lecture, provided a helpful framework for thinking about the relevance of the therapy process and how

likely it is to harness the greatest therapeutic benefit. In her lecture, Fisher examined the unique focus of occupational therapy on the use of purposeful and meaningful activity as a therapeutic agent. Further, she proposed that therapeutic occupation and adaptive occupation are the legitimate activities of occupational therapy. She also provided a model for intervention that she called the Occupational Therapy Intervention Process Model. This model provides a framework for using occupation as a therapeutic intervention (Fisher, 1998).

Figure 10–1 builds on Fisher's work. It illustrates the four continua offered by Fisher that guide you in analyzing choices for intervention. These four continua are defined as follows:

- *Ecological relevance* is related to how naturally occurring the therapy task is in real life. For instance, "Is stacking cones something that clients typically do outside of a therapy clinic? What about stacking cups in a cabinet?"
- *Source of purpose* speaks to the degree to which the task has an inherent purpose to the client versus having meaning primarily to the therapist. For instance, if a therapist tells a mother that she must do range-of-motion exercises for her child each day, is the mother likely to sense the purpose as easily as if the therapist responds to a mother's request for ideas of how to play with her child so she moves better?
- *Source of meaning* is related to the issue of purpose just described, and addresses those underlying emotional, symbolic issues that are necessary to harness motivation. Having therapy incorporate activities that the client finds important and

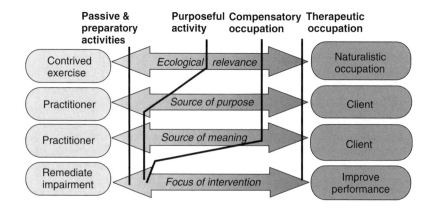

Figure 10–1 Occupation as therapy intervention choices. (Based on Fisher, 1998, and Schell, 2003.)

relevant, such as playing with a son or daughter, is very different than having a person implement a home program because the therapist says he or she must.

• *Focus of intervention* speaks to the degree to which the intervention is selected to restore an identified impairment versus to help the person develop adaptations necessary to promote participation in desired occupations.

Within occupational therapy, various terms are used to describe types of interventions that fall along the continua of ecological relevance, source of purpose and source of meaning, and intervention focus. The vertical lines on Figure 10–1 show how four types of common interventions relate or "map out" to the four continua just described. For each type of intervention, you can follow the line from the intervention name down across the four continua to see how the intervention relates to each continuum.

For example, passive and preparatory activities (such as stretching, exercises, and therapy paper and pencil drills) are interventions that are not very ecologically relevant, whose purpose and meaning reside primarily in the therapist, and that are focused on impairment. Activities of this sort don't typically occur in daily life, but rather are invented as therapy routines. An example of a preparatory activity might be having a homemaker lift a cone from a chair to a shelf in a therapy gym, while trying to convince the person it will help her to increase her strength and coordination. Research suggests that these approaches are less effective than ones that are more ecologically relevant and client centered (Trombly, 1995).

A purposeful activity is a therapy choice that is primarily different from passive or preparatory activities because it is a more naturally occurring activity in daily life. Therefore, it is a bit more ecologically relevant, but still has initial purpose and meaning coming from the therapist. For instance, a therapist might encourage a client to engage in a group activity in which everyone takes part in making a meal. Even if the person doesn't usually cook or prepare food, the therapist might encourage the person's participation, because the therapist thinks this might be a good way to encourage socialization, help the person improve his

or her ability to follow directions, and also help him or her to improve arm and hand coordination. Therefore, this activity is mostly still mapped on the left side of all the continua except for ecological relevance.

In contrast to passive, preparatory, and purposeful activities, occupational interventions are more ecologically relevant, and draw both their purpose and meaning from the client. The major difference between therapeutic occupation and compensatory occupation is the focus of the intervention. Therapeutic occupation is focused on remediating impairment and compensatory occupation is focused on adaptive approaches to improving occupational performance. For instance, a therapeutic occupation might involve having a homemaker work on improving coordination by lifting dishes from the dishwasher to a kitchen cabinet, which is a much more naturalistic occupation, but one that requires her to move in a coordinated fashion. Alternatively, that same homemaker may be taught how to cook one-handed so that she can return to helping to care for her grandchildren, a role that brings with it great pride. That would be an example of compensatory occupation. The choice of focus depends on what is realistic, given the person's diagnostic condition, personal goals, and length of therapy.

Taking the challenge to lead practice so that it is most effective can be difficult. As mentioned earlier, you may encounter roadblocks that are tied to "how things have always been done." Box 10–5 lists some of the most common roadblocks encountered in many settings to changing and innovating practice, and provides suggestions grounded in policies, procedures, and the simple managerial actions for overcoming them. These examples show how routine departmental policies and practices can directly affect the practical ability of staff members to actually implement desired practice innovations.

What Are the Implications for Staff Roles, Productivity, and Billing of Any Changes Made?

One of the biggest challenges for managers and staff alike is to articulate appropriate role expectations and relate them to productivity expectations and billing procedures. In Chapter 5, approaches to measuring productivity were discussed. The rele-

Box 10-5: Roadblocks to Leading Occupation-Based and Evidence-Based Practice and Strategies for Overcoming the Obstacles

ROADBLOCKS TO OCCUPATION-BASED ASSESSMENT AND INTERVENTION	STRATEGIES FOR PROMOTING OCCUPATION-BASED ASSESSMENT AND INTERVENTION
• Absence of items used in daily occupations, such as irons, pots and pans, or vacuums.	• Have staff develop a prioritized list of items they desire that can be purchased over time to support occupation-based assessment in context. • Have clients bring in the items they are having difficulty using.
• Staff members are resistant to giving up assessment of components.	• Develop written clinical guidelines for how components can be assessed in context (e.g., you can evaluate functional range of motion by watching a patient put dishes away or reach into a refrigerator). • Sequence initial evaluation forms so that client concerns and occupational performance issues are addressed first, along with performance context. Next, have only those impairments that appear to actually be affecting performance assessed in more detail. Point out how this increases efficiency because time is not wasted doing assessments that are not needed.
• Staff members feel they first have to restore impairments, and then they can get to occupation.	• Have supervisors or more expert clinicians model how to blend occupational and restorative techniques.
• Forms and policies and procedures do not support contextually based assessments.	• Revise forms and policies and procedures to cue staff to focus on occupational performance by focusing on occupations rather than components.
• Staff members worry that they do not have the time to find and evaluate evidence.	• Organize partnerships to facilitate literature reviews and interpretation of evidence by having other staff cover for some staff members, freeing them to search the literature or review and synthesize articles.
• Physicians or other disciplines have set expectations that you focus on impairment-related issues or remediation of performance components rather than occupational performance.	• Educate other staff to the use of therapeutic occupation through in-services, one-on-one meetings, Occupational Therapy Month activities, posters in lunchrooms, stories in newsletters, or sharing key articles or research emphasizing the value of occupation.

vant point for this chapter is that changes in practice may affect both staffing patterns and productivity expectations. For instance, Barbara shifted her approach to staffing to one that ended the del-

egation of activities of daily living (ADL) assessment and intervention solely to occupational therapy assistants and included the occupational therapists who were used to working only in the clinic in these staff activities. Although occupational therapy assistants are often used to contribute to the evaluation process by assessing ADL performance, that practice was no longer thought to be consistent with the developing understanding of occupational functioning. Occupational therapists and occupational therapy assistants were teamed, and occupational therapists assumed more responsibility for conducting ADL assessments personally. Occupational therapists started to use that time to obtain an occupational history related to self-care, as well as to observe how the individual's abilities to perform self-care tasks were affected by neurologic impairments and environmental variables. As a result, patients received more customized care directed to their particular concerns, rather than a more standard approach based primarily on the person's diagnostic condition.

PRODUCTIVITY EXPECTATIONS

In this reorganized approach used by Barbara and her staff, occupational therapists and occupational therapy assistants shared more directly in patient care routines, shifting among their patients depending on the needs of the patient and the skills of each team member. Rather than have productivity standards for individual occupational therapists and occupational therapy assistants, team productivity was measured. Although this sounds easy, it was a difficult switch, because two licensed practical nurses had to be relocated back to the nursing staff, and occupational therapy assistants and occupational therapists who had not been in the ADL group had to be refreshed, and in some cases trained, on clinical skills related to these more integrated approaches. Finally, both physicians and nursing staff had to be oriented to the new departmental procedures, and concerns and objections overcome.

Issues related to productivity expectations will vary greatly from setting to setting and as the volume of referrals increases or decreases. As pressure to meet productivity standards increases, it can sometimes become difficult for staff to feel that they have adequate control over the level and quality of care they wish to provide their clients. Helping to establish reasonable expectations and limits on what staff can hope to achieve within your setting is an important function for the occupational therapy manager. For example, managers in

an acute care setting can often help staff problem-solve what they can most effectively address given that one point along the continuum of care. Reminding staff that many of their patients will continue to receive occupational therapy at a rehabilitation hospital, at a skilled nursing facility, or at home can help them to focus on occupation-based intervention in the context of a length of stay that is often only a few days. As with many of the suggestions in this chapter, there are simple but important and effective ways to incorporate structures to support staff. For instance, one acute care manager found that simply adding two questions to the initial assessment form helped staff to focus on occupation-based and client-centered goals appropriate for the setting: "What is the patient's estimated length of stay?" and "What would the patient like to achieve in that length of time?"

BILLING AND REIMBURSEMENT

Once Barbara and her staff identified the improved practice approaches, the billing structure was reviewed to be sure that it accurately reflected the current practices. In general, the billing system was kept very simple, allowing for maximum flexibility of the staff to perform assessments and interventions appropriate to the client's needs and the mission of the institution. In this particular setting, all of the therapy billing was part of the per diem rate of the institution, and therefore few data were available to check for issues in reimbursement. However, in subsequent settings, reimbursement has actually improved as the contribution of occupational therapy's uniquely customized approach to helping people regain life skills became more apparent to insurance companies and other payers from initial evaluations, progress notes, and discharge summaries, which had been revised to permit an occupational focus.

In medical-model settings, "coding" of services (e.g., assigning codes to charges based on diagnosis of the patient and the intervention performed within a treatment setting) is partly the responsibility of the occupational therapy assistant or occupational therapist and partly the responsibility of the occupational therapy manager. Often the codes associated with different types of interventions (referred to as Current Procedural Terminology [CPT] codes) are built into a charge system so that staff members indicate a type of occupational therapy intervention, such as "ADL" or "neuromuscular facilitation," and the appropriate CPT code is automatically attached in the electronic billing system. Although this makes submission of the correct CPT code more likely, it also distances the staff from the process, and it is easy for the staff and the occupational therapy manager to become complacent as a result of the automation. This complacency can lead to problems, including denials for payment by payers such as Medicare, when CPT codes do not match the diagnosis code (e.g., the International Classification of Diseases, 9th Edition [ICD-9] code). When rendered services do not clearly match the diagnosis (e.g., you make a splint for a patient living with acquired immunodeficiency syndrome [AIDS] who has upper extremity neuropathy, but the diagnosis code for AIDS is used rather than that for neuropathy), or when the same CPT code is used repeatedly (e.g., you bill for multiple sessions of home management rather than combining codes for self-care with those for cognition and neuromuscular facilitation), payment may be denied.

Working with staff to better understand how to code services to maximize reimbursement not only benefits the organization's financial health but can also sustain other efforts described in this chapter to support occupation-based and evidence-based practice. Proper coding requires staff members to apply the same logic to billing for services that they apply during occupational analysis when planning intervention. Just as we understand that an occupation such as unloading a dishwasher has not only the physical aspects of range of motion, strength, and coordination but also the cognitive aspects of planning and sequencing, we need to understand that payers wish to see that multiple factors are being addressed in treatment. By relating a daily activity such as deciding what to mark on a charge slip to principles you are promoting within your community of practice, you can reinforce multiple concepts at the same time.

How Can We Communicate the Nature and Value of Our Services?

Because most of us do indeed function within a larger community of practice, it is important to consider how to communicate with this larger community not only about what we do on a daily basis but also about practice changes, and, over time, how to reinforce new practice patterns and related expectations. Initially, as in any change process, key players must be informed and feedback opportunities provided. However, equally important is the recognition that it is in the everyday practices of team reporting, documentation, and communications with referring parties, payers, and the like that people form their opinion of the contributions of occupational therapy and their understanding of what we do. Appendix 10–2, provided at the end of this chapter, is an example of a matrix that poses some questions that can be used to assess how well such communications reflect occupation-based, client-centered, and evidence-based practice. Appendix 10–2 examines the MOHO, but similar matrices could be developed for any conceptual practice model.

As managers, we can help staff members examine how *what* they say in everyday interactions can have dramatic effects on the understanding of others about occupational therapy in their practice setting. An example would be considering how staff members introduce themselves to new clients and how they explain to the client what it is that they do. When an occupational therapist or occupational therapy assistant explains occupational therapy to a patient who is in the hospital for a total hip replacement by saying "I'll work with you on things like bathing and dressing," he or she becomes in the patient's mind the "bathing and dressing therapist." Why would that patient explain that his or her biggest worries are how he or she is going to care for a pet and if he or she can still baby-sit for a grandchild to a bathing and dressing therapist?

Likewise, we can help staff reconsider everyday practices such as reporting on client progress in a team meeting. Rather than reporting changes in performance components, such as stating that a child is "demonstrating improved hand coordination and manipulation skills," the same information might be conveyed by stating that the child "was able to pick up finger foods and small toys for the first time." In this manner, we not only communicate the same progress, but we also ground those to whom we are communicating solidly to our role with clients, thereby increasing the likelihood of continued and appropriate referrals. Integrating occupation-based and evidence-based practice does not always mean major shifts in what we do. Rather, the principles of occupation-based and evidence-based practice can be integrated into common everyday practices in simple ways such as how we explain what we do to others.

These examples are just a few of the ways that occupational therapy managers can turn theory into practice by integrating occupation-based and evidence-based practice in daily tasks. Other simple ways to integrate theory and evidence into communication and documentation include the following:

- Include terms such as *roles*, *occupation*, and *occupational performance* with examples so that others understand the terms found on paper forms and on drop-down menus in electronic documentation.
- Integrate occupational therapy terminology on referral forms (paper or electronic) by grouping common occupations together under headings such as "occupations of daily living."
- Review discharge forms, patient education materials, and home programs and look for ways to replace language referencing performance components with language referencing occupations and "doing."

How Will We Know if All This Is Working for the Patients as Well as for the Staff?

This question takes us back to the whole notion of using evidence to guide practice. In the real-life management scenario described at the beginning of the chapter, Barbara used several strategies, ranging from institutional to departmental practices:

- Program evaluation was mandated by the facility's accrediting agency, and therefore the department was able to monitor overall patient outcomes by program. These included patient satisfaction surveys, comparisons of functional outcomes to national aggregate data, and the like.
- Staff evaluations routinely included an "upward appraisal" in which staff members identified personal, programmatic, and departmental strengths, weaknesses, and opportunities for improvement. Ongoing analyses of these factors provided trends.
- Staff morale and the respect accorded by other departments were less measurable but very apparent.
- Specifically designed questionnaires were used before and after consultation to determine the staff's ability to identify those theoretical frameworks that they were using in practice.
- Staff members succeeded in being selected by peer groups (such as state and national conferences) to present their own clinical findings.

All of these provided indicators that patients and staff were pleased with departmental efforts and outcomes.

Chapter Summary

Experiences such as those shared by Barbara throughout this chapter demonstrate that managers must place a priority on advancing their knowledge as occupational therapists or occupational therapy assistants, as well as managers. When they do this, they will be better positioned to challenge the system when evidence suggests that better outcomes can occur. Additionally, managers must be prepared to negotiate with administrators, staff, and payment sources to facilitate practical approaches to integrating best practices into the day-to-day activities of the staff. Creating and supporting excellence in your community of practice is the essence of good management.

Finding, understanding and evaluating evidence and information are the first steps of developing a community of practice focused on occupation-based and evidence-based practice. Managers need to take an active role in *leading* practice by becoming involved in these activities and further by supporting the staff they supervise to become involved by creating structures and systems that support staff. Managers can use everyday structures such as documentation forms, billing forms, policies and procedures, meeting agendas, staff development plans, and purchasing systems to build communities of practice focused on the effective use of occupation and the most current evidence in practice.

Real-Life Solutions

The information provided in this chapter spans a several-year period in which Barbara and her staff focused on developing a community of practice in which the members focused on using evolving evidence to guide their integration of occupation-based practice into their daily work. Perhaps the most telling outcomes were those that were identified from measures taken prior to and after the intensive 6-month staff development process described earlier. There were four major areas in which changes were measured or observed:

- Staff "pre" and "post" surveys showed a dramatic increase in the staff's awareness of and use of theory to guide their practice. For instance, 100% ($n = 22$) of the participants stated that they used theory to guide their practice, versus 78% ($n = 27$) prior to the activity. Further, there was a significant jump in the use of occupational behavior frames of reference (i.e., from 11% to 100%, for those using the MOHO), although staff continue to use neurodevelopmental approaches routinely, and even more than they had before the training (i.e., use of Bobath techniques went from 70% to 80%). This suggested that staff had indeed begun to integrate approaches in a manner that was more consistent with occupational therapy standards.
- Evaluation forms were changed:
  - Space was added to include patient life roles and time use.
  - Space for routine reporting of body function/structure was reduced, but appendices were

developed in which the staff could add the initial evaluation form for those persons whose impairments required detailed assessment to understand the impact on performance.
  - There was an increase in the use of data relating to physical and social environments.
- Environmental changes were made:
  - Staff requested the purchase of more home-like furniture and resources for use in the clinic (even though there was an ADL apartment), because they wanted to incorporate these into activities designed to restore function.
  - There was more individualized treatment time for simulated and community experiences.
  - More time was spent with clients' families.
- Verbal reporting was changed:
  - Staff members made a point of integrating their findings about impairments with information about the impact on performance.
  - Overall reporting was more performance-based.

It was particularly rewarding for Barbara to return to this facility several years later as part of an extensive clinical reasoning study she was conducting. It was apparent that practitioners there had continued to develop their strategies for blending occupation-based approaches with other intervention techniques in such a way as to maximize their patients' restoration of life skills and adaptation to new demands.

Resources for Learning More About Turning Theory Into Practice

Journals that Often Address Occupation-Based Practice or Communities of Practice

OTJR: OCCUPATION, PARTICIPATION, AND HEALTH

The *OTJR: Occupation, Participation, and Health* is published by the American Occupational Therapy Foundation, Inc. Articles published in the journal

include original research of interest to the occupational therapy personnel. In addition to reports of quantitative and qualitative research the journal includes briefs, book reviews, letters to the editor, and commentaries.

JOURNAL OF OCCUPATIONAL SCIENCE

The *Journal of Occupational Science* publishes articles by authors from around the world and promotes discussion of topics related to the emerging discipline of occupational science. The journal focuses on the unique experiences, concerns and perspectives of the study of humans as occupational beings.

ORGANIZATION SCIENCE

Organization Science publishes reports of research on the processes, structures, technologies, identities, capabilities, forms, and performance of organizations. This multidisciplinary journal addresses issues including organizational behavior and theory, strategic management, psychology, sociology, economics, political science, information systems, technology management, communication, and cognitive science. Research at different levels of analysis, including the organization, the groups or units that constitute organizations, and the networks in which organizations are embedded is published.

OD PRACTITIONER (JOURNAL OF THE ORGANIZATION DEVELOPMENT NETWORK)

This journal includes articles on a wide range of organizational development issues, including communities of practice.

Associations That Are Concerned with Occupation-Based Practice or Communities of Practice

THE ORGANIZATION DEVELOPMENT NETWORK

http://www.odnetwork.org/index.html
Members of the Organizational Development Network (OD Network) are practitioners representing a range of professional roles in a wide variety of organizations. The OD Network seeks to develop, support, and inspire practitioners and to enhance the body of knowledge in human organization and systems development. Members of the network are employed by private industry, nonprofit organizations, and government agencies or are private consultants, entrepreneurs, researchers, or academicians.

Other Resources

JOBDESCRIPTIONS.COM

www.jobdescriptions.com
This commercial site allows you to pay for a single use (under $20) or 1 year of unlimited service (approximately $130). You can create single, customized job descriptions for your organization that meet the requirements of the Americans with Disabilities Act compliance. The site guides you through selection of a template selected from thousands of job descriptions and uses your responses to write a custom job description that reflects your unique situation. The site also helps you create an interview form that contains suggested interview questions from the competencies in the job description.

MANAGEMENT ASSISTANCE PROGRAMS FOR NON-PROFITS

www.mapfornonprofits.org/
The mission of the Management Assistance Programs for Non-Profits (MAP) is to build the capacity of nonprofit organizations to achieve mission-driven results. Since 1979, the group has provided quality, affordable management consulting and board recruitment services to thousands of nonprofit groups. MAP primarily works with nonprofit organizations in the greater Twin Cities metropolitan area of Minneapolis and St. Paul, Minnesota. However, this organization has an excellent Web site that has information on a large range of topics, including job descriptions, in its free management library, found at *http://www.managementhelp.org/*.

Reference List

American Occupational Therapy Association. (2002). Occupational therapy practice framework: Domain and process. *American Journal of Occupational Therapy, 56*, 609–639.

Bodiam, C. (1999). The use of the Canadian Occupational Performance Measure for the assessment of outcome on a neuro-rehabilitation unit. *British Journal of Occupational Therapy, 62*, 123–126.

Darragh, A. R., Sample, P. L., & Fisher, A. G. (1998). Environment effect on functional task performance in adults with acquired brain injuries: Use of the assessment of motor and process skills. *Archives of Physical Medicine and Rehabilitation, 79*, 418–423.

Fellin, P. (1993). Reformulation of the context of community-based care. *Journal of Sociology and Social Welfare, 20*, 57–67.

Fisher, A. G. (1998). Uniting practice and theory in an occupational framework. *American Journal of Occupational Therapy, 52*, 509–522.

Gilmore, P. E., & Spaulding, S. J. (2001). Motor control and motor learning: Implications for treatment of individuals post stroke. *Physical & Occupational Therapy in Geriatrics, 20*, 1–15.

Mathiowetz, V., & Bass-Haugen, J. (2002). Assessing abilities and capacities: Motor behavior. In C.A. Trombly & M. V. Radomski (Eds.), *Occupational therapy for physical dysfunction* (pp. 137–158). Philadelphia: Lippincott, Williams & Wilkins.

McCormack, G. L. (2003). Occupational therapy skills and management skills. In G. L. McCormack, E. G. Jaffe, & M. Goodman-Lavey (Eds.), *The occupational therapy manager* (4th ed., pp. 23–34). Bethesda, MD: AOTA Press.

McCormack, G. L., Jaffe, E. G., & Frey, W. F. (2003). New organizational perspectives. In G. L. McCormack, E. G. Jaffe, & M. Goodman-Lavey (Eds.), *The occupational therapy manager* (4th ed., pp. 85–126). Bethesda, MD: AOTA Press.

Minar, D., & Greer, S. (1969). *The concept of community: Readings with interpretation.* Chicago: Aldine.

Moyers, P. A. (1999). *The guide to occupational therapy practice.* Bethesda, MD: AOTA Press.

Park, S., Fisher, A. G., & Velozo, C. A. (1994). Using the assessment of motor and process skills to compare occupational performance between clinic and home settings. *American Journal of Occupational Therapy, 48,* 697–709.

Pedretti, L. W., & Umphred, D. A. (1996). Motor learning and teaching activities in occupational therapy. In L. W. Pedretti (Ed.), *Occupational therapy: practice skills for physical dysfunction* (4th ed., pp. 65–75). St. Louis: Mosby–Year Book.

Poole, J. L., & Whitney, S. L. (2001). Assessments of motor function post stroke: A review. *Physical and Occupational Therapy in Geriatrics, 19,* 1–22.

Richardson, J. (2000). The use of a simulated environment (Easy Street) to retrain independent living skills in elderly persons: A randomized controlled trial. *Journals of Gerontology. Series A: Biological Sciences and Medical Sciences, 55,* 578–584.

Schell, B. A. B. (1994). *The effects of practice context on occupational therapists' clinical reasoning.* Unpublished doctoral dissertation, University of Georgia.

Schell, B. A. (2003). Clinical reasoning and occupation-based practice: Changing habits. *OT Practice,* ce article, 1–8.

Schell, B. A. B., Crepeau, E. B., & Cohn, E. S. (2003). Professional development. In E.B. Crepeau, E. S. Cohn, & B. A. B. Schell (Eds.), *Willard and Spackman's occupational therapy* (pp. 141–149). Philadelphia: Lippincott, Williams & Wilkins.

Trombly, C. A. (1995). Occupation: Purposefulness and meaningfulness as therapeutic mechanisms. *American Journal of Occupational Therapy, 49,* 960–972.

Wenger, E., McDermott, R., & Snyder, W. M. (2002). *Cultivating communities of practice: A guide to managing knowledge.* Boston: Harvard Business School Press.

Appendix 10–1: Sample Job Description

Title: Job Description for Occupational Therapist I

I. Function

To provide standard occupational therapy services to inpatients and outpatients as determined by the therapist's specific team assignment. To supervise fieldwork students assigned to the unit on which they work. To assist in administrative responsibilities, including patient record keeping, billing, daily and monthly team statistics, and maintenance and inventory of unit equipment and supplies.

II. Organizational Relationship

Reports directly to the Team Leader for the team to which s/he has been assigned as designated by the Director of Clinical Services. Receives clinical supervision and patient assignment from the Occupational Therapist II and the Team Leader for the team on which s/he works.

III. Key Performance Expectations

A. Patient Care

1. Evaluates, under a physician's referral, patients of age ranges for which s/he has appropriate training and prior experience in regard to their need for occupational therapy services as assigned by the Occupational Therapist II or Team Leader on her/his team. Administers and interprets clinical and functional assessments to determine the patient's present level of physical, psychosocial, developmental, and functional status. Documents the results of these assessments appropriately. Orders and fabricates assistive and adaptive equipment.
2. Plans and implements individual and group patient treatments in accordance with strengths and deficits documented in clinical findings and appropriate to the age of the client based on principles and theories of occupational therapy.
3. Orients patients and families to objectives and functions of occupational therapy.
4. Schedules, plans, and carries out individual treatment of patients, with focus on prevention of ill effects of separation from home, hospitalization, and restoration of maximal occupational performance.
5. Provides indicated home programming and patient follow-up in conjunction with the interdisciplinary treatment team.
6. Communicates orally and in written form at the interdepartmental and intradepartmental levels regarding patient status and discharge planning. Attend rounds and conferences as assigned by the supervisor.
7. Participates in outpatient clinics as assigned by the supervisor to provide occupational therapy consultation, evaluation, treatment, and follow-up.
8. Functions as an integral member of the health care team and develops and maintains working relationships with peers and members of other disciplines within the medical center local communities as appropriate to his/her job responsibilities.
9. Coordinates treatment objectives and procedures with other disciplines, services, and/or agencies, both within and outside the hospital.
10. Assists other teams with patient care as necessary and assigned.
11. Participates in continuous quality improvement activities.

B. Administration

1. Patient related:
   a. Recommends the scheduling of patients for evaluation/treatment on a weekly basis, with awareness of the specific milieu of their team unit, to the Occupational Therapist II/Team Leader.
   b. Records patient attendance and statistical data required by the unit and programs in which s/he works.
2. Unit related:
   a. Assists with inventory of supplies and equipment and other related duties as delegated by the supervisor.
   b. Assists in reporting of productivity or other statistics as delegated by the Team Leader.

C. Education

1. Provides supervision to Occupational Therapy and Occupational Therapy Assistant students as assigned by the Team Leader.

2. Assists in undergraduate teaching (labs and lectures) as assigned.
3. Assists in the orientation of students and residents from other departments and/or representatives from interested community groups to occupational therapy as assigned by the Team Leader.

D. Professional

1. Participates in unit and departmental meetings and in-services.
2. Participates in patient-related meetings.
3. Participates in hospital and departmental committees as appropriate.
4. Participates in in-service education, workshops, and other continuing education experiences as appropriate to the ages and types of patients treated.

IV. Qualifications & Knowledge Required

To qualify for the position of Occupational Therapist I, an employee must be eligible for licensure by the State Department of Professional Regulation. No minimum period of experience is required. The employee is required to have a sound basic knowledge of occupational therapy theory, evaluation, and treatment with specific skills related to the patients treated by the team to which s/he is assigned. This includes familiarity with age-specific occupational roles and needs. Knowledge of departmental policies governing patient care, charting, billing, and confidentiality of patient-related information and/or records is necessary.

V. Supervision

A. Direct and Indirect Supervision Received

Work is assigned, reviewed, and approved by the Team Leader, or by the Director of Clinical Services. After orientation and training, the employee is expected to complete routine work independently. Instructions are both oral and written (memos, departmental policies and procedures, physicians' orders).

B. Guidelines

Performance is guided by departmental protocol, patient care standards, university policies and procedures, and American Occupational Therapy Association standards.

VI. Complexity

A. Employee Qualities

The employee is expected to become an integral member of the patient care–related team and the occupational therapy department. Initiation and independence are necessary qualities. The employee is expected to provide all aspects of patient care for those patients assigned to his/her care. The employee is expected to act as a role model for, and provide direct supervision to, Occupational Therapy and Occupational Therapy Assistant students. Good interpersonal skills must be promoted to ensure proper patient care and a good working environment for both the employee and others.

B. Guidelines

Patient care services must be provided in accordance with all departmental and hospital guidelines to ensure comprehensive patient care. Administrative duties must be performed as assigned to permit the department to be properly recognized for its efforts.

VII. Contact with Others

Patients, staff, students, and visitors within the Departments of Occupational Therapy, Physical Medicine and Rehabilitation, and Physical Therapy, and the University Medical Center.

VIII. Essential Functions/Environmental Demands

A. Physical Requirements

Refined motor skills in treatment techniques and general endurance for manual work beyond the sedentary level are necessary. Strength is needed to roll, lift, and transfer immobile patients. Must be able to perform all other essential physical, social, and cognitive aspects of occupational therapy treatment with patients of all ages treated by the team that s/he supervises.

B. Work Environment

1. There is frequent exposure to communicable diseases, such as active pulmonary tuberculosis, hepatitis, and respiratory infections, and to wound infections. There is exposure to patient secretions and drainage during the course of care.
2. There is increased risk for personal injury (shoulder, wrist, and back are common sites) when moving immobile patients and guarding against patient falls.

Appendix 10–2: Documentation and Reporting Matrix

Model of Human Occupation

Think about the typical documentation and reporting expectations in your practice. To what degree do they fit with current occupational therapy theories?

	INITIAL EVALUATIONS	PROGRESS NOTES	ORAL REPORTS	DISCHARGE SUMMARIES
Volitional Issues • Personal causation • Values • Interests • Life story				
Habituation • Roles • Routines				
Performance Capacity • Musculoskeletal • Neurologic • Perceptual • Cognitive				
Environment • Physical • Social • Cultural				

Occupational Performance			
• Motor skills			
• Process skills			
• Communication/interaction skills			
Person–Environment Interaction			
• Skills and physical context			
• Skills and social context			
• Skills and cultural context			
Goals for Intervention			
• Client/patient generated			
• Focused on occupational outcomes			
Goal Attainment			
• Meaningful to client			
• Evaluated by client			
• Evaluated by therapist			

From Schell, B. A. (2003). Clinical reasoning and occupation-based practice: Changing habits. *OT Practice*, ce article, 1–8. Bethesda, MD: AOTA, with permission.

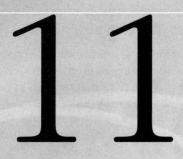

11

Brent Braveman, Ph.D., OTR/L, FAOTA
Debra Krause, M.A.

Evaluating and Improving Occupational Therapy Services

Real-Life Management

Joan has accepted a position as a regional leader for a company that provides therapy services within skilled nursing facilities. She is returning to work after several years away to raise a child. One of her new responsibilities will be to lead the continuous quality improvement (CQI) efforts for occupational therapy, physical therapy, and speech-language pathology. She worked for many years as the assistant director of an occupational therapy department and remembers being frustrated with the quality assurance (QA) activities with which she was involved.

From what Joan remembers, it seemed that a lot of effort went into collecting information and writing reports that never resulted in any real changes or improvement in services. Her new boss has informed her that the company uses a CQI approach focusing on customer satisfaction and process improvement that is very different from the old QA approach. As part of her orientation, Joan has been asked to attend a 5-day CQI Leadership Course that her new company runs each year for new supervisors, and she is interested to see if there really is a difference between QA and CQI.

Key Issues

- CQI is considered to be both a management philosophy and a management method for structural problem solving.
- Meeting or exceeding customer requirements for quality products and services through process improvement is the key to success in a CQI approach.
- Making decisions with data is the CQI equivalent of basing practice decisions upon evidence.

- Common CQI concepts, strategies, tools, and techniques can be incorporated into a conceptual CQI "tool kit" so that you choose the right tool for the right situation.
- A CQI approach calls for balancing "tasks," or process improvement, with people and their concerns and development as employees.

Over the last two decades, approaches to evaluating and improving health care services have undergone considerable change. Many health care organizations have shifted from focusing on gathering data on stable processes to *control* or *assure* quality to a focus on improving the efficiency and effectiveness of processes and on improving customer satisfaction by using a *continuous quality improvement* approach. Also referred to as *total quality management*, this approach to improving quality is a structured process for continually evaluating and improving the full range of an organization's or department's outcomes.

As you read this chapter, you should keep in mind that, although most health care organizations will address quality in some manner, the specific approaches will vary a great deal. Some organizations have fully adopted a CQI approach and use it on a grand scale. Others may have begun to integrate use of some of the strategies, tools, and techniques commonly associated with CQI but have not fully adopted a management philosophy completely consistent with CQI. This chapter will provide you with an overview of the history of CQI and its key concepts as applied at the level of the organization. However, you should consider that, as a leader, you may introduce some of the key concepts, strategies, tools, and techniques within your own department even if the organization as a whole has not adopted a CQI approach. Also, you may find a CQI approach helpful in settings such as a community-based organization in which addressing quality improvement is not mandated by an outside source, as it is in many health care settings.

Although the implementation of CQI efforts may vary from organization to organization, there are some key features that commonly are found in organizations that have fully adopted this approach. These key features are highlighted in Box 11–1.

True believers in CQI will advocate that CQI is both a management philosophy and a management methodology for solving structural problems within an organization (Kaluzny, 1994). The factor that distinguishes CQI from other management philosophies is a focus on customer requirements that change over time as the key to customer satisfaction. Because customer requirements are continually changing, organizations must continually examine the processes that comprise their work and seek new ways of improving quality.

Box 11–1: Key Features of a CQI Approach

- A commitment to quality by the organization's top leadership to provide vision and guidance for CQI efforts early in the process of adopting a CQI philosophy and methodology
- Training for staff at all levels in CQI concepts, strategies, tools, and techniques
- Methods for identifying processes for examination and opportunities for improvement throughout the organization
- Quality improvement teams composed of key stakeholders of the processes chosen for improvement
- Policies, procedures, and a system of rewards and recognition that support full participation of all levels of staff in the CQI process

---

Kaluzny (1994) noted that the primary mechanisms by which CQI is implemented within an organization are actually quite consistent with what is cited as good management techniques in general. These mechanisms include:

- Empower clinicians and managers to analyze and improve processes.
- Adopt a norm that customer preferences are the primary determinants of quality and that the term *customer* includes patients, payers, referral sources, and others as external customers and the providers or key stakeholders in critical processes, who are internal customers.
- Support a multidisciplinary approach that crosses traditional departmental and professional lines and brings all stakeholders in a process together to work toward improving the process.
- Provide the motivation for a rational, data-based, cooperative approach to process analysis and change.

To say that CQI is both a management philosophy and a management method indicates that strategies for managing both people and information are employed together. Strategies to meet the needs of employees and facilitate their active involvement, satisfaction, and success include developing effective teams, managing conflict and agreement, running productive meetings, and designing recognition and reward programs that provide meaningful incentives for employees. These types of *people* skills are combined with strategies to manage information, such as recognizing and documenting the steps of a common work process, designing effective data collection tools, benchmarking against internal or external targets, statistical analysis, and making decisions with data. Table 11–1 provides examples of elements of both the philosophy and the methods often used in CQI.

Although the focus of a CQI approach to management is customer satisfaction, the profitability, success, and survival of the organization remains the primary objective. George and Weimerskirch (1994) noted that CQI contributes to the long-term success of organizations because

- Products and services that exceed customer requirements are of greater value to customers than competitors' products and services. Increasing numbers of customers are likely to pur-chase such quality, and that improves market share and grows revenues.
- Less waste and greater productivity result in lower costs, which in turn improve profit margins, asset utilization, and competitive position.
- Higher revenue and more favorable margins, asset utilization, and competitive position improve the bottom line, which delights shareholders or key supporters.

Successful introduction of CQI as a management philosophy and an approach to quality improvement at an organization-wide level is a major endeavor and can be viewed as a developmental process. Such wide-scale use by an organization takes advanced planning, requires the investment of a great amount of organizational resources in terms of time and money, and must evolve over time. Integration at a smaller scale, such as the introduction of CQI as a management philosophy and approach for managing occupational therapy services within a larger organization or within a small business, may take less time and resources but still requires advanced planning and preparation.

Table 11-1 Philosophical Elements and Managerial Methods of CQI

PHILOSOPHICAL ELEMENTS

- A focus on internal and external customers is primary.
- Decisions are more reliable when based upon data.
- All stakeholders in a process are involved in process improvement.
- Most problems have multiple causes, therefore, blaming individuals should be avoided.
- Improvement is a continuous, never-ending cycle.
- The role of management is to facilitate process improvement rather than to make decisions about the processes, i.e., micromanage.
- Organizational learning occurs when those involved in process improvement share lessons with others in the organization, fostering personal and organizational growth.

MANAGERIAL METHODS, USE OF:

- Process improvement teams to involve stakeholders in redesigning a process.
- Process improvement tools such as flow charts, histograms, or cause-and-effect diagrams.
- A quality council early in the process of adopting a CQI approach that functions parallel to but separate from existing management to oversee quality improvement efforts.
- Statistical analysis to differentiate common cause from special cause variation.
- Measures of customer satisfaction.
- Benchmarks against historical data and against competitors.
- Process redesign so that processes may be scrapped and re-engineered from scratch if necessary.

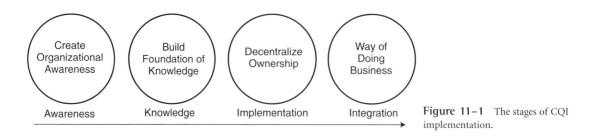

Figure 11–1   The stages of CQI implementation.

Full integration of CQI may be conceptualized in four stages, as illustrated in Figure 11–1.

First, organizational or departmental leadership must begin to create readiness for CQI by building awareness of the need to operate differently. Highlighting current problems with organizational or departmental effectiveness or efficiency can help to create a state of readiness for process improvement. Providing specific examples of customer dissatisfaction, customer complaints, or the negative impact that waste and rework has for organization or department members is also an effective strategy. Other strategies for creating a state of readiness would include presentation of CQI success stories in health care or other industries. Using examples easily found in the CQI literature that highlight companies and products familiar to most employees might be particularly effective. For example, the CQI practices of the Ritz-Carlton Hotels have often been related to health care because both hotels and hospitals share the need to "admit" guests, move them quickly and efficiently to a clean room, provide meals and services during their stay, and "discharge" the guests efficiently while assuring accurate billing.

After awareness is raised and the organization or department is ready to explore CQI as a new approach, a second step is to work with employees to build a foundation of knowledge and skills by providing education and training in CQI basics. Careful planning for both the order and the extent of initial training is important. CQI is sometimes referred to as both a *top-down* and a *bottom-up* philosophy. It is considered a top-down philosophy because it is believed that CQI cannot be successful in an organization if the top leadership does not fully buy into a CQI approach and does not role-model the use of the key concepts, strategies, tools, and techniques for employees at lower levels of the or-

ganization. For this reason, it may be best to provide training to organizational or departmental leadership or supervisors before training line staff. CQI is also considered a bottom-up philosophy because of its focus on involving those closest to the work or process in the actual process improvement, regardless of the employee's level in the organization. Providing education that focuses on the basic philosophy of CQI and presents key concepts, strategies, tools, and techniques at an introductory level is a wise first step. More in-depth training on specifics can be reserved until later, and often can be provided just before the specifics are needed (e.g., "just-in-time training").

Once a foundation of knowledge and skills is built through education and training, the first stages of decentralizing ownership of CQI from organizational leadership to all levels of the organization may begin by carefully choosing initial projects that are relatively simple and might be accomplished in a reasonable period of time. Beginning with the organization's or department's most pressing problem may be tempting, but choosing a complex and high-stakes project first may contribute to frustration and disappointment if things don't go exactly as planned. Given that the use of CQI concepts, strategies, tools, and techniques may be new to everyone, you might expect problems and errors in the first attempts at their application. Beginning with a small demonstration project may also foster further integration when employees start to see the value of CQI by experiencing a success. Another common pitfall early on is forming more CQI teams than you can properly train and facilitate. Early excitement can lead to diffused efforts in too many directions with few results, resulting to frustration and skepticism.

Finally, once a strong foundation of skills and knowledge has been established, initial projects have been carefully implemented and supported, and all levels of the organization or department are involved, the focus can shift to ongoing support of processes to fully integrate CQI into daily life. The ultimate goal is that CQI becomes *a way of doing business*. Indicators that this goal has been achieved include

- A constant focus on *customers and customer satisfaction* by employees at all levels
- Constant readiness for change and process improvement
- Use of CQI concepts, strategies, tools, and techniques within and outside of formal CQI efforts or teams as matter of daily organizational life
- A belief that taking longer to make the right decision based on data is better than making a fast decision based on speculation
- A commitment to balancing tasks with the needs of people as standard operating procedure

A Word About Evidence and Continuous Quality Improvement

Before proceeding with an overview of how health care organizations have dealt with the issue of quality, it is important to address the issue of evidence as it relates to improving quality and the CQI process. Evidence is the theme that has tied all the topics in this book together. Chapter 1 discussed approaches to finding and evaluating evidence. When you think of evidence as it relates to *evidence-based practice*, you might typically consider evidence generated via the administration of a research study intended to prove the effectiveness of an intervention or that an intervention will result in a desired or an improved outcome. In a *continuous quality improvement* approach, you will also be very concerned about evidence. Collecting and analyzing data before making changes in processes and making *data-based decisions* is primary in CQI. However, in a discussion of CQI, the term *evidence* will be used differently than it is in regard to clinical questions. Still, the underlying premise is very much the same. In both evidence-based practice and CQI, you seek to gather the best information and the strongest proof available that taking certain actions will result in desired or improved outcomes.

A Short History of Continuous Quality Improvement

A short overview of the history of CQI and its evolution and movement from industry to health care will provide a useful context for discussion of the current focus on CQI by health care organizations. Most histories of CQI credit Walter Shewart of Bell Laboratories with several major contributions in the early 1900s that are still used today in CQI, including the control chart and the Plan, Do, Check, Act (PDCA) cycle, shown in Figure 11–2 (Kaluzny, 1994).

Shewart introduced and promoted the important concept of *value*, or the relationship between cost and quality, emphasizing that considering one without the other is meaningless. Regardless of how inexpensive a product or service might be, customers will not be satisfied if the quality is poor. Similarly, regardless of high quality, products and services can be overpriced so that again customer satisfaction is negatively affected. When you stop to think about it, you are already well familiar with the concept of value in regard to products of varying cost. An example would be having dinner in a restaurant and comparing the value of a meal purchased in a fast-food restaurant to that of a meal purchased in an upscale formal dining restaurant. In both cases, you may feel that, given the relationship between cost and quality, both meals were of high value even though there may have been a great difference in the cost of the two meals. The relationship between cost and quality is represented in Figure 11–3.

One of the most familiar and recognized names in CQI is that of W. Edwards Deming. Deming's fame in the United States came many years after he began to implement a statistical approach to quality improvement in Japan during efforts to rebuild that country's economy and industry after World War II. Deming's approaches are widely credited with turning an industrial economy known for low-tech, low-quality, and low-priced goods into one that now is known for producing goods that are high tech, high quality, and often high priced. Deming introduced what he called the *quality chain reaction* that drew a direct connection between improved quality and improved financial status of an

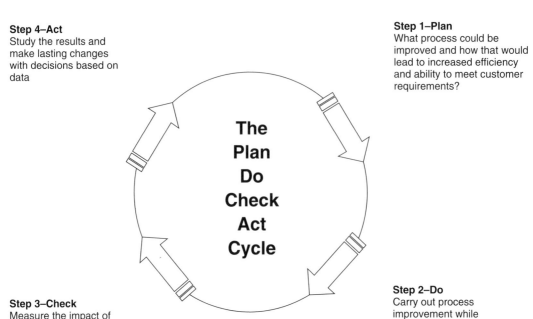

Step 4–Act
Study the results and
make lasting changes
with decisions based on
data

Step 1–Plan
What process could be
improved and how that would
lead to increased efficiency
and ability to meet customer
requirements?

The
Plan
Do
Check
Act
Cycle

Step 3–Check
Measure the impact of
the improved process

Step 2–Do
Carry out process
improvement while
collecting data

Figure 11–2   The Plan, Do, Check, Act (PDCA) cycle.

$$\text{Value} = \frac{\text{Quality}}{\text{Cost}}$$

Figure 11–3   Value: the relationship between cost and quality.

organization. Figure 11–4 illustrates Deming's quality chain reaction.

Deming is also well known for identifying what he referred to as "four areas of profound knowledge." These domains of knowledge were those that Deming felt were critical for organizational leader-

ship to master in order to effectively steward an organization through change and efforts to improve quality. Deming stressed that these domains are integrated and must be used together; they should not be treated as discrete areas of knowledge. Deming's four areas of profound knowledge are listed in Box 11–2.

In addition to the four areas of profound knowledge, Deming developed a 14-point program of recommendations to improve quality (Box 11–3). These recommendations are commonly still integrated into most formal CQI programs today and have implications related to both the philosophy of management and the day-to-day work of managers.

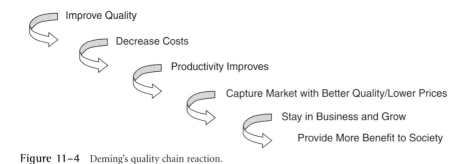

Improve Quality

Decrease Costs

Productivity Improves

Capture Market with Better Quality/Lower Prices

Stay in Business and Grow

Provide More Benefit to Society

Figure 11–4   Deming's quality chain reaction.

Box 11-2: Deming's Four Areas of Profound Knowledge

- Appreciation for a *system*, including an understanding of the components of man-made systems, the boundaries of the system, and the interaction among components within the system and that between system components and influences from outside the system. Think globally about the big picture before taking action locally.
- Knowledge about *variation*, or how performance within a process and within daily work can vary, the types of influences on processes within organizations, and how managers can reduce unwanted variation.
- *Theory* of knowledge, including the scientific method and how theory is developed and utilized in the daily work of an organization.
- *Psychology*, or an understanding of intrinsic and extrinsic factors affecting motivation and of the process of empowering employees to participate in organizational change.

Box 11-3: Deming's 14-Point Program to Improve Quality

1. Create constancy of purpose toward improvement of product and service, with the aim to become competitive and to stay in business, and to provide jobs.
2. Western management must awaken to the challenge, must learn their responsibilities, and take on leadership for change.
3. Cease dependence on inspection to achieve quality. Eliminate the need for inspection on a mass basis by building quality into the product in the first place.
4. End the practice of awarding business on the basis of price tag alone. Instead, minimize total cost.
5. Improve constantly and forever the system of production and service, to improve quality and productivity, and thus constantly decrease costs.
6. Institute training on the job.
7. Institute leadership. The aim of supervision should be to help people and machines and gadgets to do a better job. Supervision of management is in need of overhaul, as well as supervision of production workers.
8. Drive out fear, so that everyone may work effectively for the company.
9. Break down barriers between departments. People in research, design, sales, and production must work as a team, to foresee problems of production and in use that may be encountered with the product or service.
10. Eliminate slogans, exhortations, and targets for the work force asking for zero defects and new levels of productivity. Such exhortations only create adversarial relationships, as the bulk of the causes of low quality and low productivity belong to the system and thus lie beyond the power of the work force.
    - Eliminate work standards (quotas) on the factory floor. Substitute leadership.
    - Eliminate management by objective. Eliminate management by numbers, numerical goals. Substitute leadership.
11. Remove barriers that rob the hourly worker of his right to pride of workmanship. The responsibility of supervisors must be changed from sheer numbers to quality.
12. Remove barriers that rob people in management and in engineering of their right to pride of workmanship.
13. Institute a vigorous program of education and self-improvement.
14. Put everybody in the company to work to accomplish the transformation. The transformation is everybody's job.

From Deming, D.E. (2000). *Out of the Crisis.* Cambridge, MA. The MIT Press, pp. 22-23, with permission.

Although CQI was accepted and largely successful in Japanese industry, it did not gain popular acceptance in the United States until the 1980s. The Japanese, particularly Kaoru Ishikawa, also contributed to developments in CQI that continue to have an impact today (Kaluzny, 1994). One commonly used tool, the cause-and-effect diagram that assists with identifying potential root causes of problems, is often also referred to as an Ishikawa diagram.

Between 1950 and 1980, American industry lost major market share for products such as automobiles and electronics. After a documentary entitled *If Japan Can, Why Can't We?* was aired on national television, Deming was hired as a consultant for Ford and used CQI principles that eventually produced the Ford Taurus, the car that is credited with turning Ford around. Since that time, companies including Xerox, Federal Express, L. L. Bean, Motorola, and Ben and Jerry's Ice Cream have adopted and profited from a CQI approach. After decades of being ignored, CQI caught a foothold in American industry and was eventually introduced in health care settings in the late 1980s. Since that time, CQI has caught on and has been adopted as a management philosophy and approach in many hospitals and health care organizations. The adoption of CQI approaches in health care has been fostered by inclusion of standards related to customer satisfaction and quality in the standards of accrediting bodies such as the Joint Commission on the Accreditation of Health Care Organizations and the Commission on Accreditation of Rehabilitation Facilities.

The shift to a CQI approach has also been a move away from what had been referred to as *quality assurance*. In a QA approach, the focus was typically on gathering data on what were assumed to be stable processes and taking action only when major problems were noted or when outcomes fell below predetermined target levels. If targets were being met, no action was taken, even if there may have been opportunities to improve or to exceed targets. This approach was consistent with the *management by exception* approach described in Chapter 4. Carey and Lloyd (1995) described the difference between a QA and a CQI approach and provided a useful diagram to illustrate the difference in emphasis (Figure 11–5). The upper part of Figure 11–5 shows the traditional approach to QA. For any procedure, action will only be taken when the process mean exceeds a predetermined threshold. When the process average is below the threshold, there is complacency. When the threshold is exceeded, however, there is often blaming and finger pointing. The lower part of Figure 11–5 depicts a CQI approach. In this approach, the entire output of a process is the basis for action, not just those occurrences that exceed a threshold. Taking action on the entire process allows you both to reduce unwanted variation and to shift the outcome mean in a desired direction.

You should recognize that there is some overlap between strategies used in a QA approach and a CQI approach (e.g., not all of the CQI methods for collecting and analyzing data are new), and you should also be aware that what is often referred to as *quality control mechanisms* are still relevant in many instances. For example, if you have a common process that is repeated over and over, and you have examined this process and are confident that it is typically stable and produces desired results, you may wish to apply a *quality control indicator*. A quality control indicator is a consistently monitored measure that indicates a problem and the need for action when the measure falls below a predetermined level (refer back to Chapter 5 for a more thorough discussion of control indicators). Control indicators are used in health care organizations for monitoring compliance with routine processes, such as informing patients about their rights as a patient upon admission to a facility, or assuring that documentation is placed in a medical record in a timely manner. Control indicators are frequently used in many areas related to safety and daily operations, such as completion of annual education on fire safety or blood-borne pathogens, or checking the temperature daily in a refrigerator that stores food for use with patients to assure that it does not spoil. Even the most successful CQI program does not eliminate the need for quality control and the use of quality control indicators.

To this point, the term *quality* has been used numerous times without entering into any specific discussion of what the term means. A brief discussion of ways of conceptualizing quality products and services would be helpful before going further into discussion of specific CQI concepts, strategies, tools, and techniques for process improvement.

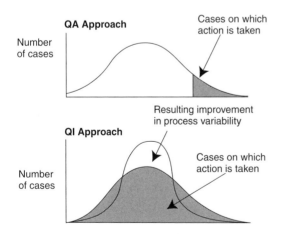

Figure 11–5   The difference between quality assurance (QA) and quality improvement (QI). (Adapted from Carey, R. G., & Lloyd, R. C. [1995]. *Measuring quality improvement in healthcare: A guide to statistical process control applications.* New York: Quality Resources.)

What Is Quality?

When you ask someone to define quality, he or she will likely begin by asking for further clarification of what you mean. This is because the definition of quality is typically context dependent. For example, how might you define quality in relation to the following products and services?

- Purchasing a piece of clothing
- Buying a meal at a restaurant
- Having service provided to your car by an auto mechanic
- Checking in to a hotel for a vacation weekend

Undoubtedly your definition will vary for each context, and likely you will want more information before providing the definition, such as

- "What sort of clothing?"
- "Is it a fast food restaurant or an upscale eatery?"
- "Is it routine auto service or is there a special problem?"
- "Is it a discount hotel or a four-star resort?"

In addition to the characteristic of *value* (the relationship between cost and quality) introduced earlier, you likely would also consider other aspects of each of the previously listed products or services in determining whether the good or service you purchased was of high quality. Aspects of customer service (e.g., performance characteristics) such as speed and accuracy of the transaction, whether the staff members were polite, and specific qualities of the product such as color, surroundings, or noise level would also affect your evaluation of whether the service or product you received met your requirements as a customer for a quality product or service. A list of sample performance characteristics

that can help to define quality in regard to products or services can be found in Box 11–4.

It has already been mentioned that customer satisfaction is the primary focus in CQI, and that customer requirements for quality are continuously changing over time. If this is true, how might you determine what your customers want today? The answer to this question may be obtained by using the "five Cs" of valid customer requirements. The five Cs of valid customer requirements include meeting requirements that are current, calculable, "completeable," consensus based, and consistent with your organization's goals. The word *valid* is used to qualify a customer requirement because sometimes you may not be able to meet these requirements because of limitations in resources or because the customer may have unrealistic expectations that you may not be able or want to meet. The five Cs of valid customer requirements are summarized in Box 11–5.

For example, the process of admitting a patient to a hospital can be measured from the time it takes from the moment the patient arrives at the admitting desk until he or she is in an assigned hospital bed. Preparing hospital beds to be "clean" and ready for a new patient is a complex process involving multiple departments. If you have ever arrived at a hotel to hear that there are no clean rooms available

---

Box 11–4: Sample Performance Characteristics to Help Define Quality

- Timeliness
- Courtesy
- Availability
- Price
- Technical support
- Safety
- Accessibility
- Professionalism
- Reliability
- Ecological impact
- Accuracy
- Waste
- Durability
- Flexibility
- Follow-up

Box 11–5: The Five Cs of Valid Customer Requirements

- **Current:** Are consistent with *today's* competitor benchmarks.
- **Calculable:** Can be *measured*.
- **"Completeable":** Those that can be reasonably accomplished.
- **Consensus-based:** Identified and supported by stakeholders in the process, including customers and resources and limitations are considered.
- **Consistent with organization's goals:** Consistent with the mission and purpose of your organization.

and felt annoyed, you can imagine how much more complicated it may be to prepare a room in a clean environment, and how a patient who may be in discomfort would react if he or she had to wait much longer than expected for a room to be ready. So, how long is it appropriate for a patient to wait? The answer would of course vary depending on the nature of the customer needs (e.g., whether the patient is arriving for a planned admission or appointment, whether there is need for urgent care based on the patient's condition). You might arrive at an answer by applying the five *C*s for valid customer requirements.

The target time for completing the admitting process should be *current* with similar processes conducted in other facilities. The process of benchmarking (comparing a current level of performance with previous performance or the performance of competitors) will be discussed in more detail later in the chapter, but organizations will often freely share information about common processes such as admitting. You can also benchmark against yourself by collecting data over time and monitoring improvement. This process of collecting data on the time it takes to admit a patient indicates that the requirement is *calculable* or *measurable*. Even qualitative elements of a process, such as whether a customer perceives staff to be friendly, can be quantitatively measured by the use of scales such as a customer satisfaction survey. Valid and reliable surveys are complex to design. You are encouraged to seek guidance or use a resource for developing surveys in order to be assured that your results are valid and can be used to guide change in your processes. Your goal should be able to be reasonably accomplished, or be *completeable*. A particular patient might expect that he or she be taken immediately to a room without stopping at the admitting desk, and that any information needed, such as insurance validation, be collected in his or her room. In this case, it might not be possible to meet the expectation of *no* waiting time, so that customer requirement would not be considered valid. However, it might be valid for the patient to expect that minimal information be collected at the admitting desk and that forms that can easily be filled out in the room be brought there to minimize waiting time. A *consensus-based* customer requirement would be identified by involving all internal stakeholders in the process (e.g., representatives from departments such as admitting, who must collect information;

housekeeping, who must clean the patient rooms; and patient transportation, who must move patients from place to place in the hospital) and by collecting information from patients on their expectations. Gaps between the expectations of customers and those of staff for performance must be examined closely so that targets for improvement are perceived as realistic and motivating for staff rather than becoming a source of discouragement. Finally, in this case, the goal of getting patients to their rooms as quickly as possible is clearly *consistent with the organizational goals* of a hospital. At times, however, a patient may request a product or service that, although desirable to the patient, falls outside the organization's goals or mission. For example, a patient might wish to receive home care services from the hospital where he or she had an inpatient stay, but if providing these services is not within the organization's mission and vision, it is a customer request that may not be valid and may go unmet.

It may be evident from the previous example that, in CQI, we are interested in measuring and improving the outcome of processes or the repeatable elements of daily work. Of course, almost everything that is accomplished is done through a process, but not every process is mission critical to the productivity of an organization. However, in every organization—in fact, within every department or product line of an organization—there are processes that are central to the productivity of the work unit. These *critical processes* (such as the previous example of the process of getting a patient from admitting to his or her hospital bed) become the focus of CQI efforts.

Many critical processes, such as the example of admitting a patient, cross department lines or require staff from more than one department to be involved to complete the process. In the remainder of the chapter, the most common CQI concepts, strategies, tools, and techniques, will be introduced (some have already been mentioned) using the PDCA cycle introduced earlier as a framework. The use of the primary concepts, strategies, tools, and techniques is discussed in the following section. Brief instructions for their use and samples are provided throughout the case example that constitutes the remainder of this chapter.

Table 11–2 categorizes some of the most common and critical CQI concepts, strategies, tools, and techniques. You may find additional concepts,

Table 11-2	Common CQI Concepts, Strategies, Tools, and Techniques
	Use/Importance/Summary
Core Concepts	
The Plan, Do, Check, Act (PDCA) cycle	The overarching framework for guiding and ordering CQI activities.
Critical processes	The important processes repeated again and again to complete the organization's or department's work.
Operational definitions	A quantifiable description of what to measure and the steps to follow to measure it consistently.
Customers and customer requirements	Identifying internal and external customers or persons who receive the output of your work and their valid requirements using the 5 Cs.
Quality indicators	Quantitative measures of compliance with valid customer requirements.
Variation	The spread of process output over time. Discriminating between natural "common cause" variation that is inherent in a process and the uncommon "special cause" variation you want to eliminate from a process or emulate if positive.
Stages of team formation	Forming, storming, norming, and performing are the four stages of team development.
Pareto principle (80/20 rule)	The largest percentage of the problem (80%) is typically caused by a small percentage of the causes (20%).
A CQI tool kit	Different tools are used at different times and used in combinations to fit the current need of the team.
Strategies	
Ground rules for meetings	Explicit agreements about how a team will work together and behave as team members, sometimes called team values.
Roles for effective meetings	Assigning roles such as the leader, scribe, facilitator, and timekeeper can lead to more effective meetings.
Consensus	A method for reaching agreement whereby all members agree to fully support a decision even if it is not how they would act if they were acting alone.
Tools	
Process flow charts	A visual representation of the steps in a process used to highlight redundancies, rework, or bottlenecks.
Run charts	A display of data in the order that they occur, highlighting variation.
Control charts	A run chart with statistically determined upper and lower control limits used to determine if a process has changed and to highlight variation.
Cause-and-effect diagrams	A tool to assist in determining possible root causes to a problem.
Proposed options matrix	A tool for comparing possible options for action against a set of predetermined criteria.
Techniques	
Data stratification	Methods for categorizing collection of data; it is important to decide how to stratify data before you collect them.

(continued)

Table 11-2	Common CQI Concepts, Strategies, Tools, and Techniques (continued)
	Use/Importance/Summary
Designing an effective data collection tool	Tools to gather facts on how a process works or its effectiveness that allow for accurate collection of data in the simplest manner.
Balancing tasks and people	Attending to both the needs of team members and the work to be completed to maintain team motivation.
Icebreakers	Short activities to help team members learn about each other or to become more comfortable interacting with each other.
Nominal group technique	A method for generating a large number of ideas through contributions of team members working individually.
Brainstorming	A method for creatively generating lists of possible causes of problems, solutions, or processes to improve.
Multivoting	A decision-making method to narrow a larger number of options to a number that can be reasonably discussed individually.
Rewards and recognition	Individually tailored methods of thanking teams for their contributions to the success of the organization.

strategies, tools, or techniques cited in other sources, and some may be referred to by different names (e.g., an Ishikawa diagram is also called a fishbone diagram or a cause-and-effect diagram). You may also find that some resources will break the PDCA cycle down into additional steps or use other acronyms to summarize the steps; however, most incorporate the PDCA cycle within their frameworks. The goal of this chapter is to introduce you to CQI at a basic level with the hope that, if you find yourself in the position of working as a member of a CQI team or become part of a CQI initiative, you will explore the concepts, strategies, tools, and techniques in more depth. As with each chapter, a list of resources to aid you in that process is provided at the end of this chapter.

The Plan, Do, Check, Act Cycle

Step 1: Plan—What Do You Want to Measure?

The first step in the PDCA cycle is to plan for action by determining the critical process or processes that you want to measure. This can be done in a number of ways. A process may have come to your attention because it is resulting in rework, wasted time, or lowered productivity. The process may come to your attention because of complaints by internal or external customers. You may choose to examine a process because it is *high risk* (when it goes wrong, there are serious implications for productivity or customer well-being), *high volume* (it is completed often, and for this reason may have a serious impact if it is less efficient than it could be), or *problem prone* (the process has a tendency to break down). You may use "idea-generating tools" from your conceptual CQI tool kit, such as *nominal group technique* or *brainstorming*. A nominal group technique is a group decision-making technique designed to generate a large number of ideas through contributions of team members working individually. Brainstorming is a technique to foster creativity and to generate a list of processes to examine. Nominal group technique or brainstorming may be used in other steps in the PDCA cycle, such as generating a list of potential causes of a problem or a list of potential options for fixing a problem. These two techniques appear similar, but, when using nominal group technique, you have team members generate ideas individually before sharing them, whereas in

Box 11–6: Steps for Nominal Group Technique

1. Clarify the group objective.
2. Individually list as many ideas as possible.
3. Go around the group and have each member state one idea on his or her list. Individuals may pass if they don't have an idea that has not already been stated.
4. Record each idea on a flip chart.
5. After all ideas are listed, clarify each idea and eliminate exact duplicates.

brainstorming you have members generate ideas by taking turns. Although the results may be similar, the differences in the techniques should be considered when examining power relationships in the group or the amount of time that you have. You can equalize power in the room by using nominal group technique because members generate ideas before beginning to share them, but it also can take longer than brainstorming. The steps for nominal group technique and for structured brainstorming are listed in Boxes 11–6 and 11–7, respectively.

Finally, a critical process inventory form may be completed (see Figure 11–7, presented later in this chapter in the case example). A critical process inventory is a tool to identify a department's *critical processes*, the *customers* for a process, the *valid customer requirements*, and *quality indicators*.

Box 11–7: Steps for Structured Brainstorming

1. Clarify the brainstorming objective.
2. Take turns calling out ideas one at a time.
3. Record each idea on a flip chart.
4. Build on and expand on the ideas of others.
5. Pass when it is your turn and you cannot think of an idea.
6. Resist stopping immediately when ideas slow down to foster creativity.
7. After all ideas are listed, assure that everyone understands all the ideas and eliminate duplicates.

An important part of planning for a CQI effort is pulling together the right members for a CQI team. As noted before, a CQI team includes representatives from all of the key stakeholders in a process (because of a focus on systems thinking). In some instances, if the process to be examined is intradepartmental (does not cross departmental lines), all the team members may be of the same discipline (e.g., all occupational therapists). However, many critical processes cross over departmental lines, and representatives from each department should be included on the team. Clearly identifying the scope of the improvement initiative and the process boundaries before beginning will help you determine who needs to be involved on the CQI team. Group dynamics change based upon the size of the group, and teams larger than six to nine members may be more difficult to lead. To help limit the size of the group, some members may function as consultants to the team and only be called in to attend meetings when needed.

Because CQI teams may be created for the sole purpose of examining and improving a process and then be disbanded when the work of the team is done, training in CQI principles is critical for the team leadership and its members. Many organizations have formal ongoing training programs for employees, but another common approach is to provide *just-in-time* training for team members. In other words, training is provided on an as-needed basis and just prior to the team beginning its work or when the team needs new concepts, strategies, tools, or techniques. The training may be provided either by the team leaders or by staff with organizational responsibility for training and facilitation. Team leaders may rely upon a conceptual *CQI tool kit*, or the idea that different key CQI concepts, strategies, tools, and techniques may be of use at different times in process improvement, and the same tools may be used at different times. Just as you may use a hammer in once instance and a screwdriver in another, once you become familiar with CQI concepts, strategies, tools, and techniques, you will choose the right tool(s) for the right time from your CQI tool kit.

To maximize the effectiveness of CQI teams, a number of different team roles are often identified and utilized. These roles are the *team leader*, a *facilitator*, a *timekeeper*, and a *scribe*. The roles of team leader and facilitator typically remain relatively stable for the life of the team, but team members typically take turns acting as timekeeper or scribe. The functions of these roles are summarized in Box 11–8. These roles are flexible and may be combined or omitted, or may overlap, in different organizations.

Having a team facilitator in addition to a team leader is sometimes viewed with skepticism, especially when there is already concern over the time commitment of team members. However, the function that the team facilitator serves is critical, especially on new teams. The amount of facilitation needed for a team typically decreases as the team begins to develop and gel, and experienced teams can become self-facilitating.

Effectively leading a team can be difficult, and some organizations or departments that have fully adopted a CQI approach may invest considerable resources in training team leaders. An in-depth discussion of strategies for developing and leading teams effectively is beyond the scope of this chapter. However, you may find a brief introduction to the stages of team development helpful. Teams do not always immediately begin to function efficiently and effectively. There are four commonly identified stages of team development: (1) forming, (2) storming, (3) norming, and (4) performing. As with any staged model, not all teams may go through each stage. Teams may revert to an earlier stage, and some teams may progress quickly to performing whereas others may take considerably longer. Keeping the stages of team development in mind, however, may assist you to lead a team, to be less frustrated with teams that are not yet at a performance stage and with planning appropriate team activities or meeting agendas with the current developmental level of the team in mind, and to move a team toward performing. The stages of team development are briefly summarized in Box 11–9.

Box 11–8: Standing Roles for a CQI Team

- **Team Leader:** guides the team through the CQI process, sets meeting agendas and leads meetings, provides "just-in-time" training to the team, liaises with organization leadership
- **Team Facilitator:** assists team leader with his or her role; monitors group process and shares observations with the team to improve effectiveness; reminds the team of the PDCA cycle and critical concepts, strategies, tools, and techniques; helps the team stay focused within the boundaries of the process being investigated; advises which CQI tools to use and provides training in tool use and CQI application.
- **Timekeeper:** helps to keep the team on track by helping to assure that meetings begin and end on time, gives warnings to the team if they are running over time for an agenda topic or if the meeting is nearing the end
- **Scribe:** takes notes or minutes of the meeting to document team progress, distributes notes to team members for review, writes on a board or flip chart during activities such as brainstorming

---

Box 11–9: Stages of Team Development

- **Forming:** Members are learning about each other and trust levels may be low. There is testing of team leadership by members and higher dependence on leadership. Team roles are unclear and expectations are tested, and minimal work is accomplished.
- **Storming:** Intrateam conflict may intensify. Members may demonstrate resistance to leadership, disruptive group behavior may occur, trust remains low, and minimal work is accomplished.
- **Norming:** Cohesion begins, a common team spirit develops, information is shared more freely. More time can be spent on task. Trust levels begin to rise, and moderate work is accomplished.
- **Performing:** Functional roles are established, team relies on facts and data, a strong sense of team cohesiveness develops, trust in each other is high, and much work is accomplished.

For more information on leading teams and running meetings (such as the use of *ground rules* to guide member behavior in meetings), you are encouraged to refer to the resources at the end of the chapter. An especially helpful resource is *The Team Handbook*, a "how to" manual for inexperienced managers (Scholtes, Joiner, Streibel, & Mann, 2002).

Step 2: Do—Collect Data on Quality Indicators

Once a critical process for improvement is identified and the appropriate team is pulled together, the team members must proceed to come to agreement on how the process they are seeking to improve actually works. This might seem like it would be simple, but it can actually be very complex, especially when the process crosses department lines. To go back to the previous example of admitting a patient to a hospital, you should recognize that various departments "owned" different parts of the process and that probably no single department was aware of all of the steps that people in other departments took to complete the process. It is likely that the extent to which the departments relied on each other also was not recognized. This is why the concept of *internal customers* is important. In organizations, most departments provide some service to another department, and that department is an internal customer. Each department also relies on other departments in order to be able to accomplish its work, and therefore is a customer of the departments upon which it relies. In our example, the admitting department relies on patient transportation to arrive in a timely manner and is therefore an internal customer of the patient transportation department. In turn, patient transportation may rely upon the scheduling department for advance notice of patients who must be moved about the hospital, and therefore is an internal customer of the scheduling department. Some processes also have *external customers*, such as patients, consumers, or payers, who receive the output of a critical process. Critical processes may have internal customers, external customers, or both.

A tool to help identify all of the parts of a process as it works from its starting point to its end point is a *process flowchart*. A process flowchart is a graphic representation of a critical process showing the beginning and end of a process, its major steps, and decision points in the process. Process flowcharts can either be *macro* diagrams that show only the major steps (typically six to eight and usually with no decision points) or *micro* diagrams that break a part of the process out into more detail for closer examination. Figure 11–6 is an example of a simplified micro process flowchart. It shows the process of starting one's day, which is a process that all of you are familiar with. In this example, it is assumed that the start of the process is the alarm clock going off and that the end of the process is driving to work. Many common activities associated with the process are left out of this simplified example. As you can imagine, micro process flowchart for processes such as admitting a patient to a hospital can be quite complicated, with a large number of steps and decision points.

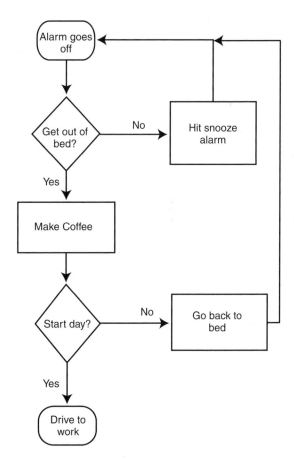

Figure 11–6 Simplified process flow diagram for the process of starting one's day.

There are two purposes for completing a process flowchart. The first is to aide you in identifying the major parts of the process, including the beginning, the middle, and the end, and the order in which these major steps are accomplished, so everyone has a common understanding of the process. Second, an overall goal of CQI that is facilitated by completing a process flowchart is to assure that a process is standardized to best practices.

Variation is a key concept in process improvement. Process improvement in fact can be said to have two objectives related to improving outcomes. The first is to decrease variation and standardize the process. The second is to shift the mean outcome in a positive direction. However, you cannot improve a process until you standardize it.

When considering variation and how it affects the mean, you must identify two types of variation. The first type of variation is *common cause variation*. Common cause variation is the naturally occurring and expected variation in any process. An example would be determining the average time it takes a pool of experienced occupational therapists to construct a resting hand splint. You would expect that, if the same therapist made 10 resting hand splints under normal circumstances, he or she would not complete each of the splints in exactly the same time and that some might take a slightly shorter amount of time and some a slightly longer time. With enough instances, the fabrication time could be averaged and the mean and a standard deviation could be determined. However, the same therapist might need to make a splint for someone with greatly increased flexor tone in the hand and elbow, which would be a lengthier process, or a new practitioner might take more time to make his or her first splint compared to an experienced therapist. These differences could also be described as variation but of a unique type known as *special cause variation*. Before determining the baseline mean or value against which you are going to compare outcomes after process improvement (e.g., benchmarking), you want to eliminate as much special cause variation as possible. In some cases, such as in the example of a new practitioner making a first splint, you may not be able to eliminate the variation but you may choose to account for it separately and not include it in the data you use to determine your baseline mean. It is important to note that occasionally, rather than eliminating special cause variation, you may want to *emulate* it when someone has stumbled upon a method of improving a process and you want others to adopt that method.

After the process had been described through the process flowchart, the team can organize to collect and analyze data. This should be a thoughtful process to avoid wasted time and energy by either collecting data elements that are not needed or going about a data collection process only to discover that you did not collect data on an important part of the process. Data are collected ultimately so that you can measure a *quality indicator*, or a quantitative measure of compliance with valid customer requirements. You need to determine what quality indicators would best measure the key customer requirements for the process you are improving. It is also critical that everyone develop a common understanding of the process that you are going to measure and how you are going to measure it. Throughout the PDCA cycle, teams develop *operational definitions*, or a description in quantifiable terms of what to measure and the steps to measure it consistently. Operational definitions are *critical*. You cannot begin to measure without having a clear understanding of what is to be measured. You must keep the following simple, but important definition in mind:

> Operational definitions are clear and concise descriptions of what to measure in quantifiable terms and include the steps to measure it consistently.

An important rule is to complete data stratification *before* you begin to collect data. *Data stratification* is the process of separating data into the types of categories that will be used to evaluate the data in a logical manner. For example, instances of transporting a patient could be stratified by day of the week on which the transport occurred, by shift (e.g., day, evening, or night), by the individual transporter who transported the patient, or from point of origin for which the transport began. Or, if you were to stratify physicians' referrals to occupational therapy, you could stratify them by referring physician, by specialty, by day of the week received, or by the type of referral. Categories for stratification can be determined by brainstorming, by examining the process flowchart, or by collecting data on a trial basis to determine if you have data points that do not easily fit into a predetermined category before continuing with data collection in earnest.

Once you know what data you wish to collect (by stratification), you can determine how to collect the data. Typically, this involves the use of some data collection tool. Data collection tools do not need to be complex. In many instances, a simple tally or check sheet in which each data point is noted in the appropriate category is sufficient. A sample data collection tool is shown in Figure 11–13 of the case example later in this chapter. In some instances, a process flowchart can be used as a data collection tool. If it is thought that a process may be breaking down at multiple points or that rework is occurring in the process, but you are unsure of the frequency at which this is occurring, a process flowchart could be used. Each time a process error is noted or a step in the process is repeated (e.g., rework is required), a mark or number could be placed next to the corresponding step of the process on the process flowchart. Some key factors for consideration in planning and designing data collection are listed in Box 11–10. Answering these questions before you begin collecting data will save you time and help to assure that the data collected are meaningful.

Box 11–10: Key Factors in Planning Data Collection for Quality Indicators

- What are your primary data sources, or where will your data come from?
- How will you collect your data for your quality indicators?
  - Can data collection be automated or distilled from some computerized system, or must it be manually collected?
  - Are your data sources reliable?
  - Have clear definitions of categories for stratification been determined and data distributed within these categories?
- What will be the frequency with which you collect data, and for how long?
- Who will collect the data?
- How often will data be reported?

Step 3: Check—Analyze Data and Identify Areas for Improvement

Once you have collected sufficient data on your quality indicators, you are ready to analyze the data and determine the need and opportunities for performance improvement. Analysis can range from simple deduction based on a frequency count to complex statistical analysis of variance using computerized statistical software. Resources for analyzing data are included at the end of the chapter. In many instances, decisions can be made by a face examination of the distribution of data collected if adequate effort was put into stratifying the data prior to collection. In addition, if the right team has been assembled and all the key stakeholders have been involved, you can usually trust their decisions about the data because they are the persons who know the most about the process. However, you must remember that a key premise of CQI is making informed decisions with data! Care should be taken to assure that you have adequate data (sufficient sample size) upon which to draw valid conclusions.

The data to be analyzed at this point will provide information about variations in the process and the frequency of instances of rework, bottlenecks, or poor outcomes in the critical process being investigated. The goal is to identify the sources of variation contributing to a lower than desired mean and to determine the extent to which each cause is contributing to the problem. It is highly unlikely that any problem has a single cause or that the multiple causes are contributing equally to the problem. It is also unlikely with complex processes that you will have the time or resources to address all the possible contributing factors.

During the process of data analysis, a team often begins to anticipate the type of improvements that they may be able to make. It is still often difficult to imagine the extent to which improvement may be reasonably expected. Earlier the term *benchmarking* was introduced. Benchmarking is an approach to evaluating your competitive position in the marketplace that has long been used in business and industry. A *benchmark* is a quantifiable measure of the outcome of a process that can be used as a comparison to current performance or as a target for improvement. Benchmarks may be determined in a variety of ways. Some benchmarks may be obtained from competitors through participation in formal benchmarking databases, for which organizations pay an access fee. At the departmental level, managers may freely share benchmarks, even with managers at competing organizations, and such benchmarks may be as close as a phone call to a colleague. A cautionary note about using external benchmarks, however, is that you can never be sure if others are collecting data in the same manner as you; therefore, the data you collect may not provide an accurate comparison. It is recommended that external data be used as a guideline rather than an absolute standard. Historical data from your own department may be also used as a benchmark. Sometimes, benchmarks may not be available and a team may set a target for improvement based upon a common-sense assessment of what the team hopes to achieve. Finally, some CQI leaders believe that it can be counterproductive to set targets and that in fact a target or benchmark may artificially limit the progress a team may make, and suggest that teams simply aim to achieve the maximum improvement they can.

A commonly used CQI principle, referred to as the *Pareto principle* or the *80/20 rule*, is helpful here. The Pareto principle is named after Vilfredo Pareto, an Italian tax collector who noticed that, within his town, the largest percentage of wealth (80%) was spread among a small percentage of residents (20%) (Carey & Lloyd, 1995). Applied to problems with a critical process, it is interpreted to mean that a large percentage of the problem is often caused by relatively few of the contributing causes. It has also been said that the Pareto principle assists you in separating the *vital few* (causes) from the *common many*. The exception to the Pareto principle is to deal with what has been referred to as "*low-hanging fruit.*" This metaphor implies that, just as you might pick an apple within easy reach first because it is less difficult than reaching better quality fruit high up on the tree, sometimes you may decide to fix a contributing cause to a problem because it is easy and inexpensive to do so even if it is not part of the 80% or a major cause of the problem.

It is helpful in analyzing the data to have simple visual displays representing the data. There are a number of tools for analyzing and presenting data to team members to guide their decision making (Box 11–11). It should be noted that commonly purchased presentation or spreadsheet software often includes easy-to-learn mechanisms for enter-

---

> ### Box 11–11: **Tools Used for Analysis and Display of CQI Data**
>
> - **Run Chart:** A graphical display of data collected over time and in the order in which they occurred that displays variation and is helpful in detecting the presence or absence of special cause variation and to determine if process changes have the desired effect.
> - **Control Chart:** A run chart to which statistically determined upper and lower limits have been added to indicate when a case of special cause variation is present and to determine if process changes have the desired effect (control charts are more sensitive than run charts).
> - **Histogram:** Commonly referred to as a "bar chart"; visually represents data in frequencies or percentages by organizing the data in categories with a different vertical bar representing each category of data.
> - **Pareto Chart:** A histogram with the categories or bars reorganized so that the relative contribution of each category is shown (e.g., the bars are organized from highest to lowest percentage or frequency).

---

ing data and creating the types of displays listed in Box 11–11.

Step 4: Act—Act to Roll Out Improvements

Once data are available that indicate categories of causes or possible *root causes*, the next step is to perform a root cause analysis. It is important to understand that, before taking action to change a process, you must be certain that you have truly identified the root causes of the problems. A root cause is the cause that, if changed, will result in real improvements in the process. Sometimes it may seem that one factor is causing a problem, but when you dig deeper it becomes clear that that factor is actually caused by another factor.

In our admitting example, a contributing factor to a long wait time for patients to get to their assigned rooms might appear to be that, when the patient transportation department is called, they are slow in responding. Further, it might be easy to jump to conclusions and place blame on the transporters (personnel) because they are sometimes seen standing in groups talking when patients are waiting to be moved. However, by conducting a root cause analysis, you might determine that the reason that these personnel are sometimes slow in responding is that all transporters are assigned to transport patients in only certain areas of the hospital, and an insufficient number are assigned to serve the admitting area. By identifying this root cause, an appropriate action could be taken that would have a real impact on the process. A helpful tool for completing a root cause analysis is a *cause-and-effect diagram* (see Figure 11–12 in the case example later in the chapter for an example).

After identifying root causes that contribute to the problem and the extent to which they influence the process (remembering the Pareto principle), a team can move forward to identify potential solutions to improve the process. Teams can rely on concepts, strategies, tools, and techniques already mentioned, including brainstorming and creating a new process flowchart to illustrate a changed process that eliminates rework or bottlenecks, or other tools might be used, such as *multivoting* or a *proposed option matrix*. Multivoting is a technique for narrowing a large number of options down to a manageable few that can be reasonably discussed in detail (for directions, see Box 11–14 in the case example later in the chapter). A proposed options matrix is a tool that assists in evaluating possible options to solve a problem by comparing them against a set of predetermined criteria such as cost, feasibility of implementation, and anticipated effectiveness (see Table 11–4 in the case example for a sample proposed options matrix).

Another important CQI strategy that can be used throughout the process is that of developing *consensus*. Consensus is an approach to decision making in which the key is to come to a decision that every member of the team agrees to support and to work toward successfully implementing, even if that is not how he or she would act if acting alone. For example, after multivoting on 10 proposed options and narrowing the choices to the top 3, the team might use consensus to decide which option to implement first. Consensus and the art of *managing agreement* are used together to assure

that, when team members agree to a course of action, they will support it fully both publicly and privately. Conversely, as teams move toward the stage of performing, team members may become more reticent to disagree with each other and to disrupt the team's newfound harmony. An effective team leader may manage agreement through strategies such as asking the team to identify reasons why a course of action might fail. By making disagreement a healthy, safe, and rewarded part of the process, the leader can prevent a team from taking an ill-advised course of action when a team member actually knows in advance that a problem exists.

Typically, when an option is chosen for implementation, it is first implemented in a pilot format before making changes permanent. This is consistent with the philosophy of continuous improvement and allows the team to work out any minor problems before investing time and energy in training other personnel or communicating the new process to the organization. Beginning with a pilot intervention also suggests to others in the organization that the team is open to feedback, which may make acceptance of the process more likely. Data should continue to be collected during implementation of the pilot intervention to determine if the changes actually resulted in improvement. Finally, just-in-time training can be provided to organization members not yet involved with the process.

A final important step in the CQI process is to provide *rewards and recognition* for the members of the team who were involved in process improvement. Some CQI teams that tackle complicated processes can work for months and become very invested in the outcome of their work. Usually, being a member of a CQI team means extra work above and beyond usual daily commitments, even if the team members are meeting during the normal workday. Providing appropriate rewards and recognition can foster an ongoing sense of commitment to the organization and can help the team members feel better about the team having to disassemble. Rewards and recognitions do not need to be costly to an organization. In fact, some of the most meaningful rewards and recognition can be very low cost, such as a personal note of thanks written to each team member by the team leader or a member of the organization's leadership that

---

Box 11–12: Keys to Determining Appropriate Rewards and Recognitions

- Consider when to recognize individual contributions and when to recognize the team as a whole.
- Consider whether all team members will receive the same reward or rewards can be personalized by giving each member a different but equal reward.
- Consider whether there are ways that your reward or recognition could backfire or be considered unpleasant or punishing by members of the team.

- Consider getting feedback from others on your choice of reward or recognition.
- Consider whether there are any temporary members of the team or consultants who contributed to the team's success who should be rewarded.
- Consider whether team members can be consulted in choosing their own reward or how they wish to celebrate their accomplishments within predetermined boundaries and guidelines.

---

points out the team member's unique contribution to the team, or perhaps a framed picture of the team or a thank-you breakfast or lunch for the team. It is important to be thoughtful in choosing a reward or in recognizing team members, though, so you do not inadvertently "punish" a team member while trying to do the exact opposite. For example, one hospital discontinued the practice of recognizing teams' accomplishments by presenting them certificates at a monthly directors' meeting after learning that being called in front of a large group to receive a certificate was not a rewarding experience for some persons who felt very uncomfortable

being in front of crowds. Often leaving the choice of rewards up to the team leader, who knows the team the best, may work well. Some key principles in considering rewards and recognitions are listed in Box 11–12.

The PDCA cycle will be illustrated through the following case example. Because not every concept, strategy, tool, or technique was utilized during this one case and all the data for the example are not still available, some information has been fabricated to demonstrate application of all of the concepts, strategies, tools, and techniques discussed in this chapter.

Case Example: Occupational Therapy Referral Process at Exeter Hospital

Exeter Hospital is a small acute care hospital that provides services including orthopedic surgery, inpatient oncology, cardiac surgery, and rehabilitation and general medicine, among others. The facility employs occupational therapists, physical therapists, nurses, social workers, psychologists, and speech-language pathologists in addition to general and specialty physicians and other health professionals. The occupational therapy department received referrals from all of the medical floors but struggled to respond in a consistent manner, especially during times of short staffing or during higher levels of volume and referrals. Complaints from physicians regarding the time it

took for occupational therapy to respond to referrals were not uncommon, nor was it uncommon for an occupational therapist to get to a patient's room only to find that the patient had already been discharged, resulting in lowered productivity and rework. The director of the occupational therapy department made a number of attempts to fix this problem, but none of the attempts made a significant impact. The hospital was in the process of transitioning to a CQI approach, and the director had recently received training in CQI leadership. Because the process of receiving and responding to referrals for occupational therapy crossed department lines, the director asked for and received

(continued)

permission to form a formal CQI team. Permission was sought from the Quality Lead Council for the hospital, which, among other responsibilities, limited the number of CQI teams functioning at once to prevent staff resources from being spread too thinly. The director then began the CQI process with the first step of the PDCA cycle, or "planning."

After the "Occupational Therapy Referral Team" was approved, the boundaries of the process were tentatively defined so the key stakeholders in the process could be identified and asked to participate on the team. Initial team members or stakeholders in the process included occupational therapists who received the referrals, a physician who was responsible for writing the referrals, a nurse who was responsible for often acting as a liaison between the physicians and other services, a hospital unit clerk who was responsible for entering referrals into the computer system, and a social worker who coordinated the discharge date for patients. Other departments such as physical therapy were identified as possible consultants to the team. Because the director was concerned that he might be too close to the process, he became a member of the team, and a nurse who had been team leader for several teams and was very experienced with the CQI process agreed to become the leader for this team. The manager of the housekeeping department, who was experienced in the CQI process, volunteered to be the team facilitator. The fact that the team facilitator was not at all familiar with the referral process was seen as an advantage rather than a disadvantage because the facilitator could be objective and might not share the inaccurate assumptions of those who already participated in the process. The team leader and the team facilitator reviewed the team roles with the team members, and also reminded them of the stages of team development so they would not become frustrated by slow progress in the first few meetings. At the first meeting, the team reviewed the typical meeting *ground rules*, such as starting and ending on time, respecting other's opinions, and that disagreement was a healthy part of the process. A sample of the team's ground rules for meetings can be found in Box 11–13.

A critical process inventory helped to identify internal and external customers in the process, their requirements, and quality indicators. As opposed to some teams who might begin by brainstorming

---

Box 11–13: Ground Rules for Team Meetings

- Meetings will start and end promptly at the designated times.
- Members should arrive with between-meeting assignments completed.
- Conflict and disagreement is a healthy, respected part of the process.
- Treat others who disagree with you with respect and dignity at all times.
- Seek to listen and understand before speaking and seeking to be understood.
- Pagers and phones should be set on vibrate and only emergency calls or pages should be answered.
- It is okay to have fun, laugh, and enjoy ourselves while we work!

---

processes to address, this team began with the knowledge that its objective was to address an identified *problem-prone* process. As with many of the concepts, strategies, tools, and techniques, the team leader and the facilitator provided just-in-time training for the team before using any concept, strategy, tool, or technique for the first time. An example of the team's critical process inventory is included in Figure 11–7.

Also as a part of the first step in the PDCA cycle, the team agreed to seek to understand how the process of referring and responding to occupational therapy referrals actually worked by completing a process flowchart. The team completed a macro process flowchart of the referral process to occupational therapy. The team also developed operational definitions such as agreeing that the process began when the physician wrote the order and ended when the occupational therapist had his or her first face-to-face contact with the patient as documented in the electronic medical record. The team's macro process flowchart is illustrated in Figure 11–8. In addition, individual team members worked with other members of their departments to complete micro process flowcharts that illustrated how portions of the overall process for which they were responsible worked (not shown).

After completing the process flowcharts, the team moved into the second stage of the PDCA cycle, or "doing" (collecting and analyzing data on quality in-

(continued)

Case Example: Occupational Therapy Referral Process at Exeter Hospital (Continued)

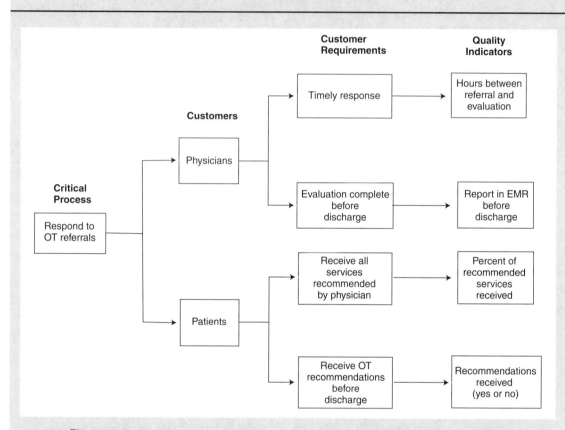

Figure 11–7   Critical process inventory. EMR, electronic medical record; OT, occupational therapy.

dicators). Because the team began process improvement with a good idea of the customer requirements that were targeted for improvement, they understood that their ultimate goal was to decrease variation in the process of responding to referrals to occupational therapy and to lower the mean response time. The team agreed to collect some baseline data on the mean length of time from entry of the referral into the medical record by the physician to the time of the first contact by the occupational therapist with the

patient as documented in the electronic medical record. The team also knew that they should identify the range of response times as well because relying *just* on the mean can mask performance problems because outliers are not identified.

The team chose categories to stratify the data before collecting baseline information and constructed a simple data collection tool. The group agreed that data should be organized according to the day of the week the referral was written, because staffing levels

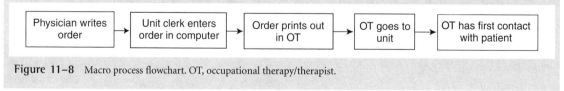

Figure 11–8   Macro process flowchart. OT, occupational therapy/therapist.

(continued)

Table 11-3	Baseline Mean Response Time* for Occupational Therapy Referrals				
Day of Week Referral Is Written	Mean Response Time (Hours)	Referring Unit	Mean Response Time (Hours)	Patient Diagnosis	Mean Response Time (Hours)
Monday	28	2 East	33	Orthopedic	27
Tuesday	26	2 West	54	Cardiac rehabilitation	22
Wednesday	30	3 East	35	Oncology	53
Thursday	27	3 West	24	General medicine	51
Friday	34	4 East	58		
Saturday	53	4 West	26		
Sunday	56				

*The figures reflect *average* response times. The range of response times included responses as short as 4 hours and as long as 73 hours.

varied from day to day; the hospital unit on which the patient was located, in case variations in unit-based processes might be impacting the outcome; and the referring service for each referral, because not every therapist was trained to respond to all types of diagnoses (e.g., therapists had to demonstrate advanced competencies before beginning to work with cardiac rehabilitation patients). They followed the suggestion of the facilitator to conduct a pilot collection of data first to see if it became evident that other categories or methods of stratifying the data should be added.

Data were collected for a period of 8 weeks to obtain an adequate sample size for data analysis. For each referral, the date and time that the referral was entered into the electronic medical record and the date and time of the first contact of the occupational therapist with the patient were noted to allow the team to identify the mean response time for response to referrals in hours and minutes. Initial data collected are shown in Table 11–3.

The overall mean response time to referrals was close to 38 hours from the time the referral was written by the physician until the responding occupational therapist saw the patient for the first time to begin the evaluation process. Although the overall mean was within the target of less than 48 hours identified in a department policy, the range of response times included response times as short as

4 hours and as long as more than 70 hours for some referrals. The team identified one case of *special cause variation* that would have shifted the mean even further in a negative direction. This case was one time period when 2 days of severe snowstorms had prevented all but one of the occupational therapists from getting to the hospital, resulting in extraordinarily long response times to referrals written on those two dates. The team agreed not to include this data point in the data analysis so they could have a more realistic view of their starting point and the impact of their work on the mean response time. The team noted from the baseline data that referrals written near the end of the week or on the weekend took notably longer to respond to than those written on days earlier in the week. They also noted that referrals from two of the units and from two of the services had longer mean response times than referrals from other units or services. *Pareto charts* were constructed to reorder the data to highlight the problem areas. These charts are shown in Figures 11–9, 11–10, and 11–11.

The Pareto charts highlighted a number of issues. Although the overall mean time for responding to referrals was actually below the stated time in the department policy of 48 hours, the response time was above target for referrals written on the weekend, for referrals coming from two units (2 West and 4 East), and for referrals from two services (oncology and gen-

(continued)

Case Example: Occupational Therapy Referral Process at Exeter Hospital (Continued)

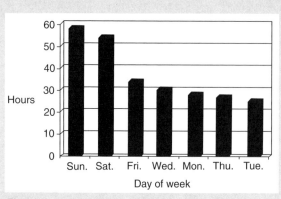

Figure 11–9   Pareto chart of data stratified by day of week.

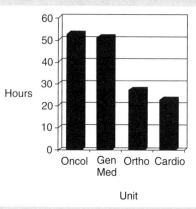

Figure 11–11   Pareto chart of data stratified by service. Cardio, cardiology; Gen Med, general medicine; Oncol, oncology; Ortho, orthopedics.

eral medicine). The team noted that 2 West and 4 East were units that primarily contained patients who were admitted to either oncology or general medicine services. Although the Pareto charts gave an indication of where the primary problem was, they gave no indication of the potential root causes of the problems.

To identify potential root causes of the long response time to referrals for the units and services with the greatest response times, the team brainstormed potential causes and then organized their ideas by categories on a cause-and-effect diagram. The team's

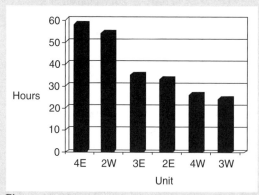

Figure 11–10   Pareto chart of data stratified by unit. E, East; W, West.

diagram is shown in Figure 11–12. Some cause-and-effect diagrams can get to be quite large. For the sake of simplicity, only a sampling of the potential causes of the problem that were identified is shown in Figure 11–12.

To construct the cause-and-effect diagram, the team began by using four common headings for the major "bones" of the diagram (the diagram is sometimes referred to as a *fishbone diagram* because it resembles the spine and bones of a fish when completed). The four headings served as categories of potential causes for the problem under investigation: (1) *materials*, or problems related to materials used in the referral process; (2) *machines*, or problems related to machines such as computers; (3) *methods*, or problems related to the parts of the process used to refer patients to occupational therapy; and (4) *man*, or problems related to personnel performance. Other strategies for identifying the headings could have been used, such as using key segments of the process flowchart. Once the headings were agreed upon, the team began to brainstorm potential causes of the problem by discussing one heading or category of potential causes at a time. (If such headings are used, it is important to assess the category re-

(continued)

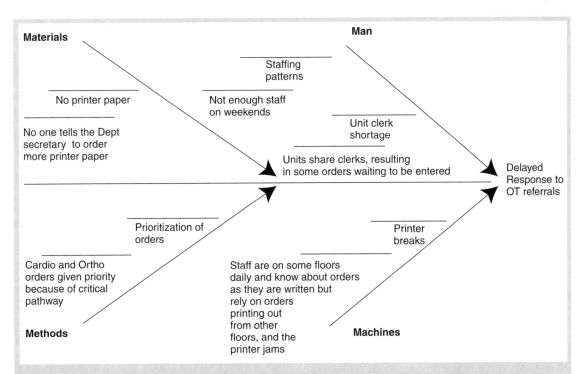

Figure 11–12 Cause-and-effect diagram of suggested causes for problems related to occupational therapy (OT) referrals. Cardio, cardiology; Ortho, orthopedics.

lated to personnel last so that you don't reinforce blaming behavior.) Although the rules for brainstorming, including not censoring suggestions as they are made, were followed, the team also only suggested possible causes that they thought were realistically contributing to the problem. After the team was finished with generating ideas, they examined the list of potential causes, noting where there were duplicates because this suggested what might be the most significant problems.

Following identification of possible causes of the problem, the next step in the cause-and-effect analysis was to verify *root causes*, or causes that were actually contributing to the problem and that, if fixed, would result in an improvement. In other words, the team needed to determine which problems, if fixed, would result in *decreasing variation* and in *shifting the mean* in the desired direction. To accomplish this, they had to return to the process of data collection and analysis. The team decided to modify the cause-and-effect diagram that they had completed so that it could be used as a *check sheet* or simple data collection tool. They simplified the diagram, removing much of the text so

that what remained was clearly understood by each team member and the staff members who would be involved in collecting data (an operational definition), even though what remained on the check sheet might not be the root cause. For example, although the root cause of the printer being out of paper might have been that no one informed the department secretary that paper was running low, the check sheet noted only those things easily counted, or, in this example, that the printer was out of paper. In each case in which the response to a referral exceeded their new target for responding to referrals, it was noted on a copy of the cause-and-effect diagram that had been distributed to all team members. Data were collected for a 2-month period. An example of a check sheet showing the results of this phase of data collection is shown in Figure 11–13.

The data showed that most cases of delayed response to referrals could be clearly tracked to two root causes. The data collected were organized in a Pareto chart that illustrated the relative contribution of each of the root causes. This Pareto chart is provided in Figure 11–14.

(continued)

Case Example: Occupational Therapy Referral Process at Exeter Hospital (Continued)

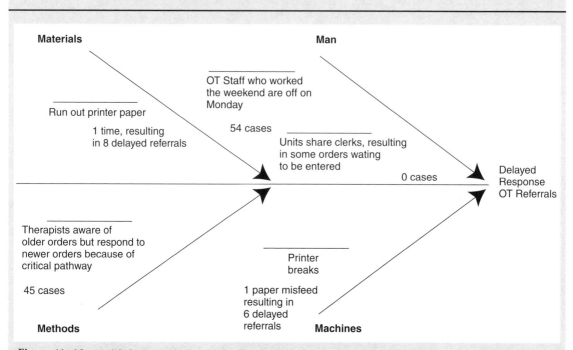

Figure 11–13 Modified cause-and-effect diagram for data collection. OT, occupational therapy.

After reviewing these data, the team had to decide how to move forward to address the root causes that they had verified. Based on the data, the team agreed

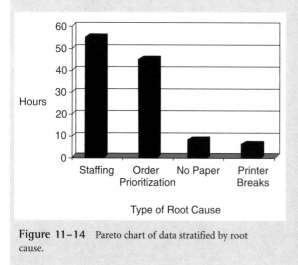

Figure 11–14 Pareto chart of data stratified by root cause.

that OT staff members who had worked the weekend being off on Mondays and the practice of prioritizing orders from orthopedics and cardiac rehabilitation above other orders appeared to be the main contributors to the problem. They noted that some potential causes were shown to not be a contributing factor to the problem. For instance, it had been thought that the practice of sharing unit clerks resulted in orders being entered into the computer more slowly at some times than others, but this delay was not documented. In other words, this potential root cause was not verified. The team applied the Pareto principle and initially agreed that they needed to focus on two of the four contributing root causes (for purposes of simplicity, some verified root causes have been removed from the example). However, before moving forward, the team leader asked the team to consider taking two steps. First, although two of the contributing root causes accounted for a small percentage of the problem, they were both related to a cause that seemed

(continued)

easy to fix (i.e., they were examples of what may be called "low-hanging fruit"). During an earlier team meeting, one member had noted that the occupational therapy department continued to rely on an old printer that utilized a continuous feed mechanism that often jammed, and that they sometimes ran out of the special paper it required. The team leader wondered if replacing the printer was a case of "low-hanging fruit." The occupational therapy director verified that he had access to funds to replace the printer with a new high-volume printer that would store large amounts of paper and operated using plain photocopy paper. He agreed to proceed with purchasing a new printer so that the team could focus on the primary contributing root causes they had identified.

Second, to identify possible courses of action, the team discussed both of the primary root causes that were contributing to the problem in a series of meetings. For each cause, they brainstormed possible actions that could be taken to address the root cause. They were surprised at the number and the variety of suggestions that were generated. To limit the suggestions to a small number that they could discuss and compare reasonably, they used the CQI technique of *multivoting*. The steps involved in multivoting are listed in Box 11–14.

When the team finished the process of multivoting, four proposed options remained to be discussed. The team considered trying to move directly to making a decision about what actions to take by reaching consensus, but instead agreed that they needed a more objective manner of comparing the options. To do this, they utilized another CQI tool, a *proposed options matrix*, to compare the four possible options for action against a set of predetermined criteria. The team's proposed option matrix is illustrated in Table 11–4.

After completing the proposed options matrix, several things became clear to the team. Two of the proposed options were rated as likely to be highly effective; however, they were also rated as being not at all feasible. The suggestion to hire a therapist to work the weekends in addition to existing staff would have clearly helped lower response time, but the salary cost for this action was estimated to be over $24,000. Given that the hospital had recently laid off employees in some departments, this option did not meet the criteria of being budget neutral and was eliminated. The suggestion to begin treating all orders the same

---

Box 11–14: **The Steps in Multivoting**

1. Agree on the criteria for selecting ideas to prevent the team from diverging, which will waste time and frustrate members, rather than converging.
   a. Begin by generating suggestions for criteria on a flip chart.
   b. Through discussion, agree on criteria that all members will use.
   c. Try to hone your list to three to five criteria.
2. Identify each idea by listing them on a flip chart beside a letter of the alphabet.
3. Agree on the number of ideas for which each member will vote (a general guideline is 25% of the ideas generated).
4. Vote individually on paper, listing the letter of each selected idea.
5. Take turns calling out the letters of selected ideas.
6. Record and add the votes on the flip chart.
7. Decide which ideas should receive further consideration (eliminate ideas with no votes, keep those with many votes, and consider keeping ideas for which some members felt very strongly).
8. Repeat the voting if too many ideas remain to reasonably discuss and compare.
9. Vote until you have two to four ideas and use consensus to make decisions from that point.

---

way and to end the practice of prioritizing orders from orthopedics and cardiac rehabilitation was also perceived to be an idea that could be effective. However, based on the anticipated reaction from the medical directors of the orthopedic and cardiac rehabilitation services, this idea was also rated as not likely to be feasible and the team agreed to end pursuit of that option.

In comparing the remaining options, the team noted that the option of changing the staffing pattern so that some staff members would work a Wednesday-through-Sunday schedule on a perma-

(continued)

Case Example: Occupational Therapy Referral Process at Exeter Hospital (Continued)

Table 11-4 — Proposed Options Matrix for Occupational Therapy (OT) Referrals

Root Cause	Proposed Option	Methods	Cost of Option	How Effective? (A)*	How Feasible? (B)*	Overall Rating (A × B)*
Staff members who work weekends take Monday off	Change staffing pattern	Have staff permanently assigned to weekends	$0.00	4	2	8
	Supplement staff	Hire a weekend therapist	$24,360	5	1	5
Orthopedic and cardiac orders are prioritized	Treat all orders the same	End practice of prioritizing orders on critical pathways	$0.00	3	2	6
	Collaborate with PT on cardiac patients	Have PT evaluate as many patients as possible on the weekend so that OT can see patients on general medicine	$0.00	3	4	12

*1 = Least effective/feasible; 5 = Most effective/feasible.
PT, physical therapy.

nent basis was expected to be effective because it would assure that roughly the same number of staff members were available every day of the week and would eliminate the problem that they were often short staffed on Mondays. However, even though no additional salary costs were associated with the option, it was rated as somewhat unfeasible based on the expectation that it would receive a very negative reaction from the staff, and staff turnover was already a great concern of the occupational therapy director. In contrast, the option of collaborating with physical therapy on the treatment of cardiac rehabilitation patients was rated as slightly less effective but more feasible, and received a higher overall rating. The team posited that, if occupational therapy focused on self-

care sessions on days when they had more staff in the hospital and allowed physical therapy to provide more weekend treatment to the cardiac rehabilitation patients, it would allow them to keep up with orders from oncology and general medicine on those days. Although they were not positive that this would truly be effective, the team agreed that it would be a very feasible option because the senior physical therapist who provided services on cardiac rehabilitation had been consulted and had agreed to fully support the plan if implemented.

After further discussion, the team agreed to proceed by first implementing the option of collaborating with physical therapy as a pilot intervention for a 2-month period and measure the impact this change

(continued)

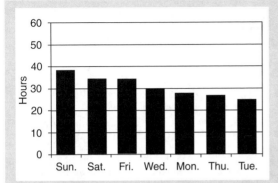

Figure 11–15 Pareto chart of post–pilot intervention data stratified by day of week.

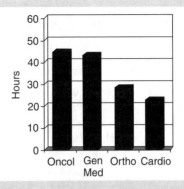

Figure 11–17 Pareto chart of post–pilot intervention data stratified by service. Cardio, cardiology; Gen Med, general medicine; Oncol, oncology; Ortho, orthopedics.

had before implementing a change in the occupational therapy staffing pattern. All members of the occupational therapy and physical therapy departments were educated to the planned pilot intervention. The medical director for cardiac rehabilitation was also consulted before the pilot intervention was implemented, and, although she expressed some reservations, she agreed to support the change for a 2-month pilot period. Data were collected during the pilot intervention and organized in Pareto charts (Figures 11–15, 11–16, and 11–17). The team agreed to stratify the data according to the original categories of data utilized, which were by day of the week that referrals were written, the referring unit, and the referring service.

Upon examination of the Pareto charts constructed using data from the pilot intervention, the team noticed positive results. First, the overall mean response time to referrals dropped from approximately 38 hours to approximately 33 hours. More importantly, the mean response time for referrals written on Saturdays and Sundays (the two most problematic days) also dropped. The mean response time on Saturdays dropped from 53 hours to 34 hours and the mean response time on Sundays dropped from 56 hours to 38 hours. In addition to these means now meeting the targets established within the occupational therapy department policies, the team also noted an additional change. The occupational therapy department routinely tracked the number of "missed referrals," or occasions when an occupational therapist responded to a referral to find that the patient had been discharged without being evaluated. The director of occupational therapy reported that, concurrent with the team's pilot intervention, he noticed a dramatic drop in the number of missed referrals. This was assumed to also be a result of the faster response rate to referrals.

After examining the results of the pilot intervention, the team agreed that the option they had implemented in pilot form had been successful. The team re-examined the other potential options to consider if even further improvement might be made, but agreed to end their intervention given the level of concern over the feasibility of the other options. This decision points out the importance of the relationship between making decisions with data, and sound judgment by management. Although the use of data in decision

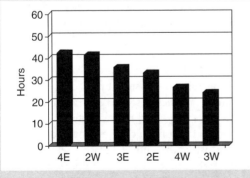

Figure 11–16 Pareto chart of post–pilot intervention data stratified by unit. E, East; W, West.

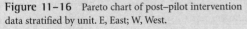

(continued)

Case Example: Occupational Therapy Referral Process at Exeter Hospital (Continued)

making is key, data analysis cannot become a replacement for leadership or decision making based on appreciation of an organization's culture or the current priorities. Data analysis should be thought of as a strategy that is used in combination with other leadership and management strategies to support effective decision making.

Before disbanding, the team sought to fully integrate the revised process by documenting the new procedures and educating staff on the units as to the revised procedures. The procedures were specifically reviewed with the director of cardiac rehabilitation to assure that there was full support.

Finally, the team leader and the team facilitator discussed methods of providing recognition of the team's success and to reward the team members and the consultants to the team for their hard work and contributions. They agreed on several steps. First, a brief summary of the team's accomplishments, a listing of the team members and consultants, and a thank-you note were printed in the "Quality Corner," an article that appeared regularly in the hospital's monthly newsletter. Second, the team leader wrote individual thank-you notes to each team member, with a copy to his or her direct supervisor recognizing a unique contribution that each team member brought to the team. Finally, the team agreed to arrange a potluck lunch to celebrate their success, and the occupational therapy department provided a cake for dessert. The team leader arranged for the hospital chief operating officer to drop by for dessert and to thank the team members in person.

Chapter Summary

In this chapter you were introduced to continuous quality improvement as both a management philosophy and an approach to process improvement. CQI was contrasted with quality assurance and quality control, and the focus of CQI on meeting and exceeding valid requirements of customers was emphasized. You were provided with an introduction to the basic concepts, strategies, tools, and techniques to begin to develop your conceptual CQI tool kit.

Although it might seem that the case example provided was "in depth," it is important to keep in mind that CQI initiatives in organizations that have mature programs can be extraordinarily complex. Further, learning how to effectively balance the tasks at hand with the people involved requires a wide range of managerial skills, from data collection and statistical analysis to managing agreement and solving conflicts. In Chapter 1, you were introduced to the strategy of evaluating different types of evidence, and it was noted that evidence-based practice requires a manager to utilize good judgment in applying evidence to a problem. Gathering and analyzing data as evidence in a CQI approach also requires sound managerial judgment. The emphasis of CQI on making decisions with data does not release the manager from his or her responsibilities for coaching and nurturing staff.

You are encouraged to remember that this is an introductory management text, and many excellent resources exist that provide more detailed guidance on each of the CQI concepts, strategies, tools, and techniques introduced in this chapter, a few of which are provided in the resources list at the end of the chapter. These concepts, strategies, tools, and techniques are useful in many aspects of routine management, including planning, running effective meetings, problem solving, and decision making outside of a formal CQI initiative.

Real-Life Solutions

Joan attended the CQI Leadership Course and learned that, in opposition to the outdated model of quality assurance, CQI was both a management philosophy and a set of management methods. She really liked the focus on customer satisfaction and appreciated that the leadership course had focused on concepts, strategies, tools, and techniques related to both managing people and managing tasks.

Joan was impressed with the strong emphasis on making decisions based on data, and that attendees were encouraged to take their time in making decisions by involving all the key stakeholders in a process in process improvement. Joan felt a little overwhelmed by the sheer number of concepts, strategies, tools, and techniques to which she had been introduced. However, she had been encouraged by the number of easily accessible resources that had been shared with her, including books and Web sites that provided clear directions for each concept, strategy, tool, or technique. Most importantly, Joan was excited that CQI focused on process improvement because she could see how this approach might lead to real changes in the way things were done. By focusing on *critical processes*, she thought that real improvements in customer and staff satisfaction might be achieved.

Resources For Learning More About Continuous Quality Improvement

Journals That Often Address Continuous Quality Improvement or Quality

QUALITY MANAGEMENT IN HEALTH CARE

Quality Management in Health Care provides a forum to explore the theoretical, technical, and strategic elements of total quality management in health care. The journal addresses key issues in health care quality management by providing a forum for the interchange of varied perspectives. In-depth interviews with prominent individuals in health care quality management and educational tutorials on basic quality management tools and processes are also provided in each issue. An information clearinghouse promotes informal communication among those involved in the field of health care quality management, and a reference center reviews books, journal articles, seminars, and videos of interest.

TOTAL QUALITY MANAGEMENT AND BUSINESS EXCELLENCE

Total Quality Management and Business Excellence is an international journal that publishes articles related to all aspects of total quality management. The journal seeks to provide a forum for discussion and dissemination of research results. The journal encourages interest in all matters relating to total quality management and is intended to appeal to both the academic and professional community working in this area.

JOURNAL FOR HEALTHCARE QUALITY

The *Journal for Healthcare Quality* is a professional forum that advances quality in a diverse and changing health care environment. The journal addresses an audience of professionals who are responsible for promoting and monitoring quality, safe, cost-effective health care. Topics often addressed in the journal include continuous quality improvement, risk management, utilization review, and the latest in regulations from the Joint Commission on Accreditation of Health-care Organizations, peer review organizations, and payment systems. The journal also publishes reviews of publications in the field and updates on pertinent legislation. It offers coverage of state-of-the-art technology, total quality management techniques, and practical applications of quality improvement systems and innovations.

Professional Organizations Concerned with Continuous Quality Improvement or Quality

NATIONAL ASSOCIATION FOR HEALTHCARE QUALITY

http://www.nahq.org
The National Association for Healthcare Quality NAHQ is committed to developing and promoting professional expertise in the art and science of

health care quality. NAHQ members include professionals in general, acute, managed, long-term, home, rehabilitation, mental health, and ambulatory care settings as well as consultants whose responsibilities include quality or risk management in a wide area of health professions.

AMERICAN SOCIETY FOR QUALITY

http://www.asq.org/

The American Society for Quality (ASQ) is a professional association that seeks to create better workplaces and communities worldwide by advancing learning, quality improvement, and knowledge exchange. Officers and member experts of the ASQ provide consultation and advice to the U.S. Congress, government agencies, state legislatures, and other groups and individuals on quality-related topics. Representatives of The ASQ have provided testimony on issues such as training, health care quality, education, transportation safety, quality management in the federal government, licensing for quality professionals, and more. The society also works with the media on quality-related matters, providing informational resources and referrals to qualified experts from its broad member base.

MISCELLANEOUS RESOURCES

- Carey, R. G., & Lloyd, R. C. (1995). *Measuring quality improvement in healthcare: A guide to statistical process control applications.* New York: Quality Resources.

http://qualitypress.asq.org/

This book provides an excellent introduction to the statistical process control applications that are most frequently used to analyze data in process improvement initiatives. Key concepts, including variation, use of critical tools (including run charts and control charts), and statistical thinking, are examined through the use of case examples.

- Biemer, P. P., & Lyberg, L. E. (2003). *Introduction to survey quality.* New York: Quality Resources.

http://qualitypress.asq.org/

As more and more professionals who are not trained as survey researchers take on tasks associated with surveys, the need has arisen for a basic introduction to current survey methods and quality issues associated with them. The authors review both well-established and recently developed principles and concepts in the field and examine important issues being currently researched. Topics include common errors in interviewing, data collection methods, and practical survey design for minimizing total survey error.

- Scholtes, P. R., Joiner, B. L., & Streibel, B. J. (2003). *The team handbook* (3rd ed.). Madison, WI: Oriel.

http://orielinc.com/

This comprehensive resource book provides resources on creating high-performance teams. Information is included on different types of teams, tools, and strategies for leading change, and a variety of CQI tools and techniques.

Reference List

Carey, R. G., & Lloyd, R. C. (1995). *Measuring quality improvement in healthcare: A guide to statistical process control applications.* New York: Quality Resources.

Deming, D. E. (2000). *Out of the crisis.* Cambridge, MA: The MIT Press.

George, S., & Weimerskirch, A. (1994). *Total quality management: Strategies and techniques proven at today's most successful companies* (2nd ed.). New York: John Wiley & Sons.

Jaeger, B. J., Kaluzny, A. D., & McLaughlin, C. P. (1994). TQM/CQI: From industry to health care. In C. P. McLaughlin & A. D. Kaluzny (Eds.), *Continuous quality improvement in health care* (pp. 11–32). Gaithersburg, MD: Aspen.

Kaluzny, A. D. (1994). Defining total quality management/continuous quality improvements. In C. P. McLaughlin & A. D. Kaluzny (Eds.), *Continuous quality improvement in health care* (pp. 3–10). Gaithersburg, MD: Aspen.

Scholtes, P. R., Joiner, B. L., Streibel, B., & Mann, D. (2003). *The team handbook: How to use teams to improve quality* (3rd ed.). Madison, WI: Oriel.

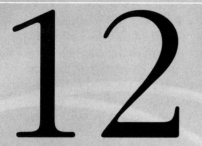

CHAPTER 12

Brent Braveman, Ph.D., OTR/L, FAOTA

Communicating Effectively in Person and in Writing

Real-Life Management

Charlotte is a level II fieldwork student completing her fieldwork in a large mental health setting that provides services ranging from an inpatient unit to a variety of day treatment options. She has always known that she wanted to work in psychosocial practice and has typically excelled academically. She entered her fieldwork expecting that she would excel there as well but has encountered some difficulties. Much to Charlotte's surprise, she has received constructive criticism from a number of the occupational therapy staff on her style of interpersonal communication with staff and with clients. What is most concerning to Charlotte is that the feedback she has received seems to indicate that there is often a mismatch between what she hopes to communicate and how her message is being received.

Charlotte's clinical fieldwork educator has been very supportive and has suggested to Charlotte that she take advantage of a fieldwork assignment to develop and present an in-service education session for unit staff by exploring strategies for improving the effectiveness of interpersonal communication. Charlotte begins by visiting the library to find some resources on communication theory and strategies for improving her verbal, nonverbal, and written interpersonal communication.

Key Issues

- There are a large number of theories of communication related to interpersonal communication, communication to the public and groups, communication in the mass media, and intercultural communication.
- Resources for improving communication are widely available to address verbal and nonverbal aspects of vocal communication, whether communicating with an individual or a group, as well as improving written communication.
- Planning your communication and paying conscious attention to aspects of communication that are often unconscious, such as rate of speech, facial expressions, or body orientation, can help you become a more effective communicator.
- Managers communicate for many reasons in many forms, including conversations, presentations, memos, business letters, business plans, and grant proposals.

The topic of communication is one that has become exponentially broader in scope and depth in the last few decades. Communication theory and research have moved far beyond focusing on the transmission and receipt of an idea between people in the same room. In little more than a decade, we moved from needing to mail information to a collaborator and wait for a period of several days for it to arrive to being able to have a document arrive in moments as an "e-mail attachment" and have live "online chats" with someone on the other side of the country or world. Communication has become a major challenge for organizations and is a central competency for the effective occupational therapy manager.

The range of communication theories that might be useful to the occupational therapy manager will be summarized in this chapter. Strategies for increasing the effectiveness of communication in person and in various written and electronic formats will be also presented.

A Short History of Communication Theory

Communication as a subject of inquiry is as old as civilization itself. We know that it was a major area of interest to the ancient Greeks and Romans. In the fifth century B.C., Plato and Aristotle developed the first recorded communications theories in the West. They were followed by others such as Cicero, Seneca, Quintilan, and Loinginus (Trenholm, 1991). The ancient Greeks focused their theories on persuasive argument and public communication.

Modern rhetoric is the body of communication study occurring roughly between 1600 and 1900 A.D. The primary work during this time reversed earlier "prescriptive" approaches to communication. Modern rhetoric raised questions about how humans come to know, be, believe, and act. In addition, it focused on aspects of delivery, including verbal and nonverbal behaviors that a speaker could use to embellish his or her presentation. Scholarship and study related to communication during this time was both theoretical and practical.

During the 19th century, the primary focus of investigation was on how speakers transmitted ideas to a listener. A major change during the 19th century was the application of the scientific method to investigation of communication theory, including the use of experimental studies focusing on finer aspects of communication and the manipulation of specific variables such as the context, timing, or aspects of delivery. This focus continued during the 20th century, including the application of behavioral methods to the study of communication. The goal of communication theory became specifying the invariant laws and describing the functional relationship between different variables that could affect the delivery or interpretation of communication. In addition, as technology has rapidly progressed over the last decade, the influence of modes of transmission has been introduced to the study of communication theory. Communication research has expanded to include investigation of a wide range of issues such as communications in politics and propaganda, commercial interests and advertising, and the impact of communication on childhood development (Littlejohn, 1999).

Theories of Communication

Communication as a field of study is well developed, and there are a large number of theories intended to explain various aspects of communication. The full range and scope of communication theories is far beyond what can be covered in this book. For example, Griffin (2000), in her introductory text *A First Look at Communication Theory*, introduced 32 separate communication theories! Theories have been developed related to interpersonal communication, communication to the public and groups, communication in the mass media, and intercultural communication. Grouping theories according to the area of communication that they seek to explain is one helpful way of organizing communication theories. Another method of classifying communication theories is according to seven traditions in the field of communication theory, as outlined in Box 12–1.

Within each of these traditions, numerous theories have been developed and, to add to the complexity of understanding communication theory,

Box 12–1: Seven Traditions in the Field of Communication Theory

1. The *sociopsychological tradition* uses the scientific method to discover communication "truths" and cause-and-effect relationships through careful systematic observation.
2. The *cybernetic tradition* views communication as information processing where communication is the link connecting the separate parts of any system, such as a computer system, a family system, an organizational system, or a media system.
3. The *rhetorical tradition*, grounded in Greco-Roman history, examines communication as an "artful address" and focuses on effective verbal communication of ideas.
4. The *semiotic tradition* views communication as the process of sharing meaning through signs (a sign is anything that can stand for something else).
5. The *sociocultural tradition* views communication as the creation and enactment of social reality based on the premise that, as people talk, they produce and reproduce culture.
6. The *critical tradition* views communication as a reflective challenge of unjust discourse arising from the Marxist tradition of critiquing society, including the use of communication to control power, the role of mass media in dulling sensitivity to repression, and blind reliance on the scientific method and uncritical acceptance of empirical findings.
7. The *phenomenological tradition* views communication as the experience of self and others through dialogue, or an analysis of everyday life from the standpoint of the person who is living it through the communication process.

some theories cross more than one tradition. In addition to the theories, multiple models of communication have been developed to explain the application of the theory in everyday communication. As explained in Chapter 9, a theory provides an explanation of how or why a particular phenomenon occurs and how that phenomenon might be influenced, and a model helps to generate theory and the methods that are used to apply that theory.

As noted, trying to address all theories of communication is simply beyond the scope of one chapter, and probably beyond the need of the typical occupational therapy manager. However, as is the case with all the topics in this book, the occupational therapy manager can benefit from exploring theories, models, and evidence to improve his or her effectiveness in communication. At this point, it would be useful to comment on the *context* of communication. As managers, we communicate in varied contexts ranging from a conversation with an individual staff member we supervise or with another manager or our boss, to communicating with large groups of people, such as when we run a staff meeting, present an in-service education program, or communicate with a continuous quality improvement team. Just as we may be able to choose more than one appropriate occupational therapy conceptual practice model to guide intervention, multiple communication theories can be applied to each of these contexts of communication. Recognizing the commonalities of these situations helps to make this process less confusing.

Trenholm (1991) identified five "problems" that all communicators face regardless of the context of communication. In other words, all communicators have these problems in common no matter what the situation and what form of communication they are using to convey their message. The five problems are

1. *Communicator acceptability*, or identifying the characteristics of the audience, how they might respond, and what the likely rewards or punishments for communication might be.
2. *Signification*, or choosing the appropriate verbal and nonverbal means to create meaningful messages, accurately interpreting the signs from the communication partner or audience, and making the greatest impact on the listener.

3. *Social coordination and relational definition*, or defining the rules to be followed throughout the interaction and coming to understand how you are expected to act within the context of a specific communication.
4. *Achieving communicative outcomes*, or discovering how you can construct a message in order to most effectively achieve the goal for your intended communication.
5. *Evolution and change*, or the fact that communication occurs over time and with the context, and, therefore, goals for communicating and the demands on the communicators can change within the context of a communication.

Much of daily communication happens quickly and naturally. We could not possibly stop and examine the context of *every* communication before it happens. However, just as we sometimes stop and use our clinical reasoning skills and processes to examine interventions that aren't going "just right," that are new to us, or that are complicated for some reason, we can also use communication theory to examine new, complex, or problematic communications to more effectively solve the five problems identified by Trenholm.

The next sections of this chapter will provide a brief overview of several of the communication theories most directly related to management. Theories that have been chosen for inclusion were chosen because of the particular contributions they can make to help the occupational therapy manager understand communication in the workplace. It may be notable that there is no theory presented specific to *mass communication*, or communication to the broad public, in this chapter. Although some have identified theories specific to mass communication, others have argued that organizing communication according to a "level" or context of communication reinforces the tendency to think of these communications as a type that are different from other "levels" of communication (Littlejohn, 1999). Because occupational therapy managers have relatively fewer needs to organize mass communication without the assistance of a public relations department, I have chosen to follow Littlejohn's suggestion that mass communication is simply a type of communication to which you can apply appropriate communication theories. Therefore, the theories chosen for review are

- *Cybernetics and information theory*, because of their relationship to the area of *health informatics*, including written communication in the form of e-mail or documentation
- *Dramatism and narrative*, because of their focus on the analysis of discourse through examination of metaphors and stories, and their applicability to understanding how clinical and interpersonal stories play out in the workplace
- *Proxemics and expectancy violation theory*, because of their contribution to aiding us in seeing how nonverbal communication, space, and distance impact relationships and understanding

Each of these theories will be briefly reviewed, and then the remainder of the chapter will focus on the pragmatic strategies for communicating more effectively in the workplace.

Cybernetics and Information Theory

Cybernetics is the study of regulation and control in systems (Handy & Kurtz, 1964). The term *cybernetics* is a translation of the Greek word for "steersman" or "governor," and describes the way feedback makes information processing possible in our heads and on our computers (Griffin, 2000). Cybernetics deals with the ways a system gauges its effect and makes the necessary adjustments to maintain effective functioning. Cybernetics recognizes that complex systems use both positive and negative feedback to adjust and adapt during action (whereas simple systems respond to feedback only after action is complete). Although the application of cybernetics to mathematical and engineering systems may seem evident, it has also been recognized to have valuable implications in the behavioral and social sciences. Cybernetics may be viewed as a way of thinking emphasizing circular reasoning and challenging the idea that one thing causes another in a linear fashion. It has been applied not only to engineering but also to states, armies, families, and individual human beings (Littlejohn, 1999).

One of the most common and relevant theories in the tradition of cybernetics is *information theory*, as developed by Shannon and Weaver. Upon review of a number of introductory textbooks on communication, a figure representing Shannon and Weaver's model of communication was found in

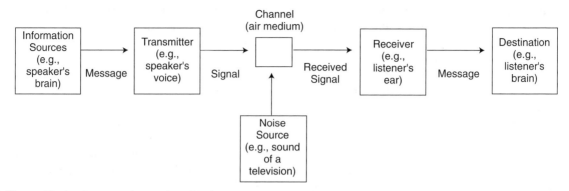

Figure 12-1   Shannon and Weaver's model of communication applied to a living room conversation. (Adapted from Griffin, E. [2000]. *A first look at communication theory* [4th ed.]. New York: McGraw-Hill.)

each to illustrate the basic process of communication as seen from a cybernetics perspective. Figure 12–1 shows Shannon and Weaver's model as applied to the conversation between two persons occurring in the living room of a home.

Shannon, a Bell Telephone Company research scientist, developed a mathematical theory of signal transmission seeking to improve the transmission of information over telephone lines with minimal distortion. His focus was on the technical aspects of communication, with little concern for the message. It might be difficult at first to see the relevance of such a "hands-off" approach for the occupational therapy manager; however, it becomes more apparent when you consider the move toward electronic documentation of intervention in settings where occupational therapists and occupational therapy assistants are employed, including hospitals, school systems, and even community-based settings. When moving from paper-based communication to electronic communication, we are certainly concerned with *what* is communicated; however, at first we must be concerned with *how* information is communicated. Shannon's theory views information as *reduction of uncertainty*. An example of this concept might be waking up in the morning to go to work in a New England town in January. When you first wake up, you are never completely sure of how your commute to work will be influenced by the weather; you are *uncertain*. However, by watching the weather report before you go to bed or upon getting up, you receive information through communication that reduces your uncertainty. You learn either that it is going to be a brisk but sunny day with an easy drive to work,

or that snow is on the way and you should plan plenty of extra time.

In interpersonal communication, the speaker's brain is the *information source*, the vocal system is the *transmitter*, and the air medium is the *channel*. The listener's ear is the *receiver*, and the listener's brain the *destination*. The final element in the model, *noise*, is any disturbance in the channel that distorts or otherwise interferes with the signal. Whether the message is coded in regular language, electronic signals, or some other code, the problem of transmission is the same: to reconstruct the message accurately at the destination (Littlejohn, 1999). Applied to our example of electronic documentation, the communication problem becomes building a system (of drop-down menus, checks, narrative text, etc.) that allows the therapist or assistant (the source) to transmit information to be accurately received by other staff (the destination).

Information theory has been influential in a number of ways, particularly in communication technology and engineering, which have become so much more relevant in health care in the last decade. Shannon and Weaver's model is commonly cited as a method of introducing the basic elements of communication. It has been criticized, however, for its simplicity and limited application to communication areas beyond electronic means. Littlejohn (1999) identified three common problems with information theory:

1. Information theory is designed as a measurement tool based on statistical procedures, and human messages are not easily broken down into observable and measurable signals.

2. Information theory plays down meaning, which is critical in the degree of shared understanding that is the goal of much communication.
3. Information theory does not account for the personal or contextual factors affecting the individual's capacity for learning (e.g., the capacity of the receiver).

Dramatism and Narrative

Dramatism and narrative are two closely associated theories that both deal with stories. Stories are one of the most important ways people use symbols to create meaning and to communicate that meaning to others.

Dramatism was developed by Kenneth Burke and focuses on the use of metaphor in communication. Burke believed that "Verbal symbols are meaningful acts from which motives can be derived" (Griffin, 2000). Further, Burke held the conviction that "Action requires symbolicity and that language use must be understood as a form of *symbolic action* in which both actor and object and events are defined, interpreted, and acquire meaning" (Meister & Japp, 1999). Burke saw the use of metaphor and persuasion as the communicator's attempt to get an audience to believe his or her view of reality to be true.

Key to persuasion in dramatism is the concept of *identification*, or the common ground that exists between a speaker and his or her audience. The more similarity in the physical characteristics, talents, occupation, background, personality, beliefs, and values between a speaker and an audience, the greater the identification. Of course, these characteristics may be weighted such that two persons who have similar physical characteristics and occupation but come from very different backgrounds, personalities, and beliefs may not identify with each other as much as two persons who look very different and have different occupations but share similar beliefs, values, and personality. An implication of identification for the communicator is that, to some extent, he or she can attempt to alter his or her presentation to increase identification by the audience and therefore increase his or her level of persuasion. For example, when presenting an in-service education program to a group of occupational therapy practitioners, a speaker can share personal and professional information that demonstrates to the listeners how the presenter is like the audience.

The most comprehensive *narrative* theory in the communication field is that of Walter Fisher. Fisher believed that human rationality in all its forms is based essentially on narrative, and, as such, communication in all its forms can be understood as narrative. Fisher defined narration as "symbolic actions—words and/or deeds—that have sequence and meaning for those who live, create, or interpret them" (Fisher, 1989). Griffin (2000) offered an expanded definition:

> *"Narration is communication rooted in time and space. It covers every aspect of our lives and the lives of others in regard to character, motive, and action. The term also refers to every verbal or nonverbal bid for a person to believe or act in a certain way. Even when a message seems abstract—is devoid of imagery—it is narration because it is embedded in the speaker's ongoing story that has a beginning, middle, and end, and it invites listeners to interpret its meaning and assess its value for their own life."*

Fisher saw narrative as a rational approach to communication. He summarized this view on the rationality of narrative to highlight his perspective that narrative can include a broad range of types of reasoning and rationality. He stated, "In narrative, no form of discourse is privileged over others because its form is predominantly argumentative. No matter how strictly a case is argued—scientifically, philosophically, or legally—it will always be a story, an interpretation of some aspect of the world that is historically and culturally grounded and shaped by human personality" (Fisher, 1987).

Fisher offered what he referred to as a *narrative paradigm* built on five assumptions. The narrative paradigm represents a shift from the more traditional *rational-world paradigm*, which purports that people are rational beings who make decisions on the basis of arguments and who see the world as a set of logical puzzles that we can solve through rational analysis. The five assumptions of the narrative paradigm are presented in Box 12–2.

Two key concepts related to Fisher's narrative paradigm are those of *coherence* and *fidelity*.

Box 12–2: **The Five Assumptions of Fisher's Narrative Paradigm**

1. People are essentially storytellers.
2. We make decisions on the basis of good reasons.
3. History, biography, culture, and character determine what we consider good reasons.
4. Narrative rationality is determined by the coherence and fidelity of our stories.
5. The world is a set of stories from which we choose, and thus constantly re-create our lives.

Adapted from Fisher, W. R. (1989). Clarifying the narrative paradigm. *Communication Monographs, 56*, 55–58.

Narrative coherence is how probable the story appears to the listener. Stories are more likely to be perceived as probable by a listener when the listener believes that he or she has been told all of the most important details of a story and that key information has not been omitted. Listeners must also believe that the story they are told is the most likely explanation and that an alternative story is not more plausible. Narrative fidelity is the extent to which a story "rings true" with a listener's experiences. Narratives have strong fidelity when they provide sound logic for our actions.

Concepts related to narrative have become increasingly visible in the social and health sciences, and particularly in the field of occupational therapy, over the last two decades (Braveman, Helfrich, Kielhofner, & Albrecht, 2003; Boydell, Goering, & Morrell-Bellai, 2000; Bury, 2001; Helfrich & Kielhofner, 1994; Helfrich, Kielhofner, & Mattingly, 1994; Lee, 2001; Lieblich, Tuval-Mashiach, & Zibler, 1998; Nochi, 2001; Robinson, 1990). The use of narrative interviews and narrative analysis of life stories or accounts of disability experiences has been validated as an approach to understanding the experiences both of individuals and of groups of individuals who share a common illness or disability (Fredriksson & Erikson, 2001; Helfrich & Kielhofner, 1994; Robinson, 1990). Recently, Kielhofner et al. (2004) documented that the

"slope" of a narrative (e.g., did things generally get better, worse, or stay about the same) might have value in predicting outcomes within a vocational rehabilitation program for people with acquired immunodeficiency syndrome.

Narratives are important because they describe what happened, define outcomes, or present the stages of a social process. The process of integrating past, present, and future selves involves the construction of personal narratives (Ingvar, Joakim, & Ingegerd, 2000; Kielhofner et al., 2002; Mattingly, 1998). Narrative thought stresses that humans create meaning about what they encounter in everyday life by plotting or framing experiences within narrative structures (Bruner, 1986; Gergen & Gergen, 1983; Jonsson, Josephsson, & Kielhofner, 2000; Polkinghorne, 1988). Narratives create a "symbolic bridge between a person's past, present and future; they can mediate multiple—apparently disparate—elements into a heterogeneous synthesis anchored in human experience" (Ricoeur, 1991).

It may be argued that individuals not only use narratives to understand their everyday lives but also use narratives as a guide to create a particular future (Jonnson et al., 2001; Kielhofner, Borell, Burke, Helfrich, & Nygård, 1995; Mattingly, 1998). Narratives are a way of creating meaning as life unfolds and as new circumstances present themselves. As noted by Kielhofner et al. (2002), "What we do continues our stories, sometimes by accepting what we perceive as inevitable, sometimes in response to a set of external events, and sometimes by aiming to create a particular outcome." Thus, narratives are created and refined in response to experiences, or as challenges are encountered as individuals seek to meet goals they set as a way of creating an outcome. Bury (2001) stated, "Not only do narratives help sustain and create the fabric of everyday life, they feature prominently in the repair and restoring of meaning when they are threatened."

It must be noted that, because a narrative is told or retold at a particular point in time, a narrative always reflects the temporal, physical, social, and emotional context of the narrator. The process of narrating experience is always set within a historical and temporal frame that the teller brings to the story (Sanchia & Street, 2001). Thus, narratives by their very nature are susceptible to change. As noted by Ricoeur (1984), "through the recreation of a narrative, new meaning can evolve in the creative imitation of the person's experienced world." This has led to some caution regarding the value and limitations of the use of narratives in the research process, because narratives are always told within a specific context and can change when told in a different context (Sanchia & Street, 2001), because it is questioned whether some information is stored by individuals within narratives or perhaps as problems without solutions (Kluwin, McAngus, & Feldman, 2001), and because narratives can be told as an effort to convince a listener who was not present that events occurred in a particular way (Riessman, 1990).

Proxemics and Expectancy Violations Theory

Proxemics is a term that was originally coined by Edward T. Hall, who was an anthropologist at the Illinois Institute of Technology, to refer to the study of people's use of space as an elaboration of culture (Hall, 1996). There are three fundamental areas related to proxemics: space, distance, and territory.

Three types of *space* have been identified by Hall: fixed-feature, semi-fixed feature, and informal space. *Fixed-feature* space is one of the ways in which people organize activities. Houses, buildings, cities, rooms, and the like are organized spatially. Objects and activities are related to these spatial arrangements, and if objects or activities are moved, people react. *Semifixed-feature* space is of primary importance in interpersonal communication, because it can be used in many different ways to convey meaning. Hall mentioned two types of semifixed-feature space: "socio-petal" spaces are those that bring people together and stimulate involvement, whereas "socio-fugal" spaces keep people apart and promote withdrawal. Socio-fugal space transmits connotative meanings such as "large," "cold," and "impersonal," whereas socio-petal arrangements usually connote the opposite. *Informal space* is significant because it includes the distances people unconsciously maintain when they interact. According to Hall, "informal spatial patterns have distinct bounds and such deep, if unvoiced, significance that they form an essential part of culture. To misunderstand this significance may invite disaster." The three types of space identified in proxemics are summarized in Box 12–3.

A classic description of the types of *distance*

> **Box 12–3: Proxemics: Three Types of Space**
>
> 1. *Fixed-feature space* is used to organize houses, cities, and spaces where people expect the organization to remain the same and will react if changes are made.
> 2. *Semifixed-feature space* includes sociopetal spaces that facilitate involvement and socio-fugal spaces that promote separation.
> 3. *Informal space* includes the distances people unconsciously maintain when they interact.

(commonly referred to generally as personal space) for various types of interpersonal communications was first presented by Hall in 1966 and continues to be used commonly today. The categories of distance identified by Hall—public, social, personal, and intimate space—and their definitions are presented in Box 12–4.

Personal comfort with distance during interpersonal communication varies from culture to cul-

---

> **Box 12–4: Proxemics: Four Categories of Distance**
>
> 1. *Public space* ranges from 12 to 25 feet and is the distance maintained between the audience and a speaker, such as a presenter at a conference.
> 2. *Social space* ranges from 4 to 10 feet and is used for communication among business associates, as well as to separate strangers using public areas, such as beaches and bus stops.
> 3. *Personal space* ranges from 2 to 4 feet and is used among friends and family members, and to separate people waiting in lines, such as at automated teller machines.
> 4. *Intimate space* ranges out to 1 foot and involves a high probability of touching. We reserve it for whispering and embracing.
>
> Adapted from Hall, E. T. (1996). *The hidden dimension.* New York: Anchor Books.

ture. When Americans interact with people from other cultures, they need to be aware of how the other parties view space. Low-contact cultures (North American, Northern European, Asian) favor the social distance for interaction and little, if any, physical contact. High-contact cultures (Mediterranean, Arab, Latin) prefer the intimate and personal distances and much contact between people. Misunderstandings can occur when these two groups interact and either invade or avoid space and contact. Violations can also occur between people of the same culture. Differences in personality can lead to different interpretations of personal space and touching. Remaining aware of cultural and personal preferences for distance and attending to others' styles and reactions can increase your effectiveness in communicating in the workplace.

Finally, the concept of *territory* has important implications for interpersonal communication. It refers to any area controlled and defended by an individual or group of individuals, with emphasis on possession of physical space. There are *public territories*, or places anybody can enter, such as a reception area; *home territories* into which entrance is restricted to members, such as an office for one or more managers or staff members; *interaction territories*, or areas where people meet informally, such as a cafeteria; and *body territories*, or the space we use ourselves. Understanding the "rules" about entering various territories can help prevent you from unintentionally violating another person's or group's assumption about the use of a territory. In addition, as a manager you'll want to consider the impact that the verbal and nonverbal signals you send about your office and accessibility as territory have on the culture of your department. Many managers claim to have an "open door" policy but give a clear nonverbal signal that interrupting their work without an appointment is not a welcome intrusion.

Expectancy violations theory (EVT) is a theory of *personal space and nonverbal communication* that falls within the sociopsychological tradition of communication theory and is closely aligned with proxemics. Judee Burgoon defined personal space as the "invisible, variable volume of space surrounding an individual that defines that individual's preferred distance from others" (Burgoon, 1978). EVT sees communication as the exchange of information that is high in relational content and

on occasion can be used to violate the expectations of another, which will be perceived either positively or negatively depending on the liking between the two people. Violation of our expectations produces arousal, which heightens the salience of cognitions about the communicator and his or her communication behavior. Arousal mediates the violation of the expectation and the subsequent communication behavior. When a violation has been perceived and arousal is triggered, the recipient evaluates the violation and the violator. Violations initiated by highly attractive sources may be evaluated positively, whereas those initiated by unattractive sources may be negatively evaluated.

The tenets of Burgoon's theory do contradict Hall's notion that people have expectations about how close others should come but offers the counterpoint that there are times when it is best to break the rules. Burgoon believed that at times violating social norms and personal expectations is a superior strategy to conformity. In addition to proximity, EVT applies the same theoretical propositions to facial expressions, eye contact, touch, and body lean. For example, although putting one's arm around the shoulders of a coworker might normally violate the expectations of employees in a particular setting, an employee who likes the "offender" might view the violation as positive if it is clear that it is meant to show appreciation for a special achievement. The propositions of EVT are summarized in Box 12–5 (Burgoon, Stern, & Dillman, 1995).

Pragmatic Strategies for Improving Communication

Communicating effectively to individuals and groups in either verbal or written format is an important skill for any manager. Understanding communication theory helps you design what will be said to most effectively transmit your message to the receiver or listener. Unfortunately, things that we do consciously and unconsciously during the process of communicating can make it less likely that our message is going to be heard and interpreted as intended. Some of the most common problems that can limit your effectiveness when communicating, as well as strategies for making your verbal and written communication more effective, are presented next.

Box 12–5: Propositions of Expectancy Violation Theory

1. As communicators, we develop expectations about the verbal and nonverbal communication of others.
2. Violations of communication expectations are arousing and cause a shift in our attention to the communicator, our relationship with the communicator, and the characteristics of the violation and meaning we attach to it.
3. Communicator reward valence (i.e., the strength of the reward), or the reactions we give or receive to violations, moderate the interpretation of ambiguous communicative behaviors.
4. Communicator reward valence moderates how we evaluate communicative behaviors.
5. Violation valences (i.e., the degree of the violation) are a function of

    a. The evaluation of the enacted behavior
    b. The direction of the discrepancy between the expected and enacted behavior toward a more favorable or unfavorably valued position
    c. The magnitude of the discrepancy

    Enacted behaviors that are more favorably evaluated than expected behaviors constitute positive violations; enacted behaviors that are less favorably evaluated than expected behaviors are negative violations.
6. Positive violations produce more favorable outcomes and negative violations produce more unfavorable outcomes relative to expectancy confirmation.

Adapted from Burgoon, J. K., Stern, L. A., & Dillman, L. (1995). *Interpersonal adaptation: Dyadic interaction patterns.* New York: Cambridge University Press.

Box 12–6: Six Strategies for Effective Conversations

1. *Ask open-ended questions* to elicit informative answers to learn new information and to avoid giving the impression that you have already made decisions.
2. *Ask focused questions* that aren't too broad to limit extraneous information and help guide listeners to the type of information that will help them best make their point or advocate for their position.
3. *Ask for additional details*, examples, and the speaker's thoughts and impressions to show genuine interest and to indicate that you are open to the speaker's message.
4. *Paraphrase*, or restate what you heard, remembering that the real purpose of paraphrasing is not to clarify what the other person actually meant, but to show what it meant to you.
5. *Check perceptions of your impressions of another person's feelings* by describing them, being careful to avoid any expression of approval or disapproval. Objectively state what you believe the other person seems to be feeling.
6. *Describe behavior without making accusations or generalizations* about motives, attitudes, or personality traits.

members of the public, including consumers of occupational therapy. Particularly when you are busy, it is important to focus on strategies that you can use to assure your listeners that you are interested in what they have to say, so they leave your conversation sensing that you feel they are important and that you heard what they needed to say. Six simple strategies to help you be more effective in conversations with others in the workplace are listed in Box 12–6.

Simple Suggestions for Effective Conversations

Some of the most important communications you will have on a daily basis are the one-to-one conversations you have with staff, other managers, or

Paralinguistics and Nonverbal Communication

You are most likely already familiar with the experience of receiving communication in which *what* is said does not have as much impact as *how* it is said. *How* communication is conveyed may include verbal aspects such as tone or volume (e.g., paralinguistics) and nonverbal aspects, including facial expressions and body movements. Ritts and Stein (2002) provided a helpful overview of paralinguistics and major areas of nonverbal behaviors that influence the effectiveness of our communication. Paralinguistics include the following facets of verbal communication:

- *Tone*, which generally indicates the overall quality of a person's voice. Tone is often referenced to give context to the manner in which voice contributes to communication, such as indicating that a person spoke in a "conversational" or a "nervous" tone of voice.

- *Pitch*, which refers technically to the frequency of the sound waves produced and heard by the ear of the listener but generally is referenced as higher or lower, and is typically thought to communicate the speaker's emotional state and level of excitement. Raising the pitch of your voice may communicate increased emotion.

- *Rhythm*, or the pattern of speech, indicated by the extent of variation in tone and volume. Varying the rhythm of your communication can help to hold the interest of your audience and, along with other aspects of vocal communication, can intentionally or unintentionally communicate level of arousal or the nature of your emotion.

- *Volume*, or the loudness or softness of voice, which not only can communicate emotion (by increasing voice volume) but also can increase interest on the part of the listener (by lowering voice volume to "pull" the listener into the message). Lowering your voice volume to a whisper during a presentation can sometimes be more effective than speaking more loudly in gaining attention.

- *Inflection*, which is sometimes also used to reference changes in pitch or tone. In linguistics, it specifically represents the change in the shape of a word, generally by adding an affix, such as a prefix or suffix, to the root word. By doing this, a change of meaning or relationship to some other word or group of words can be indicated. Inflectional operations ground the semantic content of a root word according to place, time, and participant reference, without substantially affecting the basic semantic content of the root. They often specify when an event or situation took place (e.g., pre- or post-), who or what were the participants (e.g., non-), and sometimes where, how, or whether an event or situation really took place (e.g., -like). By means of inflection, we can creatively communicate information by inferring meaning beyond the static meaning of our words, and thereby increase listener attention.

All of us develop styles of speaking over our lives, and we may or may not be aware of the impact of the various facets of our speech. In addition, the novice speaker may be more likely to be influenced by the context of communication such that the emotions of nervousness, anger, frustration, or a deep intellectual commitment may be evident in how he or she communicates via paralinguistics. Videotaping or audiotaping yourself during a presentation is a helpful way to become more familiar with your communication style so you can identify behaviors you wish to change, including those paralinguistic elements just described. Ultimately, becoming more confident in communicating with others in the work setting is achieved through practice and conscious focus on skill development. Practicing verbal communications, especially to a group, may be fostered by looking for opportunities to make presentations in low-risk situations, such as presenting part of a lunchtime in-service, co-presenting at small conferences, or even making very short presentations such as public toasts or an acknowledgment of thanks.

It is worth noting that paralinguistics are heavily influenced by culture, and, as the workplace continues to become more diverse, recognizing cultural variations in communication becomes more important. Stephan Dahl (2001) pointed out that differences in the volume, speed, and other aspects of paralinguistics are interpreted differently in different cultures. He noted, for example, "The notion that Americans are talking too loud is often interpreted in Europe as aggressive behavior or can be seen as a sign of uncultivated behavior. Likewise, the British manner of speaking quietly might be understood as secretive by Americans." Similarly, the speed of talking is different in various cultural settings. For example, Finnish is spoken relatively slowly in comparison to other European languages. This slowness of speaking has often resulted in the Finnish being regarded as somewhat "slow" and lax. Further importance is given to the amount of silence that is perceived as appropriate during a conversation. A Japanese proverb says, "Those who know do not speak—those who speak do not know." This purposeful use of silence by individuals from Oriental cultures must come as a slap in the face to Americans, for whom even a short silence is seen as embarrassing, and hence is filled up with often random speech, something often perceived as hypermanic by persons from other cultures. Similarly, there is an avoidance of silence in Arabic countries, where word games are played and thoughts repeated to avoid silence (Dahl, 2001).

Some major areas of nonverbal communication to consider are discussed in the following sections.

EYE CONTACT

Maintaining eye contact helps to regulate the flow of communication by signaling interest in others and can increase a speaker's credibility. When you speak, your eyes involve your listeners in your presentation, and the easiest way to break a communication bond between you and the listeners is failing to look at them. By looking at your listeners, you communicate that you are sincere and are interested in them, and that you care that they hear what you have to say. Eye contact can also help you to overcome nervousness by making a connection with listeners who do care about your message.

Laskowski (2002) presented a series of tips on using your eyes effectively during presentations and communications with others:

- Know your material well so that you don't have to devote your mental energy to the task of remembering the sequence of ideas and words.
- Establish a personal bond with listeners by selecting one person and talking to him or her personally. Maintain eye contact with that person long enough to establish a visual bond (about 5 to 10 seconds). This is usually the equivalent of a sentence or a thought. Then shift your gaze to another person.
- Monitor visual feedback. While you are talking, your listeners are responding with their own nonverbal messages. Use your eyes to actively seek out this valuable feedback.

FACIAL EXPRESSIONS

Expressions are a key part of effective communication. Facial expressions such as smiling can be powerful cues that transmit friendliness and openness to communication, but might also communicate impatience, frustration, disagreement, or disappointment. It is important to be aware of your facial expressions and use them consciously so that your expressions match the context and tone of your intended communication. Nervous speakers may make unconscious expressions such as frowning. Frowning may occur when a speaker attempts to deliver a memorized speech or when the speaker is feeling frustrated because listeners do not understand what he or she is attempting to communicate. There are no rules governing the use of specific expressions. As Laskowski (2002) suggested, "If you relax your inhibitions and allow yourself to respond naturally to your thoughts, attitudes and emotions, your facial expressions will be appropriate and will project sincerity, conviction, and credibility."

GESTURES

Gestures, including head nods or arm movements, can animate a presentation and capture the attention of listeners, make the material more interesting, and facilitate learning. Like unconscious facial expressions, however, unintended gestures can be distracting and make it harder for the listener to receive your message. When you make a verbal mistake (either saying the wrong thing or using inappropriate tone or volume), it is easier to correct it because you may hear it yourself. It may be harder to discontinue distracting gestures of which you are not aware. If you are going to be giving public presentations frequently, or if giving a presentation is a particularly nerve-wracking experience for you, you might consider the previously suggested strategy for improvement of videotaping yourself giving a presentation. At first you may be very aware of the camera, but after a while you are likely to drift into your normal style of presentation, and on playback of the tape you will be able to see both effective and ineffective strategies and behaviors that you commonly use.

Some of the most common behaviors of inexperienced or nervous speakers include:

- Gripping or leaning on the lectern or podium
- Finger tapping
- Lip biting or licking
- Playing with coins in your pocket or with jewelry, such as a necklace or a watch

- Frowning when nervous or frustrated that listeners don't seem to understand
- Adjusting hair or clothing
- Head wagging or nodding and beginning to react to a question or comment from a listener before he or she is finished speaking

POSTURE AND BODY ORIENTATION

Posture and body orientation communicate numerous messages by the way you walk, talk, stand, and sit. Standing erect, but not rigid, and leaning slightly forward communicates to listeners that you are approachable, receptive, and friendly. If you are involved in a one-to-one conversation, maintaining an "open" posture with both feet on the floor, arms resting comfortably in your lap or on the arms of the chair (not crossed on your chest) with no objects between you and the person with whom you are speaking, such as a desk, can indicate your attention to the conversation. Often conversations begin without the speakers realizing the importance of the discussion, and your posture and body orientation can inadvertently communicate that you are not invested in the conversation. For example, if you continue to face a computer workstation and keep your fingers on the keyboard when someone enters your office to ask a question, you may communicate that you do not wish to take the time to fully attend to the conversation. By consciously using posture and body orientation, such as by turning to face the person to whom you are speaking and leaning forward, or standing up and coming out from behind a desk, you can indicate that you are truly invested in the discussion.

During presentations, varying your body orientation can help maintain the attention of an audience as long as it is used judiciously. Moving away from a podium or lectern and walking toward the audience can effectively communicate interest and increase the sense of the audience's participation in the presentation. Naturally, moving too much or pacing nervously can detract attention from your message. During formal presentations, you may also be limited by factors beyond your control, such as the size of the room, the placement of audiovisual controls or screens, or limited ability to move around the room because of acoustics or the need to use a microphone.

Effective Presentations

Public speaking can be intimidating for many people, but being able to give an effective presentation is a critical management skill. Speaking confidently to a group can gain you instant authority and credibility. Like many skills in life, learning to give effective presentations is simply a matter of knowledge, planning, and practice. A wide variety of available resources are easily accessible on the Internet and at your local bookstore to help guide the development and preparation of a presentation. Some basic strategies for giving an effective presentation are summarized next.

When planning a presentation, it is helpful to think about the *purpose* of your communication. Most presentations fall into one of three purposes: efforts to inform, explain, or persuade. These three types of presentations are briefly summarized in Box 12–7. Simple strategies for more successful development of content for presentations are provided in Box 12–8. The strategies in Box 12–8 apply regardless of the purpose of your presentation, although thinking about these types of presentations separately when planning your content helps you to

---

Box 12–7: Three Common Purposes for Presentations

1. Presentations to *inform* provide your audience with information. Your goal is that the audience leaves with information they did not have when they arrived.
2. Presentations to *explain* help your audience become more familiar with new information they have received. Your goal is that the audience better understands the process or procedure that is your topic.
3. Presentations to *persuade* are designed to convince your audience to think differently about an issue. Your goal for this type of presentation is to change the audience's beliefs and sometimes to get them to take action.

Box 12–8: Strategies for Developing Successful Presentation Content

- **Decide on a central message.** Write in one sentence the focus of your presentation and use this simple idea to organize the rest of your presentation.
- **Brainstorm, then focus.** Balance creativity with focusing on your topic. Begin by writing quickly the things that come to mind about your topic in any order, but stop when you need to pause for more than a moment and organize your list. Then focus on what may be missing and where it belongs in your outline.
- **Develop a strong and convincing introduction and conclusion.** Catch the attention of your audience right from the beginning. Writing your conclusion first will actually help you stay focused on where you are going and what you need to say to get you there.
- **Highlight 3 to 5 key points.** A mistake that is common and easy to make is to try to plan too much for one presentation, especially when you care very much about what you have to say. Deciding on 3 to 5 key points will help you distinguish between what *could* be said and what *must* be said. Develop supporting evidence or information for each key point, writing first in bulleted points to help you keep your message *simple*

and focused. Include statistics, facts, or stories where appropriate.
- **Write and rewrite:** Write a section of your remarks and then come back to them later. Often presenters speak from notes or in an unscripted fashion using a slide show as their notes. This can make presentations seem more conversational and less formal, but the speaker must be comfortable and familiar with the topic and the slides. Other times, even for an expert speaker, a completely scripted presentation may be more appropriate. Still, a scripted presentation does not have to boring or even sound like it is being read. If you put your presentation on paper or on note cards, be sure to number them so that, if you drop them or get lost while presenting, you can easily find your place.
- **Practice, Practice, Practice:** You've heard the adage "Practice makes perfect." Perfection may be a lot to hope for, but practice certainly can improve the quality of a presentation. Read your presentation or review your notes frequently. For formal presentations that must fit a time frame closely, be sure to read your remarks out loud. You may find that, when speaking aloud, your pace slows or quickens.

Adapted from Iowa State University. (2003). Iowa State University College of Agriculture Communications Service Web site. Available at *http://www.ag.iastate.edu/aginfo/speech.html*

---

be more on target with the goal of your communication. Table 12–1 also provides strategies for success in the three types of presentations.

A good place to start when you are planning an important presentation is by thinking about your audience. Conducting an *audience analysis* is simply a process of doing the best you can to get to know your audience so that you can tailor your presentation to the occasion. A common mistake is to try to use a "one size fits all" approach and use the same presentation materials, style, and format for very different groups and situations. I recently gave a presentation to a group of occupational therapists and occupational therapy assistants to intro-

duce them to evidence-based practice. Prior to the presentation, a colleague shared a PowerPoint presentation that she had previously prepared. Happy to save time, I removed the slides that did not apply to my presentation and printed the handouts for use with my talk. As I moved through the presentation, however, I became aware of more and more instances in which the language on the slides was not a perfect fit for that day's audience. I kept having to refer to bulleted points by saying, "That should say... ." The impact was not only that the presentation was more confusing for the audience, but it also lessened my credibility with the group. With just a little more work, I could have cus-

Table 12-1	Strategies for Successful Presentations	
Type of Presentations	**Success Strategies**

• Presentations to inform
• Presentations to explain
	• Tell them what you will tell them, tell them what you want them to know, then tell them what you told them.
	  • *"Today I'm going to introduce you to four key principles of Continuous Quality Improvement"*
	  • *"The first key principle of CQI is..."*
	  • *"To summarize, today you were introduced to the four key principles of CQI, which were..."*
	• Relate new information to something they already know.
	  • *"You are already familiar with..."*
	• Begin with simple concepts and move to complex concepts.
	  • *"The most basic CQI principle is customer service; later we'll talk briefly about more complicated strategies for meeting customer needs."*

Presentations to persuade	• Start by establishing agreement with something you have to say, or establishing a common view with which there can be no dispute.
	  • *"Can we all agree that we want to be effective as occupational therapists?"*
	• Get them in a "yes" mode (ask several questions in a row related to your point of view to which the audience will respond "Yes!")
	  • *"Do you want to improve your services?"*
	  • *"Do you care about your clients?"*
	  • *"Do you want to be more effective in meeting client needs?"*
	• Number your reasons for your point of view.
	  • *"There are four reasons you should attend the Continuous Quality Improvement Leadership Course. The first is..."*
	• Close the deal by asking for agreement.
	  • *"So, can I plan on each of you attending the CQI Leadership Course?"*
	• What will it take to convince them? Ask for a firm commitment before they leave the presentation.
	  • *"How do I convince you to sign-up for the CQI Leadership Course today?"*

tomized the presentation, given full credit to my colleague, and been more effective in meeting the needs of my audience. Some simple questions to ask yourself to *analyze* your audience are listed in Box 12–9.

Effective Written Communication

In addition to communicating verbally, managers often use various modes of written communication, including memos, business letters, e-mail, business plans, and grant proposals. Confidence in business writing, as in verbal communications, comes with practice, but can be greatly improved by conscious attention to practicing and learning specific skills. Writing effectively in the workplace can be very different than other sorts of writing because communicating ideas objectively and succinctly is highly valued. Well-written documents clarify issues, guide coworkers' thinking, and help to build agreement on courses of action.

The foundation of effective business writing is clear thinking. Grammar and style matter, but critical thinking is even more important (Alpha Books, 2002). Critical thinking starts by carefully thinking through what *could* be communicated and what

---

Box 12–9: Analyzing Your Audience

- How many people will be in the audience, and how does this affect your plan for use of audiovisual equipment, handouts, or discussion questions and exercises?
- What are the background, gender, age, careers, and interests of the audience members? Can you include references in your presentation to each major demographic group to customize your presentation?
- What do you think the audience already knows about your topic? How can you make ties to what is already familiar to them as a way of introducing new topics?
- How much more will they want to know? Are you able to tell them everything they need to know in one presentation, or do you need to plan for "unfinished business"?
- Why are the members of the audience attending? Are they there voluntarily or because their boss told them to attend?
- Will there be other speakers? If so, can you coordinate your presentations ahead of time to minimize duplication and reinforce key issues?
- How much time have you been given for your presentation, including questions and answers? Can you meet the audience's expectations in the time you have been allotted, or do you need to start by reframing their expectations?

Box 12–10: The Eight Cs of Business Writing

1. *Consideration:* focus on "you" (the reader) instead of "I" or "we" (the writer).
2. *Conciseness:* omit unnecessary words and expressions.
3. *Correctness:* give accurate facts and figures.
4. *Courtesy:* be sincerely tactful, thoughtful, and appreciative.
5. *Clarity:* be clear by using short, conversational language.
6. *Completeness:* answer all questions asked so that you accomplish your goal in one memo without needing follow-up memos.
7. *Concreteness:* use specific facts and figures so that your meaning is clear.
8. *Candidness:* being honest in all your business writings.

Adapted from Hurley, P. (2003). The 8 C's of business writing. University of Hawaii Web site. Available at *http://emedia.leeward.hawaii.edu/hurley/eng209w/ principles/intro/8cs.pdf*

---

should be communicated to help achieve your objective. Much like with a verbal presentation, identifying the purpose of written communication (e.g., to inform, to explain, or to persuade) is a good first step that will guide your decision making about what to put in and what to leave out of any document. Regardless of the form of writing, you should be able to clearly state the purpose of your writing in a single sentence before you begin. Box 12–10 includes eight factors to consider

when writing for business; these factors are sometimes referred to as the "Eight Cs of Business Writing."

Resources for specific forms of writing (e.g., memos, letters, e-mails, business plans, and grant proposals) abound and can easily be located at your local bookstore or on the Internet. The following sections briefly overview key strategies for increasing effectiveness in each form of writing. You are encouraged to find and use some of the many resources specific to the format of writing you are using.

The Business Memo

Memos are appropriately used for communication internal to your organization. They typically confirm conversations, request actions, inform others of problems, or update others on events or progress. Memos are not appropriate for communicating to outside parties and have limited use in establishing policy. They should not be used as a substitute for initial conversations or for dealing with issues that can be settled with a short telephone conversation, especially if the situation evokes strong emotions. You should never write a memo in anger; it is better to wait until the next day, when you can decide whether the communication is necessary and if a memo is the most appropriate form of communication, and you can compose the memo in a calm manner. Some additional tips for writing memos are included in Box 12–11.

Business Letters

As opposed to memos, which are written to an audience internal to your organization, a business letter is written to communicate to an outside audience. Business letters must be taken very seriously because you will most likely be considered a representative of your organization. Many of the strategies for writing an effective memo also apply to writing an effective business letter (e.g., the Eight Cs of Business Writing). As with a memo, you should be able to answer these few questions clearly before you begin to write:

- Why are you writing?
- Whom are you writing to?
- What information do you want to convey, or what do you want to ask them to do?
- Why should they care or agree?

Business letters typically include three major sections: the opening, the body, and the closing. The opening paragraph should introduce the reason you are writing to your reader, stated in clear, concise, and candid language. The reader should easily be able to understand why you are writing and what you are going to ask or convey by the time he or she has finished reading your opening. Your opening will make an impression on your reader that will set the context as he or she reads the remainder of your communication. You may ask yourself, "What do I want the reader to be feeling or thinking when he or she finishes reading this first paragraph?" and then examine your opening to see if it is likely to have the desired impact on your reader.

Box 12–11: Tips for Writing Effective Memos

- Keep paragraphs short and to the point. Be concise, yet try to be complete.
- Paragraphs should be in block form with no indentation and may be organized according the following framework:
  - Introduction: a few sentences that state the reason for the communication
  - Background: one or two paragraphs describing the context for the request or recommendation included in the memo
  - Recommendation/Request: a concise statement of what you desire to have happen
  - Rationale: two to three paragraphs proving the reasoning for your recommendation
  - Conclusion: a brief statement restating your position
- Accent or highlight major points by using underlining, bullets, or bold type, but use these approaches sparingly.
- Use short headings to separate major topics in your memo to keep things organized, provide structure, and make for smooth reading.
- The title (RE: ....) to your memo should reflect its contents and should be no more than a few words long.
- Make sure your distribution list is relevant. Send your memo or e-mail only to those who are directly concerned with the issues contained or raised in your message.
- Be considerate of the recipients' time and don't use memos or e-mails as a way to reinforce or defend your position, or to indirectly put down other people in your firm.
- Proofread carefully for errors before distributing.

In the body of your letter, you will concisely state and explain what you want or what information you are writing to share. It is important to have reasonable expectations for a business letter. If you expect that your reader will need much additional information or the opportunity for a face-to-face meeting to discuss your topic or ask questions, then the body of your letter should set the stage for the next step in the process. For example, consider a fieldwork coordinator at a university who wishes to establish a relationship with a new practice setting in order to place fieldwork students there. The ultimate goal is to get the manager of the setting to agree to take several students each year. Including all the information that might be necessary to convince the manager to make an affirmative decision in a single letter would not be an effective strategy. A face-to-face meeting is a more effective strategy, and thus the goal of the business letter would more appropriately be to ask the manager to agree to a meeting to discuss taking fieldwork students.

It is critically important that you pay close attention to the tone of your letter and that you neither write in a style that is overly "familiar" if you do not have an established relationship with the reader, or in a style that is aggressive or demanding. If you are uncertain about how a letter might be received, asking a colleague to read the letter for you and respond to the tone of the letter is always a good idea. In addition, business letters should seldom exceed one to three pages. If necessary, additional documents can be included with the business letter that provide supporting documentation or reference material. These documents can be cited in the body of your business letter or listed at the end of your letter as appendices or enclosures.

The closing or final paragraph of your letter needs to accomplish two goals. The first of these goals is to provide a concise summary of the purpose of your letter in no more than a sentence or two. This may seem like a daunting task, especially if the subject matter of your letter is of considerable importance. The most common mistake, however, is trying to "overshoot" or accomplish too much in one letter. The second goal of the closing is to request a specific action and suggest a time frame for action if appropriate. This action might be to adopt a point of view based on information provided in the letter, or it might be a task that you want the reader to agree to complete. If asking for a task to be completed, it is important to also include a time frame in which you would like the reader to act.

E-Mail

The use of e-mail has virtually exploded over the last decade. There is no doubt that it has become an extraordinary convenience that has impacted the business environment in many positive ways and has fostered communication, especially in terms of speed and ease. However, there are dangers inherent in this form of communication both in terms of what is communicated inadvertently and in terms of some negative impacts of e-mail on work productivity. E-mail is simply a communication tool that must be used wisely to remain an advantage rather than a disadvantage.

Electronic communication is different from traditional written communication in a number of fundamental ways. E-mail tends to be more conversational because messages can be exchanged very quickly. In other forms of written communication, such as the memo or business letter, you must make everything clear because your reader may not have a chance to ask clarifying questions. With e-mail, the reader can ask questions immediately, and this tends to make e-mail seem more as if you are having a conversation. Therefore, it is easy to forget key differences between a face-to-face conversation and e-mail. In e-mail, your reader won't have access to the nonverbal and paralinguistic cues described earlier that communicate emotion and help the receiver of communication interpret meaning. Therefore, meaning can easily be misconstrued. For example, efforts to be humorous that might be effective if the reader could see you smiling or hear you chuckling as you write the message might be perceived as sarcastic or rude.

Some aspects of paralinguistics can be incorporated into e-mail messages, but again can sometimes indicate unintended meaning. For example, TYPING IN ALL CAPITAL LETTERS may be understood as the e-mail equivalent of increasing the volume of your voice; this may effectively indicate a word you wish to stress but can also be interpreted as shouting. The term *emoticons* has developed to indicate the use of symbols or punctuation to indicate emotion. For example, one particular combination of symbols—written as "<G>"—may be used to indicate that you are "grinning" or saying something in jest. The word *netiquette* has been coined to describe rules of e-mail behavior that have found common acceptance. You should keep in mind that the content of messages can be guided by the same rules for effective written communication as other forms (again, the Eight Cs of Business Writing) but that strategies for adding context or emotional cues need to be considered separately. There are many easily accessible guides to netiquette and strategies for communicating emotion or other aspects of vocal speech, such as a *pause equivalent*, that can be found by conducting a simple Internet search or in books on business writing found in your local bookstore. Box 12–12 includes a short list of how to avoid the most common mistakes in the use of e-mail. Remember, once you hit the Send button, you lose complete control over where your message goes and who will see what you write.

Business Plans and Program Proposals

Writing a business plan or a proposal for a new program is an example of a specific and complex writing task faced by some occupational therapy managers. A business plan is a detailed document that describes the need and the costs and benefits of a new program or service. The written document itself actually summarizes a complicated process of collecting and analyzing a range of data, and this process may occur over many months. Full-scale business plans for the initiation of a new business enterprise may be many pages in length, whereas shorter program proposals are sometimes requested by administrators to justify the need for more discrete services, such as expanding services to an existing population. Such shorter proposals still may be difficult to write, especially if you are not provided with a lot of guidance as to how the proposal should be structured and what should be included.

Writing a business plan for the first time is not a venture that should be undertaken without preparation and assistance. The development of effective business plans requires both skilled business writing and strong organizational, financial, and data-analysis skills. Outlines for business proposals can commonly be found through organizations such as the Small Business Administration (*http://www. sba.gov/*), and these outlines can also be used to help you organize shorter program proposals. A sample outline showing the common elements of a business plan is included in Box 12–13 to highlight the complexity of what is typically included in such a plan (Baron, 1998; Small Business Administration, 2003).

Grants

Another form of business writing in which the occupational therapy manager might participate is grant writing. Although grants as a form of funding may most often be associated with research, some grants support the development and implementation of new programs. Such grants may pay for the development or evaluation of model programs, to prove the effectiveness of an intervention, to assist with capacity building of an organization to provide a service, or to cover start-up costs of new programming, including equipment and sometimes staff for a limited period of time. These types of grants are often sought by community-based organizations. Grants may be available through city, state, or federal government sources or through a wide range of nonprofit foundations. A short,

---

Box 12–12: Ways to Avoid Common Mistakes in E-Mail Use

- Never write and send e-mail when you are angry.
- Do not attach unnecessary files.
- Do not overuse the High Priority option.
- Don't reference earlier messages without including part of the "message thread."
- Read the e-mail before you send it.
- Do not overuse Reply to All.
- Be careful with abbreviations and emoticons.
- Do not copy a message or attachment without permission.
- Do not use e-mail to discuss confidential information.
- Don't send or forward e-mails containing libelous, defamatory, offensive, racist, or obscene remarks.
- Use the c: field (copying others on an e-mail) sparingly

Box 12–13: Sample Elements of a Business Plan

Executive Summary

- Short (2- to 3-page) summary of what will be presented
- Sets the context for the program you are trying to "sell"
- Appears first in the document but must be written after all other sections of the document are prepared

Market Analysis

- Describes your target market, including
  - Demographics of consumers
  - Characteristics of payers and the payer mix
  - Your market niche

Demographic Analysis

- Age, gender, nationality, educational level, etc. of consumers
- Diagnostic criteria or statistics representing challenges to activity and participation

Competitive Analysis

- Do you have competitors?
- What are their relative strengths and weaknesses?

- How do consumers view your competition?

Referral Analysis

- Do you have established referral mechanisms?
- Are there potential referral sources not yet tapped?

Financial Plan

- Projections for 3 to 5 years (often called a Pro Forma)
- Analysis of revenue, expenses, and discounts/bad debt

Marketing Plan

- Needs assessment summary
- Consumers and payers to be targeted
- Strategies for promotion
- Year-by-year plan to support growth

Operational Plan

- Organizational chart
- Description of key personnel
- Description of fit of systems such as billing and documentation with existing organizational systems

---

nonexhaustive list of various types of grants that are available is provided in Box 12–14.

Like business plans, grant writing should not be entered into without some preparation, and this will increase the likelihood of your success. The response to a *request for proposals* (RFP) issued by a

Box 12–14: Common Types of Grants

- Research (including investigator awards)
- Program or demonstration
- Training (including postdoctoral awards)
- Operating
- Technical assistance
- Publication
- Infrastructure
- Technology development

funding source can sometimes be very competitive. Often you may initially have to submit a letter of intent in which you are asked to summarize your request for funds, including the need for the program, the intervention, a brief description of how the funds will be used, and anticipated outcomes, in as little as two to four pages. Once again, using a guide such as the Eight *C*s of Business Writing to review your work can be helpful.

IDENTIFYING FUNDING SOURCES

Finding the right match for a funding source is an important first step in grant writing. Writing grants can be extraordinarily time consuming, and you do not want to invest days or weeks of work to write a strong proposal only to hear from the funding source that it does not match their priorities. Key to finding the right match is having a clear understanding of your interests and what you want to accomplish. Completing the first steps of program development and marketing, including a demographic and market analysis, will provide you with some of the information you will likely need to include in your proposal (see Chapters 9 and 13).

A helpful strategy for finding potential funding sources is to develop a network of others who are interested in the same types of programming. Although sometimes they may be your competitors in submitting a response to an RFP and might not be willing to share much information about strategy, you will be surprised how often your peers in occupational therapy and other professions will be willing to direct you to opportunities. One of the best ways to promote such behavior is by doing that yourself. As you develop a network, watch for those occasions when you find an RFP that does not exactly fit your needs or for which the timing may be wrong for you but that might be a match for someone in your network, and forward the information to him or her. Soon you will likely notice that others are doing the same for you.

Other key strategies include conducting an Internet search for foundations that relate to your interests and putting yourself on lists to receive e-mail notifications of RFPs. A number of Web sites include search engines that list funding sources. Web sites useful for searching for federal grants (e.g., *http://www.grants.gov/*) include links to allow you to receive e-mail notifications of new grant opportunities as they are announced. Another important source of grant announcements for government grants is the *Federal Register*. All federal announcements of grants are published in the *Federal Register*, and a search engine for announcements can be found on the Federal Grant Opportunities Web site (*www.fedgrants.gov/*). An excellent resource for finding opportunities with private foundations is The Foundation Center (*http://fdncenter.org/*).

Once you find opportunities for funding, you need to determine which ones are good matches. A helpful tool is to create and use a "matching worksheet" to evaluate the fit between what you want to do and what the funding source is willing to pay for. A sample matching worksheet is included in Table 12–2 for a program for children from birth to 5 years of age with a physical disability to expose them to play and social interests, for which you desire funding for equipment. Although not a perfect match on all criteria (listed along the left side of the table), funding source 1 is a better match than the other funding sources even though none of the funding sources is a strong match related to leisure or funding of equipment.

In the matching process, you need to consider the following factors:

- Do you match the eligibility criteria as stated by the funding source?
- Are there types of expenses listed as funding exclusions (e.g., indirect costs, food, etc.)?
- Can you meet the deadline for responding to the RFP?
- How quickly will reviews be conducted and a funding decision made?

Table 12-2	Sample Funding Matching* Worksheet for a Program to Introduce Children from Birth to 5 to Play and Social Options		
	Funding Source 1	Funding Source 2	Funding Source 3
Develop a direct service program	5	5	3
For children birth to 5	5	5	5
Who have a physical disability	5	3	3
To expose them to play and social options	3	3	3
Need funding for equipment	3	3	3
*1 = weak match; 5 = strong match.			

- What are the typical funding amounts and is the potential payoff worth your investment of time in writing the proposal?
- What percentage of proposals is commonly funded?

WRITING THE GRANT PROPOSAL

When preparing your submission, you must be sure to read the rules carefully and highlight the key points. It is important to pay special attention to rules about the allowable number of pages, type size, margins, and any defined sections or budget exclusions. Funding sources typically take these rules very seriously and will often not even review a proposal that does not fit the criteria. You can imagine that it would be very demoralizing to spend days, weeks, or even months writing a proposal only to have it rejected because your narrative was a half-page too long or you use too small a type size!

You need to plan your writing strategy—develop a timeline, obtain necessary support, divide the labor, and pull in experts (e.g., evaluators, statisticians). You should consider if writing alone is a wise strategy for you. Sometimes grant proposals are strengthened greatly by including other organizations as collaborators. Even though the grant dollars may have to be split between organizations, your proposal may be perceived as having a greater impact if funded. A local university is the best place to start to obtain help with complicated proposals. There you can find mentors and critics who can help along the way by reviewing your work and giving you suggestions to strengthen your proposal, but you should be sure to ask for their assistance with plenty of notice.

When writing, it is helpful to use the headings of your proposal sections to format your work and to keep track of requirements and rules for formatting your submission. Formatting your proposal in the order of any criteria provided by the funding source used to evaluate submissions is a great way to keep your writing organized and clear. You must do your research and make sure you "know your stuff." It is not uncommon for your first submission to be rejected, but often you are invited to submit your proposal again after incorporating reviewer feedback. It is important to remember that experts in your area of interest are often serving as reviewers, and you do not want to damage your credibil-

ity in the future by making factual mistakes or assertions that are poorly supported because you have not adequately prepared yourself to write a sophisticated proposal.

Your statements of purpose and outcomes should be clear, and your argument should be logical and well supported by current and appropriate references. The proposal is your "sales pitch" to a funding source, and you want them to buy your argument. In addition to describing the purpose and outcomes, there are other common components of grant proposals. These components are listed in Box 12–15.

Some errors commonly made in writing grant proposals that you will want to avoid include

- Lack of definitions for key concepts or terms that may be unfamiliar to the reviewers
- Too much jargon (words or abbreviations familiar to those in your setting but not to others)
- Inconsistencies in language across proposal (this can commonly happen if you have multiple people working on a proposal)
- Logic leaps that assume that the reviewers are familiar with your topic
- Errors in spelling and grammar
- Failing to address all points in the RFP
- Lack of current and comprehensive references
- Promising more than is possible in the time frame you have to implement your proposal or for the funds you are requesting
- Underbudgeting or overbudgeting

Other mistakes are commonly made in the process of submitting proposals to funding sources that can result in proposals being rejected. For example, you need to know who in your organization has to sign the proposal. If there is any research element to the proposal, or if you will be collecting protected health information as defined by the Health Information Portability and Accountability Act of 1996 (HIPAA), you must meet all of the requirements listed for involving an Investigational Review Board or managing the protected health information (U.S. Department of Health and Human Services, 2003). You must be very careful to note and understand correctly the due date for the proposal. Some due dates reference the "received by" date, meaning your proposal must be received by the funding source by that date, and others reference the "postmarked by" date, meaning that your

---

Box 12-15: **Common Components of Grant Proposals**

- **Statement of Need:** Why is your proposal important?
- **Objectives:** What will you accomplish if funded?
- **Literature Review:** What prior work has been done in this area, including research or other program implementations, to support the need for you to carry out your proposed work?
- **Proposal Narrative:** The portion of the proposal that includes procedures, expected outcomes, and how you will measure outcomes. This is the main body of your proposal that ties together the other pieces.
- **Management Plan:** A listing of project goals and objectives, including time frames and accountability for major project tasks.
- **Evaluation:** How will you know that your project is being implemented as planned (formative evaluation), and how will you measure its outcomes and success (summative evaluation)?
- **Budget:** A year-by-year breakdown of expenses, often presented in table format, in-cluding personnel, overhead (indirect cost recover, or ICR), and supplies and equipment.
- **Budget Narrative:** A 1- to 3-page written explanation justifying your budget proposal.
- **Institutional Resources:** Will your organization match funds and donate time or supplies, and does it have adequate space to allow you to achieve your objectives?
- **Team Qualifications:** Do you have personnel, including a project director (principal investigator), who have the skills and experience to warrant the amount of funds you are requesting?
- **Dissemination Plan:** Will you share what you learn or the outcomes of your program with others, and, if so, how will you do that?
- **Appendices:** Any documents referenced in your narrative, including letters of support from collaborators. (Sometimes you can shorten your narrative to the required length by putting some items in an appendix.)

---

proposal must be postmarked by the due date. If possible, you should plan to submit your proposal a few days early so that, if you hit an unexpected roadblock, you will have a few days to recover and still meet your deadline. Rushing at the last minute is often why writers make some of the common errors described previously.

You must be careful to submit the correct number of copies of the proposal; often the RFP states that an original (with all original signatures) and a specified number of copies must be submitted. A cover letter citing what is included with your submission is recommended, and you should check your submission against the cover letter and the original RFP criteria as you are preparing to mail or ship it. In addition, you should follow directions as to how to present your proposal (e.g., some RFPs state specifically *not* to use binders and to only use clips).

Grant proposals are typically reviewed by a panel of experts, or by a *peer review panel* in the case of many federal RFPs. As noted earlier, many first submissions are not funded, but you should not be overly discouraged if this happens to you. Many funding sources have funding rates of less than 10% of the submitted proposals. If your proposal is rejected, it may be possible to resubmit it at another time. Some funding sources only accept proposals in response to published RFPs, but others have open calls for proposals at designated times of the year. When resubmitting your proposal, you should review your feedback carefully and make revisions to address the comments. A detailed explanation of how you addressed the reviewer comments can be included in your cover letter to the agency or explained within the proposal.

Writing a successfully funded grant proposal is a very rewarding experience and can even be fun. You should approach the process as a contest and continually strategize about what you can do to make your submission stronger. Once you are funded, you are responsible to deliver the product as proposed—you have essentially established a contract with the funding source. Included in that contract is the fact that you may be committing yourself to employment at a site for a specified period of time. Many grants cannot be "ported," or moved to another organization even in the same community, and some funding sources may stop funding if key personnel cited in the proposal leave the organization and there is doubt whether those remaining are qualified or able to finish the project. Also a part of the understood contract is that you are typically not free to significantly alter your program (objectives, procedures, budget) without permission from the funding source. Additional resources for helping you with the process of finding funding sources and preparing effective grant proposals are included at the end of the chapter.

Chapter Summary

This chapter introduced you to the wide range of theories that have been developed to explain communication, including theories of interpersonal communication, communication to the public and groups, communication through mass media, and intercultural communication. You learned that the many theories of communication are sometimes organized according to seven "traditions" of communication research, and you were provided with an introduction to a number of theories that are useful for the occupational therapy manager, including cybernetics and information theory, dramatism and narrative, and proxemics and expectancy violation theory.

Real-Life Solutions

Charlotte began to prepare for her in-service for the unit staff by visiting the local university library. She was pleased to find that there was a large selection of books on communication that addressed both communication theory and "hands-on" strategies for improving various types of communication. She had difficulty understanding how some of the theories might be helpful at first, but found a number of introductory communication textbooks that organized theories using a variety of frameworks. By investigating these frameworks, she began to see that some communication theories were more easily applied to communication in the work environment than others, and that, just like occupational therapy theory, no single theory seemed to provide everything she would need for every type of communication or context.

As Charlotte read about some of the theories, she could easily see how they might be utilized to guide her communication. She was surprised to find narrative theory as a theory of communication because she had read a number of research studies in occupational therapy that used narrative approaches to explore interactions with clients. She also found that she and some of the unit staff members discussed issues related to proxemics and violation expectancy theory without realizing there was a theory that addressed issues of personal space.

In addition to including an overview of several of the most relevant theories of communication, Charlotte decided to provide staff with some handouts that listed specific strategies for improving communication during conversations, in presentations, and in written communication. She found strategies and information on paralinguistics and nonverbal communication especially helpful because much of the feedback she had received about her own style involved mismatches between the content of her communication and how it was conveyed. She chose to include resources from university communication department Web sites, from commercial Web sites, and from government Web sites (she also included information on evaluating Web sites!).

Finally, Charlotte was proud to be able to pass valuable information on business writing and grant writing on to her supervisor, who had recently suggested at a staff meeting that the occupational therapy staff should investigate possible alternative sources of funding to expand elements of their programming for the most at-risk populations.

In addition, this chapter provided you with a basic introduction to common problems in verbal and written communication and to some strategies for improving the effectiveness of your communication during conversations, in presentations, and in various forms of business writing. Although there are strategies specific to each form of communication, paying close attention to what is said or written (content), how it is said or written (delivery), and the context of the communication can help you prepare so that there is a greater likelihood that your listener or audience receives the same message that you intend to send.

Occupational therapy managers spend much of their time involved in interpersonal communication, and developing skills through conscious effort and practice is a valuable investment of time. Luckily, many resources are available to guide you in your practice. Some of those resources are listed at the end of this chapter, but many more can be found by conducting an Internet search or visiting your local library or bookstore.

At the beginning of the chapter, you were introduced to Charlotte, a fieldwork student who had received some feedback indicating that she needed to improve her communication skills. Charlotte agreed to prepare an in-service education program for the staff members of the unit to which she was assigned on strategies for effective interpersonal communication.

Resources for Learning More About Communication

Journals Related to Communication

COMMUNICATION THEORY

Communication Theory publishes original quantitative and qualitative research related to the theoretical development of communication from varied disciplines, such as communication studies, sociology, psychology, political science, cultural and gender studies, philosophy, linguistics, and literature.

WRITER'S DIGEST

Writer's Digest is a popular magazine for writers. The magazine provides a wide range of informational, instructional, and inspirational offerings for writers. Examples of such offerings include a variety of books, magazines, special interest publications, educational courses, conferences, Web sites, and more.

Associations Concerned with Communication

THE AMERICAN COMMUNICATION ASSOCIATION

http://www.americancomm.org/

The American Communication Association (ACA) is a not-for-profit organization, a virtual professional association with actual presence in the world of scholars and practitioners alike. The ACA was created to promote academic and professional research, criticism, teaching, practical use, and exchange of principles and theories of human communication. The ACA embraces researchers, teachers, businesspersons, and specialists located in North, Central, and South America and in the Caribbean.

Resources for Learning More About Writing Grant Proposals

THE FOUNDATION CENTER

http://www.fdncenter.org/

The Foundation Center's mission is to support and improve philanthropy by promoting public understanding of the field and helping grant seekers succeed. The center collects, organizes, and communicates information on U.S. philanthropy, conducts and facilitates research on trends in the field, provides education and training on the grant-seeking process, and ensures public access to information and services through its Web site, print and electronic publications, five library/learning centers, and a national network of Cooperating Collections.

THE CATALOGUE OF FEDERAL DOMESTIC ASSISTANCE

http://www.cfda.gov/public/cat-writing.htm

The online Catalog of Federal Domestic Assistance gives you access to a database of all federal programs available to state and local governments (including the District of Columbia); federally recognized Indian tribal governments; territories (and possessions) of the United States; domestic public, quasi-public, and private profit and nonprofit organizations and institutions; specialized groups; and individuals. After you find the program you want, contact the office that administers the program and find out how to apply.

THE GRANTSMANSHIP CENTER

http://www.tgci.com

The Grantsmanship Center (TGCI) was founded in 1972 to offer training and low-cost publications and other resources to nonprofit organizations and government agencies. The TGCI conducts annual workshops in grantsmanship and proposal writing. The *Grantsmanship Center Magazine*, published by the TGCI, is mailed to the staff of 200,000 nonprofit and government agencies in the United States and 58 other countries. TGCI's *Winning Grant Proposals Online* collects the best of funded federal grant proposals annually and makes them available on CD-ROM. The TCGI proposal-writing guide, *Program Planning and Proposal Writing* (PP&PW) is a widely read resource for both new and experienced grant seekers.

Reference List

Alpha Books. (2002). Business writing. In J. Chisolm (Ed.), *Every manager's desk reference* (pp. 826–920). Indianapolis, IN: Pearson Education.

Baron, K. B. (1998). The business plan: A tool for program development. *Administrative and Management Special Interest Section Quarterly, 14*, 3–4.

Boydell, K. M., Goering, P., & Morrell-Bellai, T. L. (2000). Narratives of identity: Re-presentation of self in people who are homeless. *Qualitative Health Research, 10*(1), 26–38.

Braveman, B., Helfrich, C., Kielhofner, G., & Albrecht, G. (2003). The narratives of 12 men living with AIDS. *Journal of Occupational Rehabilitation, 13*, 143–147.

Brunner, J. (1986). *Actual minds, possible words.* Cambridge, MA: Harvard University Press.

Burgoon, J. K. (1978). A communication model of personal space violations: Explication and initial test. *Human Communication Research, 4*, 130–146.

Burgoon, J. K., Stern, L. A., & Dillman, L. (1995). *Interpersonal adaptation: Dyadic interaction patterns.* New York: Cambridge University Press.

Bury, M. (2001). Illness narratives: Fact or fiction? *Social Health and Illness, 23*, 263–285.

Dahl, S. (2001). Communications and Culture Transformation. Stephweb.com Web site. Available at *http://www.stephweb.com/capstone/*

Fisher, W. R. (1987). *Human communication as narration: Toward a philosophy of reason, value, and action.* Columbia: University of South Carolina Press.

Fisher, W. R. (1989). Clarifying the narrative paradigm. *Communication Monographs, 56*, 55–58.

Fredriksson, L., & Erikson, K. (2001). The hidden disability dilemma for the preservation of self. *Journal of Occupational Science, 2*(1), 13–21.

Gergen, M. M., & Gergen, K. J. (1983). Narrative of the self. In T. R. Sarbin & K. E. Scheibe (Eds.), *Studies in social identity* (pp. 254–272). New York: Prager.

Griffin, E. (2000). *A first look at communication theory* (4th ed.). New York: McGraw-Hill.

Hall, E. T. (1996). *The hidden dimension.* New York: Anchor Books.

Handy, R., & Kurtz, P. (1964). A current appraisal of the behavioral sciences: Communication theory. *American Behavioral Scientist, 7*, 99–104.

Helfrich, C., & Kielhofner, G. (1994). Volitional narratives and the meaning of therapy. *American Journal of Occupational Therapy, 48*, 318–326.

Helfrich, C., Kielhofner, G., & Mattingly, C. (1994). Volition as narrative: An understanding of motivation in chronic illness. *American Journal of Occupational Therapy, 42*, 311–317.

Hurley, P. (2003). The 8 C's of business writing. University of Hawaii Web site. Available at *http://emedia.leeward.hawaii.edu/hurley/eng209w/principles/intro/8cs.pdf*

Ingvar, F., Joakim, O., & Ingegerd, B. (2000). On the use of narratives in nursing research. *Journal of Advanced Nursing, 32*, 695–703.

Iowa State University. (2003). Steps to giving an effective speech. Iowa State University College of Agriculture Communications Service Web site. Available at *http://www.ag.iastate.edu/aginfo/speech.html*

Jonsson, H., Josephsson, S., Kielhofner, G. (2000). Evolving narratives in the course of retirement: A longitudinal study. *American Journal of Occupational Therapy, 54*, 463–470.

Kielhofner, G., Borell, L., Burke, J., Helfrich, C., & Nygård, L. (1995). Volition subsystem. In G. Kielhofner (Ed.), *A Model of Human Occupation: Theory and application* (2nd ed., pp. 39–62). Baltimore: Williams & Wilkins.

Kielhofner, G., Borell, L. Freidheim, L., Goldstein, K., Helfrich, C., Jonsson, H., et al. (2002). Crafting occupational life. In G. Kielhofner (Ed.), *Model of Human Occupation: Theory and application* (3rd ed., pp. 124–144). Baltimore: Williams & Wilkins.

Kielhofner, G., Braveman, B., Finlayson, M., Paul-Ward, A., Goldbaum, L., & Goldstein, K. (2004). Outcomes of a vocational program for people with AIDS. *American Journal of Occupational Therapy, 51*, 64–72.

Kluwin, T. N., McAngus, A., & Feldman, D. M. (2001). The limits of narratives in understanding teacher thinking. *American Annals of Deafness, 146*, 420–428.

Laskowski, L. (2002). Five effective ways to make your body speak. www.hodu.com Web site. Available at *http://hodu.com/speaking-skills.shtml*

Lee, C. S. (2001). The use of narrative in understanding how cancer affects development: The stories of one cancer survivor. *Journal of Health Psychology, 6*, 283–293.

Lieblich, A., Tuval-Mashiach, R., & Zibler, T. (1998). *Narrative research.* Thousand Oaks, CA: Sage.

Littlejohn, S. (1999). *Theories of human communication.* Belmont, CA: Wadsworth.

Mattingly, C. (1998). *Healing dramas and clinical plots: The narrative structure of experience.* Cambridge, UK: Cambridge University Press.

Meister, M., & Japp, P. M. (1999). Analyzing narratives of expertise: Toward the development of a burkeian pentadic scheme. *Sociology Quarterly, 40,* 587–613.

Nochi, M. (2001). Reconstructing self-narratives in coping with traumatic brain injury. *Social Science and Medicine, 51,* 1795–1804.

Polkinghorne, D. E. (1988). *Narrative knowing and the human sciences.* Albany, NY: State University of New York Press.

Ricoeur, P. (1984). *Time and narrative.* Chicago: The University of Chicago Press.

Ricoeur, P. (1991). *From text to action: Essays in hermeneutics, II.* Evanston, IL: Northwestern University Press.

Riessman, C. K. (1990). Strategic uses of narrative in the presentation of self and illness: A research note. *Social Science and Medicine, 30,* 1195–1200.

Ritts, V., & Stein, J. R. (2002). Six ways to improve your nonverbal communications. Honolulu Community College

Web site. Available at *http://www.hcc.hawaii.edu/intranet/committees/FacDevCom/guidebk/teachtip/commun-1.htm*

Robinson, I. (1990). Personal narratives, social careers, and medical courses: Analysing life trajectories in autobiographies of people with multiple sclerosis. *Social Science and Medicine, 30,* 173–186.

Sanchia, A., & Street, A. (2001). From individual to group: Use of narratives in a participatory research process. *Journal of Advanced Nursing, 33,* 791–797.

Small Business Administration. (2003). Business plan basics. Small Business Administration Web site. Available at *http://www.sba.gov/starting_business/planning/basic.html*

Trenholm, S. (1991). *Human communication theory* (2nd ed.). Englewood Cliffs, NJ: Prentice Hall.

U.S. Department of Health and Human Services. (2003). Medical privacy-national standards to protect the privacy of personal health information. U.S. Department of Health and Human Services Office for Civil Rights Web site. Available at *http://www.os.dhhs.gov/ocr/hipaa/*

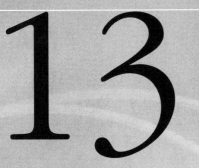

CHAPTER

13

Brent Braveman, Ph.D., OTR/L, FAOTA

Marketing Occupational Therapy Services

Real-Life Management

Patrick is the new Director of Occupational Therapy in a community hospital. The occupational therapy department provides a range of services, including services to the acute medical and psychiatric units and outpatient services for adults and children. Patrick's supervisor, Keesha, who is the Administrative Director of Rehabilitation Services, has encouraged him to begin to explore additional services that could be developed to bring in new streams of revenue. She has stressed that any new products or services that are added cannot be focused on simply providing more service to existing populations because most of those patients are insured under some form of capitated reimbursement, such as a Medicare Diagnosis-Related Group or negotiated discounts. However, Keesha is also concerned that the needs of occupational therapy's customers, such as nurses and physicians, are not being met and has requested that Patrick investigate whether existing services are adequate to meet the needs of these various customers.

Patrick was introduced to the marketing process in the management course that he took as part of his entry-level occupational therapy education. As such, he is aware that marketing is a process of assessing the needs, resources, and limitations of both an organization and the target populations served by the organization. He remembers that it was stressed that the marketing process can be very complicated but can also be applied in simpler ways and used by occupational therapy managers for the development and promotion of occupational therapy services. Patrick also remembers that making connections with others in the organization who are concerned with aspects of marketing or with meeting the needs of the same target populations is an important first step. To get the ball rolling, Patrick sets up appointments with the director of physical therapy, and with an associate in the publications and promotions department who he knows is involved in the organization's strategic planning activities.

Key Issues

- Marketing is more than just advertising a product or service; the marketing process includes assessment of the needs, resources, and limitations of your organization and its target populations.
- The complexity of the market-

ing process should not be underestimated; however, the process can be applied and adapted for use by all levels of managers within an organization.
- Much of the data, information, and other forms of evidence

used in the marketing process may be readily available from primary and secondary data sources already identified by your organization and may be used in other key management functions, such as planning.

333

Over the last few decades, our dualistic health care system has become increasingly complex. As a result, the profession of occupational therapy has been faced with both challenges and new opportunities. Among other challenges, we have faced the continued need to explain who we are and what we do while competing with others for limited resources and reimbursement. Consumers have become more sophisticated in their understanding of health services and have increased expectations of health care providers. Both traditional health care organizations and organizations in emerging practice settings have faced difficult economic times. Many organizations have flattened their administrative structures, often decreasing resources devoted to staff functions such as planning and marketing. The remaining resources are typically focused on an organization's major revenue-producing products and service lines. Although occupational therapy services are often part of these service lines, it may be difficult to garner resources specifically for the development and promotion of a new occupational therapy product or service.

At the same time that the occupational therapy profession has been challenged, there have been opportunities to expand into new areas of practice. We have seen a return of many occupational therapists and occupational therapy assistants to community-based practice, and practice has expanded in areas such as work rehabilitation and school-based practice. Moreover, an increasing number of occupational therapy practitioners have become successful entrepreneurs and business owners. As noted by Jacobs (1999), the tendency for the novice occupational therapy manager might be to respond to emerging opportunities by designing a program and then looking for customers. However, principles of effective marketing dictate that this process be reversed and that you closely examine target populations and design programs to match the needs, resources, and limitations of potential customers.

Although traditional occupational therapy entry-level curricula have focused on preparing graduates to provide holistic, occupation-based intervention, they have understandably fallen short of preparing practitioners in managerial skills beyond the basics. The marketing process can be extraordinarily complex. Occupational therapy managers and business owners who want or need to assess the needs of the target populations they serve and to

design, develop, and promote new products and services to meet those needs will likely need some education or training beyond their entry-level education. Luckily, in many larger organizations there are professionals who have made marketing products and services their career and can guide you in the process.

The complexity of the marketing process should not deter you from thinking that you can learn the necessary skills to effectively develop and promote occupational therapy services. The marketing process can be simplified, adapted, and applied in a basic manner to even existing and traditional services such as obtaining referrals for basic activities of daily living. This chapter will provide an introduction to the full marketing process and describe the synergistic relationship between marketing activities and other managerial functions described in other chapters, such as program development (see Chapter 9). The use of data, information, and other forms of evidence in the marketing process will also be discussed.

Target Populations

You may notice in this book, and in other books and resources on management, that various terms are used to refer to those who benefit from occupational therapy services as well as those who pay for services. In Chapter 11, you were introduced to the concept that it is common among persons concerned with continuous quality improvement efforts to identify both internal and external *customers*. Some customers are also the direct beneficiaries of occupational therapy services and are often referred to as *patients* or *clients*. Although these individuals often are responsible for full or partial payment for services, you are likely already familiar with the term *third-party payer*. Further, the term *consumer* is sometimes used to refer to those who buy products and services (Richmond, 2003).

There is no doubt that the many terms used to describe those who receive and those who pay for occupational therapy services are potentially confusing. This is especially true as occupational therapy practitioners move into new areas of practice that are supported by new sources of revenue and payers. As noted by Richmond (2003), buyers of oc-

cupational therapy products or services have become more diverse and today include private and
public businesses, nonprofit organizations and
charities, and managed care providers as well as
physicians, insurance companies, and our patients
and clients. Terminology is important, and it is important to distinguish between the various types of
persons who receive or pay for your services in
order to effectively implement the marketing
process. Doing so will aid you in designing specific
methods to collect data, information, and other
forms of evidence on the needs, resources, and limitations of those who are the intended targets of
your occupational therapy product or service without wasting valuable effort. Throughout this chapter, the term *target population(s)* will be used to
refer to any group of persons who receive, benefit
from, or pay for an occupational therapy product
or service.

Components of the Marketing Process

A simple way to think about the marketing process
is to view it as comprising four major components
or steps. It is easier to understand the activities and
purposes of these components if they are described
separately. However, it is important to recognize
that in reality the components are often completed
simultaneously rather than one after the other, and
that activities from one component inform and aid
with completion of other components. Also, managers use much of the data, information, and other
forms of evidence obtained in the marketing process
in other managerial functions, such as planning or
program development and evaluation activities.

Each of the four components of the marketing
process is briefly described in Box 13–1 and is outlined in the following sections of this chapter. As
you read about each component, you should recognize that in some situations, such as in the case of a
small business owner or entrepreneur, an occupational therapist or occupational therapy assistant
might be responsible for all steps of the process or
might consider hiring a marketing professional to
complete parts of the process for him or her. In
other situations, such as the case of a director of occupational therapy for a department in a large integrated health care system, an occupational therapy

> ### Box 13–1: Components of the Marketing Process
>
> - **Organizational Assessment:**
>   Examination of the factors within an or-
>   ganization that will influence the devel-
>   opment and promotion of a new product
>   or service.
> - **Environmental Assessment:**
>   Examination of the data, information,
>   and other forms of evidence, including
>   the needs of target populations, that will
>   guide the development and promotion of
>   a new product or service.
> - **Market Analysis:** Use of the information
>   gained during organizational and envi-
>   ronmental assessments to validate per-
>   ceptions of the wants and needs of the
>   target populations that will receive a new
>   product or service.
> - **Marketing Communications:** Packaging
>   and promoting a product so the target
>   populations and other key stakeholders in
>   a new product or service have a clear
>   understanding of what the product or
>   service is and how it may be accessed.

manager may collaborate with or rely on professionals in other departments such as marketing,
publications, or development to complete some of
the marketing components.

Organizational Assessment

Organizational assessment is the process of collecting data, information, and other forms of evidence
to examine the internal factors and influences that
will impact the future development of your product or service. Organizational assessments examine
factors such as your organization's reputation in
the community, the staff's qualifications, type and
quality of equipment, available space, geographic
location of your organization, and the level of administrative support for new programs (Jacobs,
1999). The desired result of this assessment will be
to have a comprehensive understanding of the resources available to aid you with development and
promotion of your product as well as the challenges
and constraints that you will face. You will also seek

to gain an understanding of the perspectives of the key stakeholders within your organization, such as other department directors or those responsible for the financial health of your organization.

The best place to start an organizational assessment is with a review of the organization's mission statement and the mission statement of your department. This review establishes the context for evaluating the extent to which your planned product or service matches the objectives of your organization. There is not always a perfect match between each and every product offered by organizations and their missions, but starting with a mission review will give you some indication of how a new product or service proposal might be received. If the relationship between your proposal and your organization's mission is not clearly evident, you should be prepared to provide an explanation of why valuable time and resources should be used to carry out your proposal. Similarly, as an occupational therapy manager, you may find yourself in the position of being asked to develop services for members of target populations that are not a good match for your department. In this case, a mission review will aid in preparing a sound rationale for why you should not respond positively to such a request.

Organizations sometimes end up involved in delivery of products or services that are not a good match with their mission for a number of reasons. At times, influential members of an organization can be successful in moving forward agendas or projects that are not good matches for the mission. At other times, an organization may knowingly take on projects that are not reflective of its mission because of perceived advantages to the organization, such as a new source of revenue. However, although such products and services may bring benefits to the organization, they may also pull valuable and needed resources from other products, services, or activities that are more closely aligned with the needs of those that the organization serves. It is important to recognize the *opportunity costs* involved in such ventures. You learned in Chapter 5 that opportunity costs are those things you cannot accomplish secondary to lack of resources because you are investing your time and other resources in another effort. All decisions to develop a new product or service have opportunity costs associated with them. Most successful organizations develop new products and services in a planned and thoughtful manner. This means that we must be prepared to accept that a new product or service idea that we value highly may not be enough of a priority for others to devote the necessary resources to move forward on its development.

It is beneficial and important to coordinate organizational assessment activities with others in the organization who may be able to assist you and who will also benefit from information that you may learn. In addition to marketing or development departments, those involved in strategic planning in any way, such as other department directors, may be important allies in the marketing process. Other department managers may already have or might benefit from the information that you will need to assess your organization's needs, resources, and limitations.

One common marketing activity that assists with both the organizational assessment and the assessment of the environment is what is referred to as a *SWOT analysis*. This acronym stands for *strengths, weaknesses, opportunities, and threats*. A SWOT analysis was previously described in Chapter 5 as part of organizational and environmental assessments in the planning process. It was suggested that often SWOT analyses can be conducted by combining a review of key documents or reports (financial reports, outcome statistics, program evaluation, or accreditation reports) with staff interviews, discussions, or structured brainstorming exercises. SWOT analyses may also be completed with a focus toward development of a particular product or service.

Large organizations routinely collect various forms of data, information, and other evidence that are used in planning and marketing activities. Information on referral rates, payer mix, geographic location of target populations, space utilization, and staff turnover are just some examples of such information. Occupational therapy managers may find this readily available information helpful in planning new products and services as well as to aid with the evaluation of existing products. Sometimes, however, the information that you need may not be available, especially if you are seeking information related to a specific occupational therapy product or service that might not catch the attention of those concerned with larger organizational

Box 13–2: Simple Strategies for Organizational Assessment

- Conduct informational interviews with other department directors over coffee or a meal to learn more about the skills, resources, and needs of other disciplines.
- Obtain your boss's permission to make an announcement about a potential product or service that you are considering in a directors' meeting, in a newsletter, or on a Listserv and ask for input or concerns from your peers.
- Ask your boss and representatives from departments such as planning, marketing, publications, or business affairs if routine reports are produced that might be helpful to you that you are not currently receiving.
- To obtain information from physicians, nurses, or other internal customers, conduct a short survey of needs, resources, or limitations by visiting other departments' staff meetings.
- Complete a SWOT analysis with your department; enlist other department directors to do the same and share the results.
- Spend some time reviewing your own organization's Web page and make a note of relevant services offered by other departments that might have some synergy with one of your existing or future products or services.

needs. A sample list of simple strategies for organizational assessment is presented in Box 13–2.

Environmental Assessment

An environmental assessment focuses on examination of external data, information, and other forms of evidence, such as demographic characteristics, cultural trends, health care utilization patterns, political and regulatory issues, new technologies, or socioeconomic status of the target populations served by your organization, to help determine their needs and resources. Identification of existing products and services offered by your competitors and their strengths and weaknesses is also completed as part of the environmental assessment.

One way to think about the types of data, information and other forms of evidence that you will collect is that market research data can be divided into two categories. These two categories are referred to as *primary data sources* and *secondary data sources* (Doman, Dennison, & Doman, 2002). Primary data sources are those that generate data that are specific to your product or service. Such data sources can include existing customers or potential customers from your target markets, referral sources, payers, employees, suppliers, consultants, or other sources involved in your product or service. Primary data usually cost some money to generate, ranging from a few dollars for a simple in-house survey to tens of thousands of dollars for a sophisticated survey of the needs of a large target population. Secondary data sources are those that already exist and may provide data, information, or other forms of evidence for free or may charge for use of the data. Such data sources might include government census reports, economic statistics about a potential target population in a specific geographic area, information from news sources, or surveys conducted by trade associations. Your organization may already purchase or use data from some of these secondary sources.

It is interesting to note that, unfortunately, requests for some of the types of information, data, or other forms of evidence that you may wish to obtain from others in your organization, such as demographics, reimbursement patterns, and information on discounts to payers, may sometimes be met with a less than enthusiastic response. This type of response may result from concerns that you might be communicating inaccurate information about the organization to outsiders or that you might be duplicating the efforts of others, or may occur because others feel that their level of control or power in the organization is threatened. It may be unusual in some organizations for directors of smaller departments to initiate development of new products, programs, or services. By identifying early the others who have vested interests in marketing activities and who might also benefit from your success in the development of a new product or service and keeping them informed, you may be more likely to gain their true support.

Once you have identified others who play a role in assessing how your organization interacts with the community and your organization's or department's target populations, you can search the information available to learn more about their needs, resources, and limitations. Examples of the sorts of data, information, and other forms of evidence you might use in evaluating the needs and resources of your target populations include

- Population demographics (age, marital status, socioeconomic data, insurance status, etc.)
- Payer mix for particular catchment areas
- Targeted areas for expansion for your organization
- Organizational plans for future space and resource allocation

As discussed in Chapter 2, some types of secondary data, information, and other forms of evidence that you might use to describe your target populations and their needs are available from sources such as federal, state, and local agencies or from nonprofit organizations. Sources such as the U.S. Census Bureau (*http://www.census.gov*) or the Centers for Disease Control and Prevention's National Center for Health Statistics (*http://www. cdc.gov/nchs*) may provide you with information such as demographics or incidence rates of a particular disease or condition within a geographic area. Organizations such as the National Multiple Sclerosis Society (*http://www.nmss.org/*) may have state or local chapters that not only can provide you with demographic data on a target population but may have also conducted needs assessments or other surveys that describe existing services and information on their use and effectiveness. Combining evidence from several sources may be necessary to piece together a complete picture of your target population.

Conducting large-scale needs assessments of communities or target populations not already served by your organization is a major effort, and describing this process in depth is well beyond the scope of this chapter. Community needs assessments can require extensive time and resources. However, there are some efforts than can be undertaken by occupational therapy managers to collect some information about target populations that may be combined with other sources of data, information, and other forms of evidence as part of an

---

Box 13–3: Simple Strategies for Environmental Assessment

- Use the Internet, phonebook, and professional association directories to identify competitors in the area who are already serving your target population and review their Web sites and brochures to learn about their products and services.
- Conduct information interviews with leaders of community-based organizations or public health officials concerned with the health and wellness of your target population.
- Conduct informal or formal focus groups* with members of your target population.
- Have a booth or a table at a health fair, community festival, or street fair or collaborate with others in your organization to offer free screenings where you can also collect information on your target population.
- Identify the physicians providing services to your target population and collect information by making appointments to visit their office, conducting a mail or telephone survey, or offering a continuing education event or meeting where you might be able to collect information on their perceptions of your target populations needs, resources, and limitations.

*Focus groups are a type of formal data collection and research strategy. Marketing professionals often use focus groups to collect information about a target population's needs or reaction to a product or service, and formal use of focus groups is a sophisticated process. To learn more about focus groups, see the list of references provided at the end of the chapter.

---

assessment of the environment. A sample list of simple strategies for environmental assessment is presented in Box 13–3.

Market Analysis

The purpose of the market analysis component of the marketing process is to use the data, information, and other forms of evidence identified during your assessment of your organization and the environment to validate your perceptions of the wants and needs of the target populations with which you interact. The desired outcome of your market analysis is a *marketing plan* that coordinates and uses information about your organization, its products and services, and its objectives and strategies to guide your activities to communicate with your target populations about your occupational therapy products and services (Richmond, 2003).

Marketing firms routinely conduct sophisticated forms of market analysis. A trial marketing of a product in target communities is one example of market analysis strategy. Few occupational therapy departments have the resources available to conduct such types of market analyses. However, lack of financial and human resources should not deter you from completing this vital stage of the marketing process or from relying on a little creativity. Some of the same strategies that can be used to collect primary data, information, and other forms of evidence from your target populations as part of your environmental analysis can be used in the market analysis to validate your perceptions of the needs, resources, and limitations of the same target populations.

As the director of an occupational therapy department in a small acute care hospital with few financial resources and little spare time, I worked with my staff to identify several inexpensive and creative ways of conducting a market analysis to compare our perceptions of the needs and resources of our various customers, including physicians, nurses, and patients. In one example, we were beginning to develop a hand rehabilitation program and had collected primary data from the sources obvious to us, such as the plastic surgeons who we knew treated patients with hand injuries. We suspected that other physicians might also see patients that they would refer to us if they understood the range of services that we could offer. To validate those perceptions, we designed a one-page needs assessment that listed common diagnoses such as arthritis and repetitive motion injuries along with the services that an occupational therapy practitioner specializing in hand rehabilitation could offer. Space was provided for the physicians to note how often their patients would benefit from the services described. On several mornings over the course of 2 weeks, we offered coffee and dough-

nuts in the physician's lounge, although, in order to get a doughnut, the physician had to complete our assessment first. Through this process, we not only validated the perceptions that we had formed during our organizational and environmental assessments but also began establishing a new relationship with potential referral sources for our hand rehabilitation program.

Marketing Communications

Marketing communications is the marketing component with which you are likely most familiar. Marketing communications consists of packaging and promoting a product. Thinking of occupational therapy services as a product may be a new way of thinking for some. It is common for new therapists who are just beginning to learn about the complexities of the health care system and confronting issues such as reimbursement and productivity demands for the first time to feel frustrated because they "Just want to treat their patients!" Yet, it is the nature of a free-market economy and of the *dualism* present in our health care system that services can never be provided without someone considering expenses and revenues (see Chapter 2). Even when care is provided for "free," as it is sometimes assumed to be in our welfare system or by a health care provider's *indigent care* funding, revenues to support those services must come from some source. Thinking about occupational therapy services as a product that can be packaged and sold will help you to accomplish that aim more effectively.

Marketing communications involves devising methods of communicating with your target populations to promote your occupational therapy products and services. As noted earlier in the chapter, it may be helpful to distinguish between target populations that are payers (those who provide financial reimbursement for your services) and those that are customers (those who are the direct recipients of your services) when involved in the marketing process for a new occupational therapy product. Sometimes the payer and the customer may be one and the same, but at other times identifying the specific concerns of payers and recipients of services and devising related but separate communications can be more effective in getting the word out about your new product or service. It is also conceptually helpful to realize that often, when providing a service, we may have one payer but multiple customers, such as the patients, referring physicians, nurses, families, and others.

Marketing communications also involves figuring out who has to be educated to what aspect of the services you provide and what will be the most successful medium to deliver your message. A helpful set of concepts to help with the marketing process, and particularly with marketing communications, is what has been referred to as the *Four Ps of Marketing*. The Four *P*s of marketing are product, price, place, and promotion. Each of these four will be briefly discussed in the following sections of this chapter.

PRODUCT

Defining your product clearly for all involved in product development, delivery, and marketing communications is important. This may sound simple, but a common mistake—and the fastest way to lose potential customers from your target populations—is to promise more than you can deliver. For example, consider the process of beginning to develop work-related services. At first you might have available staff members who are trained to conduct work capacity screenings if provided with specific job descriptions and the necessary duties of a classification of employees, such as the ability to lift 40 lbs. or the ability to bend repeatedly. Your plan might be to begin by conducting work capacity screenings only and offer additional services later as you are able to add more staff or send existing staff for training. As physicians or others become aware of the services that you are offering, it may be common to begin to receive calls about other related services, such as conducting assessments of worksites and making recommendations for worksite adaptations. In these situations, it is tempting to try to accommodate such requests to "grow your business" faster, but it is important to avoid the temptation of promising an enthusiastic customer a service that you are not prepared to deliver. Failing to deliver on such promises is the fastest way to squelch a program's potential.

Defining your product means knowing in advance exactly what you can and cannot deliver, as well as what you may be able to deliver but not want to deliver. Not only does this help prevent you

from making promises that you cannot fulfill, but it also helps you in comparing your product or service to that being offered by competitors in your area to determine the risks involved in continuing with product or service development.

PRICE

As a consumer of a wide range of products, chances are that you already understand more about the concept of *price* than you probably realize. Naturally you are familiar with the monetary cost of a product; however, with most products or services there are other less obvious types of cost to a consumer that will influence the success of a new product or service. Some of these other types of costs are described in Box 13–4.

In Chapter 11, you were introduced to the concept of *value*, or the relationship between cost and quality. It was suggested that at times we might be satisfied with lower quality if the associated costs were also lower. We do not expect the quality of a fast-food cheeseburger to be the same as a cheeseburger we buy at a nicer restaurant; however, we do evaluate the cost compared to the quality of the product or service we receive and determine whether the product or service is of good value. This evaluation of cost, quality, and value does not always hold true when it comes to our health care. In fact, seldom are we willing to accept lower quality services despite lowered costs. We need to be careful when communicating with members of our

---

Box 13–4: Costs Associated with Product or Service Use

- *Time costs*, such as the time involved in getting to or using your service, including the time away from paid employment or family
- *Emotional or psychological costs* associated with admitting the need for your service
- *Physical costs*, such as pain associated with a treatment
- *Monetary costs* beyond direct charges for services, such as costs for parking or travel to and from your service location

target populations about the cost and quality of our services and avoid the temptation of promising more for less. Still, even when quality is high, the perceived value of a service may be lessened when members of target populations encounter non-monetary costs such as difficult parking, long waiting periods, or unpleasant surroundings.

PLACE

Place refers to where and when your product or service is available to your target populations. Again, this may seem straightforward when it comes to most occupational therapy services. However, as competition for limited health care reimbursement has increased, health care providers are becoming more flexible and creative to meet the needs of those they serve and increase customer satisfaction. Giving consideration to providing services on days and at times when members of your target populations are available, such as weekends and evenings, may give your product or service an edge over that of your competitors. Another example might be to develop relationships and programs in which the therapist brings the program to the target population rather than expecting them to come to a clinical site. The popularity of *onsite work programs* in which rehabilitative services are provided at the workplace of injured workers is an example of such programming that has become increasingly popular. In addition to the advantage for the therapist in seeing the client's "real-world setting," the client misses less time from the workplace and costs may be saved for both the payer and the employer because they are able to have the injured worker return to light duty more quickly.

PROMOTION

New products and services may need to be promoted both within and outside of your organization depending on the organization's complexity and the target populations for the new programming. A first step to internal or external promotion is making a list of anyone else in the organization that might have an interest in your product or service, or who might have an interest in reaching the same target populations. For example, after beginning the hand rehabilitation program described earlier, I initiated visits to some local workers' compensation insurance representatives to persuade

them to refer their clients to our program. After several visits, the importance of promoting a product or service internally became evident. On one visit I encountered questions about the injury tracking system that was being marketed by my organization through direct mail brochures to insurers. On a second visit, I discovered that another representative from my organization had made a "cold call" to the insurance office just before my arrival. She had been marketing the organization's Employee Assistance Program services.

Because I was unprepared to answer the questions that I was being asked, it appeared that I was not familiar with all that my organization had to offer. In addition, as an organization we appeared disorganized, and further, we had lost an opportunity to gain some economy of effort to impress potential payers with multiple complimentary products. After these experiences, I contacted both representatives and we met and undertook a coordinated effort to promote several of our products that we thought would be attractive to a workers' compensation insurer. Often programs have to be promoted internally or to others within the organization, especially in settings in which occupational therapy is heavily dependent upon others (e.g., nurses or physicians) to identify clients who would benefit from its products and services.

External promotion also calls for a carefully coordinated effort by all stakeholders who are interested in providing products or services to the same target population. By collaborating with others in your organization, you can develop an action plan for promoting your products and services to various target populations. Answering the following questions can help you begin to develop an action plan for external promotion:

1. Who is the target population of your product or service (i.e., the consumer)?
2. Besides the consumer or direct beneficiary of your product or service, who else is either an internal or external customer (e.g., nurses, physicians, payers)?
3. What are the primary goals of your consumers and customers?
4. Who will be involved in deciding where to go for services?
5. What is the most efficient and effective way to reach your consumers and customers?

Selecting Promotional Media

There are various methods that you can select to deliver information about your product or service to members of your target populations that can be referred to as promotional media. Choosing the most effective promotional media may be straight-forward or complex depending upon whether you will be promoting your product or service inter-nally, externally, or both. Often the time and fi-nancial resources that you have available will limit your choice of promotional strategies. Recognizing the advantages and disadvantages of each form of promotional media will also help to narrow your options and to make a selection. The advan-tages and disadvantages of some of the most com-mon forms of promotional media are presented in Table 13–1. In addition to the strategies listed in Table 13–1, other methods of promoting a new product or service to a target population might in-clude exhibiting at a continuing education confer-ence; developing a free speakers' bureau; offering an in-service education program to physicians, nurses, or other target populations; or holding an open

Table 13-1	Advantages and Disadvantages of Common Forms of Promotional Media		
Communication Method	Advantages	Disadvantages
Face-to-face meetings	• Lower cost depending on number • Can customize message and alter based on response • Can evaluate customer reaction more easily	• Time intensive, can reach fewer contacts • May be perceived as an interruption
Brochures & direct mail	• Can reach larger number of contacts with one effort • Provide contact information in sustainable form for future • Time investment in develop-ment only	• Higher cost depending on num-ber and quality • Fixed message • Difficult to evaluate customer reaction and effectiveness of effort • May be difficult to reach the "decision maker"
Telephone solicitations	• Lower cost • Can customize message and alter based on response • Can reach larger number of contacts	• May be perceived as an interruption • May be difficult to reach the "decision maker"
Seminars	• Can customize message and alter based on response • Can evaluate customer reaction more easily • Establishes a relationship with attendees that can be developed	• Higher cost • Time intensive, can reach fewer contacts • Difficult to evaluate customer reaction and effectiveness of effort
TV/radio/print ads	• Can reach larger number of contacts with one effort • Provide contact information in sustainable form for future • Time investment in develop-ment only	• Higher cost • Fixed message

house in your department or program (Jacobs, 1999).

Chapter Summary

This chapter provided an introduction to the marketing process and a description of the four marketing components: organizational assessment, environmental assessment, market analysis, and marketing communications. Hopefully, you now recognize that the process of identifying the needs, resources, and limitations of your organization and of various target markets can be extraordinarily complex. However, this chapter also provided a perspective on simplifying the process and applying it to the common sorts of challenges that an occupational therapy manager may face in developing a new product or service.

Throughout the chapter, the value of developing collaborative relationships with others in your organization, community, and profession that can help you with marketing functions was stressed. Such relationships not only aid in identification of resources that can be used but are also helpful in identifying the various types of data, information, and other forms of evidence available from primary and secondary sources that will help you justify the need for a new product or service. It is also critical that you become aware of the efforts of others who might be developing and promoting complimentary products or services for the same target

Real-Life Solutions

After meeting with the director of physical therapy and the associate from the publications and promotions department, Patrick became energized about the process of exploring the needs, resources, and limitations of his department and hospital as well as those of the target populations served by the department of occupational therapy. The director of physical therapy shared some of the same concerns about whether her department was meeting the needs of physicians, nurses, patients, payers, and other target populations but had felt overwhelmed and did not know how to start investigating the situation on her own. Not only was the physical therapy director responsive but, in addition, both she and Patrick received praise and recognition from their boss, Keesha, who appreciated their collaborative efforts.

Patrick learned that he, the director of physical therapy, and the associate from publications and promotions already collected some of the same data, information, and other forms of evidence about the effectiveness of current services and the needs and resources of various target populations. However, he also discovered that they each collected some data, information, or other forms of evidence that were not being widely shared. By combining efforts, they would not only save valuable time and energy but would be able to develop a more complete picture of some of their key target populations.

Patrick was not surprised to learn that there were few available resources to support new activities or complex and costly strategies for assessing the organization and its environment. He was optimistic that he and his new collaborators would be able to identify creative and inexpensive methods of assessing their departments and their hospital and of learning more about the needs, resources, and limitations of their target populations. Patrick and the director of physical therapy each agreed to start by having their staff participate in a SWOT analysis exercise and share the results with each other. They also agreed to have their staff review existing programs and their perceptions of effectiveness and identify any potential new products and services for either discipline so they could begin to collaborate with key stakeholders in the marketing process for occupational therapy and physical therapy.

Patrick, the director of physical therapy, and the associate from publications and promotions agreed to begin meeting every 2 weeks to discuss progress. Patrick also volunteered to gather data, information, and other forms of evidence on health care marketing so that they could begin to develop a more sophisticated understanding of each of the four marketing components and strategies for success.

populations so that you share data, information, and other forms of evidence and avoid wasted time and effort.

Marketing can be complex, and the novice occupational therapy manager may feel overwhelmed when first learning about the diverse range of activities that must be completed when exploring the development of a new product or service. In some situations, such as that of a business owner or entrepreneur, it may be wise to consider hiring a marketing consultant to assist with the process, but even the novice manager can rely on skills developed in related managerial functions such as planning and program development to become an active participant in the marketing process.

At the start of the chapter, you were introduced to Patrick, who was being encouraged by his boss, Keesha, to explore and develop additional services that could bring in new streams of revenue. Although he had had some exposure to the marketing process in an administration and management course as part of his occupational therapy education, he decided to begin by reaching out to others in his organization.

Resources Related to Marketing Health Services

Journals that Often Publish on Marketing Health Services

HEALTH MARKETING QUARTERLY

Health Marketing Quarterly is a journal that targets professionals in the areas of marketing for health and human services. The journal focuses on applied strategies and resources such as "how-to" marketing tools. Each issue includes articles that demonstrate the applicability of marketing for specific health services. Health care managers and service providers will appreciate the inclusion of articles and columns devoted to such topics as how to develop a thorough marketing approach and how marketing can improve awareness of opportunities, increase customer/patient satisfaction, and improve the cost-effectiveness of programs. The

focus of the journal is broad and includes a range of contexts including:

- Group practice marketing
- Mental health marketing
- Long-term care marketing
- The marketing of ambulatory care
- Alternative care programs
- Social services
- Hospitals
- Health maintenance organizations
- Health insurance
- Health products

STRATEGIC HEALTH CARE MARKETING

Strategic Health Care Marketing focuses on news, analysis, and interpretation of events affecting the ever-changing health care services marketplace. Coverage includes

- Customer/patient satisfaction
- Wellness and prevention
- Advertising and brand management
- The Internet
- Niche marketing opportunities
- Employee recruitment/retention
- Database/relationship marketing
- Care management
- Community and public relations
- Special markets
- Report cards
- Ambulatory care development
- Market research reports
- Physician relations
- New product development

Organizations Concerned with Marketing Health Services

AMERICAN MARKETING ASSOCIATION

http://www.marketingpower.com/

The American Marketing Association (AMA) has over 38,000 members representing every area of marketing including health related fields. For over six decades, the AMA has served as a resource for providing marketing information. The AMA Web site, MarketingPower.com, offers a wide array of newly expanded information including research, case studies, and best practices in marketing. The

AMA's prestigious marketing journals provide access to the newest developments in marketing thought, while the AMA has a more practical focus on the applications of marketing strategies to address daily needs on the job. In addition, the AMA offers specialty conferences, 1-day "hot topic" seminars, bootcamps, and workshops to help marketers build the skills that keep them ahead of emerging trends, and help long-term professional development.

Suggested Resources on Focus Groups

Edmunds, H. (1999). *The focus group research handbook.* Lincolnwood, IL: NTC Business Books.

Goebert, B., & Rosenthal, H. (2002). *Beyond listening: Learning the secret language of focus groups.* New York: John Wiley & Sons.

Krueger, R. A. (1998). *Analyzing and reporting focus group results.* Thousand Oaks, CA: Sage.

Krueger, R. A., & Casey, M. A. (1998). *Focus groups: A practical guide for applied research.* Thousand Oaks, CA: Sage.

Reference List

Doman, D., Dennison, D., & Doman, M. (2002). *Market research made easy.* Bellingham, WA: Self-Counsel Press.

Jacobs, K. (1999). Marketing occupational therapy services. In K. Jacobs & M. K. Logigian (Eds.), *Functions of an occupational therapy manager* (3rd ed., pp. 27–40). Thorofare, NJ: Slack.

Richmond, T. (2003). Marketing. In G. L. McCormack, E. G. Jaffe, & M. Goodman-Lavey (Eds.), *The occupational therapy manager* (pp. 177–192). Bethesda, MD: AOTA Press.

14

Regina F. Doherty, M.S., OTR/L
Elizabeth Peterson, M.P.H., OTR/L
Brent Braveman, Ph.D., OTR/L, FAOTA

Responsible Participation in a Profession

Real-Life Management

Every day Ellyn and the occupational therapy staff with whom she works eat their lunch together and spend the lunchtime discussing a wide range of topics. Today the conversation turned to a letter that all occupational therapists in their state received from the state regulatory board informing them of changes to the state occupational therapy practice act. Some of Ellyn's coworkers were complaining about the addition of requirements for continuing education to the licensure act. They would now have to meet these requirements in order to renew their license to practice every other year. The staff members were voicing the concern that all of the benefits relating to continuing education provided by their employer had been eliminated and that they would now have to cover the cost of attending continuing education to satisfy the state's new requirements.

One of the staff, Carrie, expressed concern that the physical therapy state practice act had also been changed. It now included activities of daily living as part of the scope of practice definition for physical therapy. Further, she had heard that, although the physical therapists were not successful in gaining direct access (with which no physician's referral would be needed in the state for physical therapy), the state physical therapy association had already begun a fund-raising and lobbying effort to have it included in the next version of their practice act.

As Ellyn listened to the staff complain about the state of affairs, she became more and more frustrated. Ellyn became involved in her state occupational therapy association when she was a student and was elected as her class representative to the association. From that moment on, she had developed an intense interest in advocating for her profession and her clients at the local, state, and national legislative levels. She was still an active member of her state association as well as the American Occupational Therapy Association (AOTA). She had volunteered on the state licensure committee and had even visited her congresswoman on Capital Hill in Washington, D.C., as part of a conference sponsored by the AOTA Political Action Committee (AOTPAC).

Ellyn knew that few if any of the staff sitting at lunch were members of the state occupational therapy association and that less than half were members of AOTA. She found it frustrating that her peers complained about the outcomes of processes that they could have influenced but instead left to others. She decided that she needed to do something and left lunch early to talk to her department director about scheduling an in-service presentation on how to become involved in state and national association activities and on the responsibilities of being a "professional."

Key Issues

- Being a responsible occupational therapy service provider requires active support of your state and national professional associations as the primary vehicles to advocate for the future of occupational therapy.
- Participating fully in your profession requires that you under-

stand how your professional association and other related bodies are structured, the functions they serve, and how you can become involved to influence the future of occupational therapy.

- Ethics is a discipline or branch of philosophy that helps you

examine how to live a responsible and moral professional life. The occupational therapy manager and occupational therapy service providers must have an understanding of the resources and systems available to respond to ethical dilemmas.

Throughout this book, membership in the AOTA has been emphasized as an important strategy for finding useful resources related to data, information, and other forms of evidence. Additionally, it has been suggested that developing a network of peers at the local, state, and national levels can help you find and evaluate evidence and other resources to aid clinical and managerial decision making. This theme will continue in Chapter 14, and, further, it will be suggested that as a *professional* you have a responsibility to join and actively participate in both your state and national professional associations. Neither managers nor practitioners can fulfill their responsibilities that come with the adoption of an evidence-based approach to practice without understanding the contexts in which practice occurs, and this requires a working knowledge of the key stakeholders that seek to influence the profession.

As an occupational therapy manager, you will not only have the responsibility of taking steps to play an active role in supporting and developing your chosen profession but will also play a vital role in encouraging the active participation of those you supervise. In order to be successful at both of these tasks, you must develop a working knowledge of the key organizations and bodies that are involved in shaping how practice occurs. Many of these bodies, such as the AOTA, the National Board for Certification of Occupational Therapy, Inc. (NBCOT), state regulatory boards, and accreditation bodies, have been mentioned in other chapters. They will be briefly discussed again in this chapter, focusing specifically on how a manager can become involved in or interact with each organization or body to obtain data, information, and other

forms of evidence and to play a role in shaping the future of occupational therapy practice.

Finally, a key role of the occupational therapy manager is assuring that the occupational therapists, occupational therapy assistants, occupational therapy fieldwork students, and others whom he or she supervises practice in an ethical and responsible manner. An introduction to ethics will be provided, including a listing of common ethics theories, and supports for ethical practice both internal and external to occupational therapy practice environments will be discussed.

What Does It Mean to Be a Professional?

A profession has been characterized as "an occupation that regulates itself through systematic, required training and collegial discipline, that has a base in technical, specialized knowledge, and that has a service rather than a profit orientation enshrined in its code of ethics" (Starr, 1984). The Ontario Institute of Agrologists (2004) characterized a professional as one of a group of persons who jointly and individually assume responsibility for

- Defining the nature of the service provided to society.
- Defining the minimum base of knowledge and skills needed to provide that service.
- Defining the limits of his or her individual ability to apply that knowledge and those skills.
- Defining the code of ethics to be used to guide and evaluate his or her service to others.

- Policing himself or herself regarding his or her provision of service to others.
- Recognizing his or her obligations to society and to other practitioners by living up to established and accepted codes of conduct.
- Maintaining membership in professional groups and carrying his or her part of the responsibility of advancing professional knowledge, ideals, and practice.

In the United States, the primary vehicle for a profession to have a unified influence to promote and develop its services to society is the *professional association*. The implication for individual occupational therapists is clear. Being a responsible "professional" means we must join and sustain active membership in both our state occupational therapy association and the AOTA. State associations not only provide a mechanism for interacting with our peers on a local level but typically also play critical roles in defining the nature of the profession's service at the state level through their influence on state regulatory bodies (e.g., licensure). As our national association, the AOTA serves a range of critical functions related to the development and promotion of occupational therapy as a profession. In addition, a number of other organizations support the profession. The structure and function of these organizations and bodies will be reviewed briefly in the next section of this chapter.

Occupational Therapy Professional Associations

The American Occupational Therapy Association

Becoming involved in the AOTA becomes much easier if you understand the organization and appreciate the high value placed on membership in the organization. You may have a real impact on the association and the profession through general membership in the association and through the numerous volunteer leadership opportunities available to you. When you speak of "the AOTA" or hear others speak of it, it is important to pay close attention to whether the reference being made is to the *bureaucracy*, or the paid staff who work within an employed accountability structure; the *association*, or the members who join to have the bureaucracy

work on their behalf; or both. It is important to note that the term *bureaucracy* is not a pejorative term in this case; rather it simply refers to the type of organization that employs persons in an accountability structure. Most organizations in which workers are employed are in fact most accurately categorized as bureaucracies. Also, you should note that some paid staff members of the AOTA who work within the bureaucracy are also occupational therapists or occupational therapy assistants and are members of the association. Although it may seem to be a fine point, knowing that the AOTA hires specialists in areas such as marketing and publications who are often not occupational therapists can help you be more effective in interactions with AOTA staff.

The AOTA is governed by a structure that includes an executive director, a paid employee who is a professional experienced in running a nonprofit professional association. Often the executive director is not an occupational therapist. He or she is responsible for oversight of the activities of all paid staff and for collaborating with the volunteer sector of the association. The members of the AOTA elect a group of volunteer officers, including a president, vice president, secretary, treasurer, and directors who serve on the association's board of directors. In addition to the board of directors, the AOTA is led by a number of commissions, committees, and boards that are also often led by volunteers who are elected by the membership as a whole or a subset of the membership. One example of a subset of the membership includes the Special Interest Sections, which elect a chairperson every 3 years. These chairpersons regularly meet as a group (the Special Interest Sections Council) to advise the association on important matters, to develop products or resources to meet their members' needs, and to identify issues of importance that will affect practice. The primary bodies of the AOTA are listed with brief descriptions in Box 14–1. The major functions of the association are listed in Box 14–2.

The American Occupational Therapy Association Political Action Committee

The AOTPAC is a voluntary, nonprofit, unincorporated committee of members of the AOTA. The AOTPAC was authorized by the Representative Assembly in 1976 and has been operational since

---

Box 14–1: **The Primary Governance Bodies of the American Occupational Therapy Association**

- **Board of Directors:** The Board of Directors is composed of the elected officers of the association; directors are elected from the general membership and include at least one occupational therapy assistant and a public member.
- **Representative Assembly:** The Representative Assembly is the policymaking body (e.g., congress) of the AOTA, made up of elected representatives from each state and Puerto Rico, chairpersons of committees and commissions (e.g., the Special Interest Sections Council, the Commission on Practice, the Commission on Education), and a public member.
- **Special Interest Sections Council (SISC):** The SISC is a body of the Representative Assembly organized to represent 11 specialty areas of practice and to meet the range of member needs related to practice in these areas.
- **Commission on Standards and Ethics (SEC):** The SEC is a body of the Representative Assembly that recommends the standards and ethics of the AOTA and can review complaints and make recommendations for discipline of AOTA members for ethical violations
- **Commission on Practice (COP):** The COP is a body of the Representative Assembly and serves the AOTA by promoting the quality of occupational therapy practice and developing practice standards for occupational therapists and occupational therapy assistants relative to provider and consumer needs.
- **Commission on Education (COE):** The COE, a body of the Representative Assembly, is a visionary group that identifies, analyzes, and anticipates issues in education. The COE generates education-related policy recommendations to the Representative Assembly for deliberation. The COE works in conjunction with the Education Special Interest Section (EDSIS) and has interactions with the Accreditation Council for Occupational Therapy Education (ACOTE).
- **Affiliated State Association Presidents (ASAP):** The ASAP is comprised of state presidents from the 50 state occupational therapy associations (and Puerto Rico) affiliated with the AOTA and is a body of the AOTA Board of Directors.
- **Accreditation Council for Occupational Therapy Education (ACOTE):** The ACOTE is an associated body of the Executive Board and has the mission of fostering the development and accreditation of quality occupational therapy education programs. By establishing rigorous standards for occupational therapy education, the ACOTE supports the preparation of competent occupational therapy practitioners.

---

the spring of 1978. The purpose of the AOTPAC is to further the legislative aims of the association by influencing or attempting to influence the selection, nomination, election, or appointment of any individual to any federal public office, and of any occupational therapist, occupational therapy assistant, or occupational therapy student member of the AOTA seeking election to public office at any level. The committee is not affiliated with any political party (AOTA, 2004b).

Federal regulations prevent the AOTA as an organization from making contributions to political candidates; however, as a separate nonprofit organization, a political action committee (PAC) is free to raise money and make donations to support the political campaigns of candidates with views that favor the agenda of the AOTA. The AOTA is allowed to legally support the PAC by providing the operating expenses required for the PAC to fulfill its function.

The AOTPAC is governed by a board of directors, with a director representing each of five regions of the United States. In addition, there are nonvoting AOTA staff members who help to guide

---

Box 14–2: Major Functions of the American Occupational Therapy Association

- Promote awareness of occupational therapy in society by keeping it visible and in demand.
- Advocate for the profession at the national, state, and local legislative levels.
- Provide for the continuing education and professional development needs of the membership.
- Provide mechanisms and structures for the membership to interact with each other.
- Support the provision of quality education for occupational therapists and occupational therapy assistants by developing and maintaining a process for accrediting educational programs.
- Guide the membership in the delivery of ethical and responsible intervention.
- Support the development of knowledge and scientific inquiry to develop evidence to guide occupational therapy practice.
- Support the development of standards and guidelines to guide occupational therapy practice.

---

the PAC's activities. The majority of the money that supports the PAC's legislative activities comes from direct member contributions.

Among others, the AOTPAC cites three central criteria used in determining which candidates to support (AOTA, 2004b):

- Is the candidate sympathetic to the goals of the occupational therapy profession? Has the candidate supported specific proposals or policies advanced by the profession?
- If an incumbent, does the candidate hold a key position of responsibility (i.e., chair or member of important committee or subcommittee; member of majority or minority leadership)?
- If a nonincumbent, will the candidate pursue assignment to a key committee or subcommittee, or be likely to be in a position to assist the profession?

The American Occupational Therapy Foundation

The mission statement of the American Occupational Therapy Foundation (AOTF) is as follows: "Through the use of fiscal and human resources, AOTF expands and refines the body of knowledge of occupational therapy and promotes understanding of the value of occupation in the interest of the public good" (AOTF, 2003). The AOTF was created in 1965 to advance the science of occupational therapy and to increase public understanding of its value. The foundation has funded three centers for scholarship and research that have resulted in $3 to $5 million dollars per year in competitive grant funding, has jointly funded more than $4 million dollars of research with the AOTA, publishes a research journal (*OTJR: Occupation, Participation and Health*), and funds over 70 scholarships for occupational therapy education each year.

In 2004, the Agency for Healthcare Research and Quality (AHRQ) provided a grant to the AOTA and the AOTF to fund a conference of international occupational therapy researchers and leaders to determine the state of the art in evidence-based occupational therapy practice and to coordinate international initiatives to foster such practice. In addition, participants sought to establish a set of consensus guidelines for evaluating and reporting research evidence and to discuss mechanisms to enhance dissemination of the evidence. More information about the AOTF and its role in the promotion of the science of occupational therapy and of evidence-based practice can be found on its Web site (*http://www.aotf.org/*).

The Fund to Promote Awareness of Occupational Therapy

The Fund to Promote Awareness of Occupational Therapy was founded in 2002 as a separate nonprofit organization (501c.3) with the mission of promoting awareness on the part of the general public of occupational therapy. The Fund runs promotional campaigns that educate the public about the role that occupational therapy plays in different areas of practice and with different types of disabilities and a range of public and social issues.

The Fund develops promotional materials and public awareness campaigns of which practitioners can avail themselves to promote occupational therapy in their local communities. Examples of promotional campaigns created and directed by the Fund include efforts to educate the public about services for older drivers, increasing awareness of back injury or other problems in children caused by carrying overloaded backpacks, and publicizing other occupational therapy success stories. You can find more information about the Fund at its Web site (*http://www.promoteOT.org/*).

The National Board for Certification of Occupational Therapy, Inc.

The NBCOT plays a critical role in occupational therapy by developing and administering the certification examination for occupational therapists and occupational therapy assistants. The certification examination is one of many steps that serve to assure that persons practicing as occupational therapists have developed entry-level competence. The examination is developed by conducting an analysis of entry-level practice every 5 years (NBCOT, 2004b).

In addition to the development and coordination of the certification examination, the NBCOT fulfills several other functions. These include verification of certification for employers, and investigation of complaints against occupational therapy practitioners as a means of protecting the public. The Disciplinary Action Information Exchange Network (DAIEN) contains a listing of final disciplinary actions and nondisciplinary actions taken by the NBCOT, as well as disciplinary actions taken by state regulatory entities. Actions are posted to the DAIEN on a quarterly basis and removed after 1 year. The NBCOT communicates with other bodies that serve disciplinary functions, including state regulatory agencies. You can find additional information about the NBCOT on its Web site (*http://www.nbcot.org/*).

State Occupational Therapy Associations

State occupational therapy associations serve many of the same functions for occupational therapy professionals on a state level that the AOTA performs on a national level. In addition to being a mechanism to develop and maintain a network of peers, state associations serve the following functions:

- Providing opportunities for continuing education and professional development through state association conferences, publications, and sponsored events
- Advocating for the profession at the state level through political action and lobbying to influence outcomes of processes such as licensure and other forms of regulatory control
- Increasing public awareness of occupational therapy
- Providing a vehicle for occupational therapists to develop networks of peers to support professional development and practice
- Providing an opportunity for members to develop skills in leadership, interpersonal communication, management, and other personal and professional skills

Ethics

Being a responsible professional, whether your primary role is as a clinician, manager, educator, or researcher, includes having an understanding of ethics as a discipline and the systems in place to help occupational therapy service providers resolve the ethical dilemmas that they encounter. Ethics is a practical discipline that addresses real-world problems. It is an inherent, active part of daily clinical life that aids us in the evaluation of morality, conduct, and social practices. Skill in ethical reasoning and approaches to clinical care are of great value to managers and clinicians. Leadership and management today involve motivating staff to achieve best practices, and best practices are enhanced by ethical reflection.

Ethics is learned moral development. It is an evolution that occurs as a lifelong process. The basics of ethics must be taught, valued, and supported in practice in order for ethical reasoning to be fostered (Scanlon & Glover, 1995). As managers and supervisors, we must aid our staff and students in ethical development. Effective moral judgments and reasoning are just as important to occupational therapy practice as sound clinical judgments and reasoning. In order to best understand ethics in clinical practice, we must familiarize ourselves with ethics theory and terminology.

What Is Ethics?

Ethics is a generic term for various ways of understanding and examining a moral life (Beauchamp & Childress, 2001). Some approaches to ethics are normative, others non-normative. Normative ethics asks more concrete questions related to morality (Purtilo, 1999). Most ethics questions encountered by occupational therapists on a day-to-day basis are normative in nature. The two broad types of non-normative ethics are *descriptive ethics*

and *metaethics*. Descriptive ethics and metaethics are grouped together as non-normative because their objective is to establish what factually or conceptually *is* the case, not what ethically *ought* to be the case (Beauchamp & Childress, 2001).

The AOTA's Occupational Therapy Code of Ethics is an example of non-normative or descriptive ethics. However, individuals who ask whether or not the content of the AOTA Code of Ethics is justifiable raise issues associated with normative ethics.

Selected basic terms related to ethics principles and concepts are presented in Box 14–3. Terms related to ethics theories are presented in Box 14–4.

Box 14–3: Terminology Related to Ethics Principles and Concepts

- **Advance directive:** Also called a *living will*, an advance directive is a written statement made by an individual that indicates treatment wishes in the event that he or she becomes incapacitated. The term is often used in conjunction with *health care proxy*, the person designated by the individual as his or her representative in health care decision making when the advance directive is in place.
- **Autonomy (respect for):** A norm of respecting the decision-making capabilities of autonomous (self-governing) persons (Beauchamp & Childress, 2001).
- **Beneficence:** a group of norms for providing benefits and balancing benefits against risks and costs (Beauchamp & Childress, 2001).
- **Bias:** A preference or inclination, especially one that interferes with impartial judgment (American Heritage College Dictionary, 1993).
- **Bioethics:** A branch of ethics devoted to the study of problems surrounding medical practice, health care delivery, and medical and biological research (Bailey & Schwartzberg, 2003).

- **Conscientiousness:** Intending to do what is right; trying with due diligence to determine what is right (Beauchamp & Childress, 2001).
- **Compassion:** A trait that combines an attitude of active regard for another's welfare with an imaginative awareness and emotional response of deep sympathy, tenderness, and discomfort at another's misfortune or suffering (Beauchamp & Childress, 2001).
- **Competence:** Having the cognitive and psychological ability to make decisions that others judge to be rational; to be judged competent, it is necessary for the individual to be able to communicate these decisions to others (Hansen, 2003).
- **Confidentiality:** The practice of keeping privileged patient information within proper bounds. Confidentiality always involves a relationship, whereas privacy does not. Confidentiality is the most long-standing dictum in health care codes of ethics (Purtilo, 1999).
- **Conflict of interest:** A conflict between the private interests and the public obligations of a person in an official position (American Heritage College Dictionary, 1993).

(continued)

Box 14–3: **Terminology Related to Ethics Principles and Concepts** *(continued)*

- **Discernment:** The ability to make judgments and reach decisions without being unduly influenced by extraneous considerations, fears, personal attachments, and the like (Beauchamp & Childress, 2001).
- **Distributive justice:** A method of determining how to dispense or allocate resources (e.g., equal shares for all; first come, first served; the greatest good for the greatest number) (Hansen, 2003).
- **Duty:** An act or course of action required by custom, law, or religion (American Heritage College Dictionary, 1993). The position of "occupational therapist" brings with it a number of duties outlined by the law and the profession.
- **Ethical dilemma:** A situation marked by conflict between ethical beliefs and involving choice between alternatives that appear to be equally morally acceptable (Kornblau & Starling, 2000).
- **Fidelity:** Faithfulness to obligations, duties, or observations. The duty of fidelity (faithfulness) requires health care professions to take seriously, and act in accordance with, all the ethical mandates and opportunities that define a professional role (Purtilo, 1999).
- **Life-sustaining treatment:** Medical intervention that serves to save or restore bodily functions (e.g., mechanical ventilator, dialysis).
- **Informed consent:** Consent containing three elements: information, voluntariness, and competence (Bailey & Schwartzberg, 2003.)
- **Integrity:** A virtue that represents two aspects of a person's character: (1) a coherent integration of aspects of the self—emotions, aspirations, knowledge, etc.—so that each complements and does not frustrate the others; and (2) the trait of being faithful to moral values and standing up in their defense when necessary (Beauchamp & Childress, 2001).
- **Justice:** The principle of fairness; a group of norms for distributing benefits, risks, and costs fairly (Beauchamp & Childress, 2001).

- **Non-maleficence:** The fundamental duty that instructs us not to do anything that would injure another (Bailey & Schwartzberg, 2003).
- **Paternalism:** The intentional overriding of one person's known preferences or actions by another person, wherein the person who overrides justifies the action by the goal of benefiting or avoiding harm to the person whose preferences or actions are overridden (Beauchamp & Childress, 2001).
- **Principle:** A basic truth, law, or assumption that may serve to act as a standard for behavior. Principles may be general in nature and may rely upon rules to guide specific action.
- **Privacy:** Three types of privacy are typically identified. Physical privacy is a restriction on the ability of others to experience a person through the five senses; informational privacy is a restriction on facts about the person or persons; and decisional privacy is the exclusion of others from involvement in decisions made by the person and the person's group of intimates.
- **Rights:** Justified claims that individuals and groups can make upon other individuals or upon society; to have a right is to be in a position to determine, by one's choices, what others should do or need not do (Beauchamp & Childress, 2001).
- **Rules:** General norms that guide actions that are more specific in content and restricted in scope than principles. Detailed rules function as precise action guides (Beauchamp & Childress, 2001).
- **Shared decision making:** A process by which clinical decisions are made through shared discussion of information between the client and the care team or the family and the care team. Essential for shared decision making are listening, respect, and integrity. Inherent in the process is education and assessment of the client's understanding. Shared decision making is the basis of informed consent.

(continued)

- **Substituted judgment:** Substituted judgment begins with the premise that decisions about treatment properly belong to the incompetent or nonautonomous patient by virtue of rights of autonomy and privacy. The patient has the right to decide but is incompetent to exercise it, and it would be unfair to deprive an incompetent patient of decision-making rights merely because he or she is no longer (or never has been) autonomous. Substituted judgment requires the surrogate decision maker to make the decision the incompetent patient would have made if competent. A health care proxy is often called upon to use substituted judgment (Beauchamp & Childress, 2001).

- **Trust:** a confident belief in and reliance upon the moral character and competence of another person (Beauchamp & Childress, 2001).

- **Veracity:** Adherence to the truth; truthfulness (American Heritage College Dictionary, 1993).

- **Virtue:** A character trait and an internal disposition to seek moral perfection, to live one's life in accord with this moral law, and to attain a balance between noble intention and just action (Pelligrino, 1995).

Box 14–4: Common Ethics Theories and Approaches

- **Casuistry or Case-Based Ethics:** An approach to analyzing moral issues or problems based on a formal and systematic method of closely examining cases. Casuists hold that ultimately you can find common moral themes among cases (Beauchamp & Childress, 2001).

- **Care-Based Ethics:** Based on the assumption that a caring relationship is an ethics-based framework within which to examine ethical issues. Moral reasoning involves intertwining of emotion, cognition, and action (Benjamin & Curtis, 2001).

- **Character-/Virtue-Based Ethics:** In virtue-based ethics theory, the emphasis is on the agent, or the person. The standard is the good person, whom one can rely on to be good and to do good under all circumstances.

- **Common Morality Theories:** All common morality theories (1) are pluralistic; (2) rely on ordinary, shared moral beliefs for their starting content and make no appeal to pure reason, rationality, natural law, a special moral sense, or the like; and (3) hold that any ethics theory that cannot be made consistent with these pre-theoretical common-sense moral judgments falls under suspicion (Beauchamp & Childress, 2001).

- **Communitarianism/Community-Based Theory/"Common Good" Theories:** Theories that consider benefit to the community as a whole as the standard by which to make correct moral judgment. These theories help to set checks and balances on individual self-interest (Purtilo, 1999).

- **Consequentialism (Teleological Theory):** This theory focuses on consequences and outcomes of a deed or action as the standard by which to make correct moral judgments (B. A. Kornblau & Starling, 2000; Shannon, 1997).

- **Deductive Theories and Approaches:** Theories and approaches that propose that the human mind (usually the faculty of reason) is capable of discerning truths about moral life from a pattern of visible laws in the universe or from some set of general rules or principles that can be discerned by humans through intuition, revelation, or other reliable means. The general truths become a basis to guide action in concrete situations (Beauchamp & Childress, 2001).

(continued)

Box 14-4: Common Ethics Theories *(continued)*

- **Deontological Theories:** "Duty-driven" theories that focus on one's duties and rights in order to determine an ethical course of action. This theory focuses on strictly following rules and principles of ethics. Deontological theories require that a method of weighting duties be available to determine what to do when conflicts arise (Purtilo, 1999).
- **Individualistic Theories and Approaches:** Ethics theories and approaches that take individual well-being as the standard by which to make correct moral judgments (Purtilo, 1999).
- **Inductive Theories and Approaches:** Theories and approaches that start with a concrete experience. Some suggest that these theories and approaches are less a system for guidance and more a rejection of the belief that reliable action guides can be found (Purtilo, 1999).
- **Intuition-Based Ethics:** Ethics theory that uses individual intuition as the standard by which to make correct moral judgments. Intuitionism allows us to follow our convictions but ignores the need to deal with the contradictory opinions of others or to win them over to our side (Kornblau & Starling, 2000).
- **Liberal Individualism/Rights-Based Theory:** Theories that focus on a person's individual rights (civil, political, legal) in order to determine an ethical course of action. These rights protect the individual from societal intrusions (Beauchamp & Childress, 2001).
- **Principle-Based Theory:** Relies on ordinary shared moral beliefs to provide a basis for the evaluation and criticism of actions. General norms guide actions that often leave room for judgment, because principles are "prima facie," meaning one can trump the other (e.g., beneficence, nonmalfeasance) (Beauchamp & Childress, 2001).
- **Utilitarianism:** The doctrine that advocates doing the most good for the highest number of people (Bailey & Schwartzberg, 2003).
- **Virtue Theory:** A theory that concerns itself with the types of virtues, integrity, or character traits one should display. This theory examines the roles one plays and behavioral expectations each role encourages or requires (B. A. Kornblau & Starling, 2000; Sim, 1997).

Ethics theories such as utilitarianism, liberal individualism (rights-based theory), and communitarianism (community-based theory) attempt to identify and justify existing norms (Beauchamp & Childress, 2001). In a pluralistic society with divergent moralities, no single unifying ethics theory or vision of morality prevails. A debate over which theory is "right" and which theory is "wrong" is really beside the point. Ethics experts encourage us to focus on acceptable features in different theories, often with attention to how ethical decisions are justified, without having to choose one over the other (Beauchamp & Childress, 2001; B. L. Kornblau, 2001; Purtilo, 1999). Understanding the different theories adds depth to ethical thought and action. It is helpful to recognize that we can learn from all of the theories (Beauchamp & Childress, 2001).

Professional ethics are principles or rules intended to express the particular values of a group of providers and that serve as guidelines for professional behavior. They help to explain the profession to people served, and serve as a code of conduct. As Corbett (1993) explained, our professional ethics within occupational therapy are the rules we use to make certain that each therapist is operating in a fashion that protects the integrity of our profession, and hence the viability of all occupational therapists. Ethical practices serve as an important source of continuity of professional ideals because they embody the philosophical values of the profession (Christiansen & Baum, 1991). These rules ensure our clients' best interests and protect the profession itself and its position in the public mind (Corbett, 1993). Although professional codes of ethics are also a means of establishing trust between the professional and society, codes are only one element of professional behavior, and they do not automatically create the desired professional practice (Scanlon & Glover, 1995). Professional codes are only guides; applied ethics must be both valued and supported in practice in order for moral reasoning and clinical reasoning to be successfully integrated. Within occupational therapy, professional ethics are formally established and monitored by licensing boards and other credentialing agencies (e.g., the NBCOT), by our professional association (the AOTA), and by individual departments and organizations.

Why Do Managers Need to Learn About Ethics?

Understanding ethics theories and debating their application may seem like a philosophical exercise, but in reality, ethics theories and principles are highly relevant to daily life—especially the life of a health care provider. By definition, an ethical dilemma is a choice between two equally compelling alternatives, a predicament for which one finds no singular or clear-cut satisfactory solution (B. A. Kornblau & Starling, 2000). The nature and scope of occupational therapy practice provide plenty of fuel for ethical dilemmas. An example would be the occupational therapist or occupational therapy assistant working in acute care who constantly has to decide how to ration her time spent with patients in order to provide services to as many clients as possible, or the school-based therapist who is beginning to suspect that one of the students he is following is the victim of neglect, but is concerned about angering the parents and possibly placing the child in greater harm. Ethics aids everyone in the evaluation of morality, conduct, and social practices.

In their efforts to support delivery of high-quality services within a given occupational therapy department, managers are well served to recognize that "best practice" and "ethical practice" are inextricably linked. As noted by Christiansen and Lou (2001), ethical issues are part of every health care encounter, and moral principles such as truth, fairness, doing the right thing, avoiding harm, and respecting autonomy lie at the heart of these ethical concerns. In her 1983 Eleanor Clarke Slagel Lecture, Joan Rogers eloquently articulated the ethics question that clinicians are challenged to answer: "What among the many things that could be done for this patient, ought to be done?" (Rogers, 1983). Because the answer to this question involves a *judgment*, influenced by both facts and the client's values, the clinical reasoning process terminates in an ethical decision, rather than a scientific one. Thus, the quality of the services provided is directly impacted by a clinician's ability to negotiate the ethics questions experienced in practice.

State statutes provide a basis for practicing the best possible occupational therapy for the benefit of clients served, the occupational therapy service provider, and the profession as a whole. Not surprisingly, a strong overlap exists between "legal practice" and "ethical practice." Many state practice acts directly include a code of ethics in the regulations, and some have included the AOTA's Code of Ethics in whole or in part (Diffendal, 2002). Often, an action that constitutes an ethical violation may be a practice act violation, and vice versa. The issue of provider competency will be used to illustrate this point, and its relevance to occupational therapy managers.

Occupational therapy practitioners have a legal and ethical responsibility to be competent in the services they are delivering. Concerns related to provider competency can be quite diverse, and range from administering an assessment without proper credentialing to failing to use proper safety precautions during treatment. At the heart of all concerns related to provider competency is the recognition that failure to provide service with competence can result in harm to the patient (maleficence). Although each practitioner is responsible for knowing the laws that regulate practice, the supervisory nature of many managerial positions places increased responsibility on the individual running a department. Occupational therapy managers often evaluate the competency of students entering the field or therapists working in a new setting (e.g., the neonatal intensive care unit). Ultimately, it is often the occupational therapy manager who is held accountable for both the accomplishments and mistakes occurring within a department. In addition to failing to support best practices within his or her department, a manager who neglects supervisory responsibilities associated with establishing and monitoring provider competency can be the subject of legal and ethical conduct violations, and may face disciplinary action.

Several national trends have complicated occupational therapy practice and, in some cases, converged to increase the likelihood of encountering ethical dilemmas in practice. These trends include new regulations (e.g., the Health Insurance Portability and Accountability Act of 1996 [HIPAA]), expanding cultural diversity/differences in healing traditions, and technology advances (including the information explosion and increased public access to the Internet). Even the trend of evidence-based practice brings with it a number of serious ethical considerations. Christiansen and Lou (2001) described evidence-based practice as a "gift that comes in ethical wrapping." They advised that, from a moral and professional standpoint, the dangers of not attending to the evidence are just as significant as the ethical issues attending to its application. Among health care trends, managed care is consistently recognized as a source of ethical challenges in clinical practice. Practitioners are often expected to provide more with less, and frequently serve as advocates for clients who are unaware of managed care plan complexities. Ethical dilemmas associated with managed care often center on the conflict between business goals and the holistic commitment of our profession (Lohman & Brown, 1997). They may also require occupational therapy practitioners to develop and apply new skills to respond effectively (Braveman & Fisher, 1997).

Changes in health care regulation occur frequently, and often lead practitioners into unfamiliar territory where the luxury of drawing from prior experience is absent. In such situations, ethical problem-solving skills become all the more valuable. Consider the situation experienced by Sarah and Liz, who are both graduate students in the entry-level master's program at a private university. They had completed all their academic requirements and were now ready to begin their final fieldwork affiliations. Sarah received a call from her fieldwork site 2 weeks prior to her affiliation start date informing her that the Centers for Medicare and Medicaid Services has just issued a memorandum that outpatient occupational therapy services provided by a student will no longer be covered. The site treats mostly clients over the age of 70, so they will need to cancel Sarah's affiliation. Sarah shared this information with Liz, who called her fieldwork site. They were aware of the ruling and told her they do not foresee a problem. Sarah and Liz were left confused about the different approaches adopted by their potential fieldwork sites to the same ruling.

The overview of national trends provided here is intended to highlight the heightened need for occupational therapy managers to be prepared to address ethical dilemmas. Although dealing with ethical dilemmas is recognized as a stressful aspect of practice, Barnitt and Partridge (1997) have identified several influences that positively impact clinicians' capacity to deal with dilemmas across settings. These include previous experience with similar dilemmas, time for reflection, and support from peers. In addition to serving as role models, department managers are in a position to develop the presence of such influences within their department. Clearly, occupational therapy department managers are in a unique position to support ethical practice among staff they supervise. Managers often work in close contact with staff members, and thus have the opportunity to observe service delivery in action. Additionally, the expertise that supports professional advancement for occupational therapy managers is the same expertise that can be used to help staff members negotiate both day-to-day and unique problems that arise.

Managers' appreciation of the *contextual features* of practice may be especially valuable to staff members confronted with ethical dilemmas. Findings from a study conducted by Barnitt and Partridge (1997) suggest that the context or setting of an ethical dilemma has a major effect on therapists' reasoning. Important context-related features identified by the authors included the site of the dilemma, the work group, the patient group, and the hierarchical or power relations in operation. With respect to site-specific issues, studies point to the fact that ethical problems differ from setting to setting. In her study undertaken to identify ethical dilemmas experienced by occupational and physical therapists working in the U.K. National Health Service, Barnitt (1998) found that, among occupational therapists, dilemmas occurring in mental health settings were common and often centered around concerns related to managing difficult or dangerous behavior in patients and unprofessional staff behavior. Foye, Kirschner, Brady-Wagner, Stocking, and Siegler (2002) surveyed occupational therapists in a free-standing academic rehabilitation hospital to explore situations from their clinical practice that raised morally troubling questions. Reimbursement pressures, conflicts regarding goal setting, and patient/family refusal of team recommendations were the topics most frequently mentioned by the therapists working in that rehabilitating setting.

Barnitt and Partridge (1997) recognized that the patient group served is a very important contextual factor that influences therapists' reasoning when confronted with ethical dilemmas. Russell, Fitzgerald, Williamson, Manor, and Whybrow (2002) offered an excellent example of ethical concerns arising out of work with a specific patient group: older adults. Using a "critical incident" interview approach with 12 Australian occupational therapists, Russell et al. identified therapists' explicit and implicit understandings of independence as a value concept and practice issue. Their findings suggest a "mismatch between idealized and practice-based talk about independence." Specifically, the authors found that the therapists studied invoked concerns about safety and duty of care as a caveat to implementing their independence ideals and justifying the retention of professional control. The study highlights the need for occupational therapist practitioners to carefully examine how

their own values pertaining to independence and safety are translated into practice. Together, the Barnitt and Partridge (1997) and Russell et al. (2002) studies illustrate how the context of practice influences both the nature of ethical dilemmas encountered and therapists' reasoning in the midst of those dilemmas.

How Can Managers Actively Support Ethical Practice Within a Department?

Supporting Ethical Behaviour

Kyler (1999) has drawn from previous work (Kanny & Kyler, 1999) to provide a number of suggestions to individuals teaching ethics within occupational therapy curricula. Because the role of the manager in supporting ethical practice within a department often parallels the role of an occupational therapy educator, a number of these strategies can be used by managers to support ethical practice within a clinical occupational therapy department. The suggestions presented in Box 14–5 are adapted

---

Box 14–5: Supporting Ethical Practice Within Occupational Therapy Departments: Suggestions for Managers

- Recognize that supporting ethical practice within a department requires managers to first explore their own values and develop their own ethical reasoning skills in order to be comfortable with the topic.
- Model appropriate sensitivity to ethical issues.
- Examine ethics theories, principles, and related concepts, and incorporate discussion of ethics theories and principles into conversations about patient care.
- Identify formal and informal avenues to improve cultural competence.
- Help staff members recognize the ethical significance of their values, employer policies, individual decisions, and group decisions.
- Identify legal channels that the recipient of services or health care practitioner may utilize to resolve a problem or serve as a resource.
- Understand the formal and informal ethics dispute resolution systems that have jurisdiction over occupational therapy practice.

- Be able to quickly access resources (including internal, institution-specific documents, and AOTA documents) that can be used to guide behavior, and know the content of those documents.
- Help clinicians realize that their own positions cannot simply be a matter of opinion.
- Support discussions of explanations and clinical reasoning.
- Actively listen to others and help staff recognize that listening to others is vitally important to the formulation of cogent arguments and decisions.
- Facilitate the formulation of questions that arise out of ethically stressful situations.
- Actively involve staff members in ethical decision-making processes based on reflection and critical assessment of values as they relate to the facts of a given situation.
- Help staff explore options for action in a given situation.

Adapted from Kyler (1999) and Kanny and Kyler (1999).

from Kyler (1999) and Kanny and Kyler (1999) and should not be considered in a linear or hierarchical fashion. However, a few comments regarding the beginning and ending of the process of supporting ethical practice within a department are in order.

It is important to note that the process of supporting ethical practice among staff members begins with the creation of a clinical *milieu* that supports staff members' involvement in identification and resolution of ethical dilemmas. Within a supportive environment, an occupational therapy manager can help staff members gain an awareness of values shared by the health care team that may or may not be shared by clients and their families. The following case example illustrates this point.

In the end, the outcomes yielded by fostering attention to, and resolution of, ethical dilemmas among staff are many. In addition to being better able to manage ethical dilemmas, staff members who learn skills associated with analyzing ethical

dilemmas will be capable of more thoughtful decision making in treatment, which should influence the quality of care provided. Additionally, those clinicians will be better prepared to manage the day-to-day stress associated with patient care, and may be better equipped to avoid the "burn out" experienced by so many health professionals. When faced with difficult ethical decisions, the manager must be ever-present in the discussion, employ active listening, and ask clarifying questions. It is helpful for managers to compassionately acknowledge both the clinicians and the client's feelings and emotions. Managers can recognize that it may not be possible to provide answers to all questions. However, it is helpful to be honest and to display a willingness to further explore issues.

Occupational therapy service providers can draw from the work of several authors to learn strategies that can be used to analyze ethical dilemmas (AOTA, 2003; Jonsen, Siegler, & Winslade,

Case Example: The Case of Joe

Joe is a 12-year-old boy admitted to the hospital with visual changes and neck pain following a collision with another boy during his Little League baseball game. Joe's head computed tomography (CT) scan revealed a large left parietal brain tumor with midline shift. Emergency surgery was recommended, and Joe underwent a craniotomy for tumor removal. Postoperatively he did very well, although he needed to undergo chemotherapy to continue therapeutic treatment of the tumor. Joe's mother requested that he not be told he had cancer. She asked that she be allowed to explain to him that there was something on his brain that was removed and that he should get better. Many members of the health care team struggled with this request. They felt that Joe needed to actively participate in his health care and be fully aware of the cancer diagnosis so that he could effectively "fight it" (The tumor had been found incidentally because, if not for the collision, he may have never had the head CT scan.) In time, Joe was informed of his diagnosis in a most effective and caring way.

Communications were facilitated by ethics support staff at the hospital that helped the family and the health care team find a compromise that supported the best clinical care for Joe.

This case helps to highlight how a health care team might impose its own value of information on others. In this case, the health care team members wanted to share specific health information immediately. Joe's family felt that his spirit would be broken by the cancer diagnosis. They placed tremendous value on hope, and less value on the need to share precise health care information with Joe at the time of diagnosis.

As Jameton (1990) pointed out, discussion of ethical and moral dilemmas within a department is an important process by which a moral culture can become more tangible. The following case example builds upon the findings of Barnitt and Partridge (1997) to illustrate how an occupational therapy manager can (1) recognize an opportunity for exploration of moral culture and (2) foster supportive discussions.

Case Example: The Case of Jerry

Jerry is a 42-year-old occupational therapist who works on the geriatric rotation in a community hospital. Her mother recently passed away following a long battle with Alzheimer's disease. Jerry was asked to evaluate Joan, a 78-year-old woman who lives alone and who was admitted to the hospital with the diagnosis of "failure to thrive." Joan's medical workup revealed that she had a urinary tract infection. During the initial evaluation, Jerry observed that Joan was confused, a poor historian, and in need of moderate cueing and minimal assistance to perform basic bathing and dressing tasks. Jerry recommended nursing home placement for Joan upon discharge, and documented her assessment. Later in the week, Jerry was on vacation, and her manager, Sue, worked with Joan. Sue noted that Joan's confusion was diminished (not surprisingly, given that she had received 3 days of intravenous antibiotics) and that she required less cueing for self-care. Joan was also able to articulate her desire to return to her own home upon hospital discharge. Sue was concerned that Jerry's personal experiences with her own mother might have interfered with her ability to provide the best care recommendations. She noted that Jerry was much too conservative with recommendations for Joan, but suspected that other staff members might have recommended minimal supports for her. Sue decided to have a case discussion at the next staff meeting to assist the staff in exploring their own personal values related to autonomy and client-centered care. As a manager, she did not "teach ethics"; however, she did want her staff to be critical of their unexamined moral beliefs, and to respectfully listen to and examine the views of others.

1998; Kornblau et al., 2000; Purtilo, 1999; Scanlon et al., 1995; Trompetter, Hansen, & Kyler-Hutchinson, 1998). Scanlon and Glover (1995) identified key steps shared by many approaches to case analysis. Those steps are listed in Box 14–6. The fact that ethical dilemmas are often recurring is important to note, and underscores the importance of Step 7, as outlined by Scanlon and Glover (evaluating how the dilemma could have been prevented). Fletcher, Lombardo, Marshall, and Miller (1997) described several ethical considerations that have great weight in clinical practice, and thus deserve special attention. They are balancing burden and benefit, disclosure, informed consent and shared decision making, the norms of family life, health care provider responsibilities and professional integrity, societal norms of cost effectiveness and resources allocation, cultural and religious considerations, and considerations of power.

ETHICS COMMITTEES

When strategies to support application of ethics in clinical practice are examined, it is important to discuss the role of institution-based ethics committees.

Occupational therapy managers who ensure occupational therapy representation on organization-wide ethics committees are taking highly visible and productive steps toward bringing core values into sharper focus and enhancing practice. Ethics committees are vital internal supports to all health care organizations. Whether at the discipline-specific level or the hospital or organization level, it is essential that occupational therapists or occupational therapy assistants are prepared to participate on these committees. Ethics committees provide an environment for safe and open discussion of moral questions. These questions can range from basic to complex. Ethics committees are interdisciplinary. In this way, topics and cases can be reviewed and analyzed from many different perspectives. Morality is a culture, and ethics committees promote this culture by helping staff members with different beliefs, cultures, and professional codes observe and explore important issues. It is important to remember that different staff groups within the same institution, or even the same profession, may speak different clinical languages and be bound by different codes of ethics, hence the interdisciplinary

---

Box 14–6: Basic Elements for Making Reliable Moral Judgments

1. *Identify an ethical issue.* Describe the ethical issue clearly so that it can be addressed by all parties, even those who may have different sensibilities.
2. *Gather relevant information/facts.* Identify all the known facts.
3. *Describe values at stake.* It is crucial to determine whose values need to be considered in the ethical discourse (e.g., those of the patient or his or her designated decision maker, the family, the health care team member) and what they are.
4. *Identify a range of options.* Even when values seem to directly conflict, there may be ways to develop a variety of options that respect or balance the values of each party.
5. *Make a choice.* Sometimes choices are less than satisfactory, and ambiguity lingers. However, as with clinical judgments and the ongoing evaluation of them, one always will identify things that could have been done differently and things that are celebrated for having been done well. The same is true of moral judgments, for which reliability, not certainty, is expected. Reliability depends on the capacity and opportunity for sustained and critical discussion of choices.
6. *Give reasons to support choices.* State why a particular choice is ethically supported.
7. *Evaluate how the dilemma could have been prevented.* Each discussion of an ethical issue provides an opportunity to reflect on how organizational and professional structures, policies, and practices have contributed systematically to the issue, or how they can be changed to address it. Without this type of analysis, a pattern of ongoing crisis management of ethical issues, rather than a preventative approach, is likely to continue.

Adapted from Scanlon, C., & Glover, J. (1995). Ethical issues. A professional code of ethics: Providing a moral compass for turbulent times. *ONF*, 22, 1515–1521, with permission. ©Oncology Nursing Society.

---

approach to ethics is rich in debate and analysis. For example, an occupational therapist may be bound by his or her code of ethics to discharge a patient who is making no gains in therapy and no longer has a need for services based on his or her functional status. The nurse for the same patient is bound by her code of ethics to never desert this patient as long as he or she is hospitalized.

An interdisciplinary ethics committee should include representation from each clinical discipline in the institution. A typical committee includes a physician, nurse, social worker, occupational therapist, physical therapist, case manager, speech-language pathologist, chaplain, palliative care clinician, respiratory therapist, pharmacist, and patient advocate. Managers, volunteer services staff, patients and their family members, and laypersons may also participate as indicated.

Ethics committees in different institutions have different charges. Most serve to consult, educate, and assist with policy revision and development.

They empower staff members as they provide a process to handle difficult ethical issues and ease the potential emotional responses of staff. They also serve to encourage decisions in accordance with ethical institutional policies. Institutions with active interdisciplinary ethics committees support the best patient care possible. They are also able to provide the institution with institutional case histories so that trends and decisions can be monitored.

In today's society, most health care organizations understand the need for ethics committees and independently establish them. However, in order for a health care organization to receive accreditation from the Joint Commission on Accreditation of Healthcare Organizations (JCAHO), it must have a functioning process to address ethical issues in the areas of patients' rights and organizational ethics (JCAHO, 2004). In 2000, the Society for Health and Human Values' Society for Bioethics Consultation Task Force on Standards for Bioethics

Consultation identified the following skills required for ethics consultation: ethics assessment skills, process skills, and interpersonal skills (Aulisio, Arnold, & Younger, 2000). Ethics assessment skills are necessary to distinguish the ethical dimensions of the case and identify morally acceptable options and their associated consequences. Process skills are needed to resolve values uncertainty or conflict. Interpersonal skills are necessary so active listening and communication that is respectful, supportive, and empathetic to all parties involved occurs.

Occupational therapists and occupational therapy assistants are a natural fit for institution and organizational ethics committees. Ethics encompasses values clarification, reflecting on and optimizing quality of life, group communication, and narrative reasoning—all skills that occupational therapy professionals are highly knowledgeable in. Occupational therapists and occupational therapy assistants have unique training in understanding and applying meaningful occupation. We follow clients throughout the life span and bring a broad spectrum of care knowledge to ethics committees. Occupational therapists and occupational therapy assistants are also skilled in group facilitation, which is always needed when debating heated moral issues.

Managers who support their occupational therapy staff in participation on ethics committees will find that committee membership brings with it many benefits to their occupational therapy department. The ethics committee member undergoes intense education and training in ethics. He or she then brings this expanded knowledge base to the occupational therapy department and assists in the departmental facilitation of "difficult discussions." The committee member serves as a resource to both other disciplines in the hospital and the occupational therapy staff to promote values clarification and mentor less experienced staff in applying ethical reasoning to their clinical practice. The committee member also aids in occupational therapy– specific case analysis to assist with the clarification of ethics questions and the possible resolution of more complex moral dilemmas. In their study of physical and occupational therapists, Barnitt and Partridge (1997) found that dealing with ethical dilemmas was a skilled and stressful aspect of practice. They also found that one of the positive influences on this was support from peers. The occupational therapy representative on the ethics committee is able to provide this support. This in turn leads to improved coping skills among staff and an environment that supports moral courage and ethical practice.

In the event that you manage an occupational therapy department or service in an organization that does not have a facility-wide ethics committee, there are other resources to turn to. The facility's partnering or umbrella organization may have a broader based committee that serves to address the interdisciplinary ethics needs. Other internal facility resources include the advocacy office (or an ombudsman service), the social services department, chaplaincy services, the human resources department, and the Institutional Review Board as related to research activities. It is important to remember that ethics resources should always be readily accessible, and that staff members need to know that their occupational therapy administration is on the front line when it comes to dealing with ethics questions that arise in clinical practice. A supportive administration promotes reflective practitioners.

How Does the Profession Support Ethical Behavior?

A number of strategies that department managers can use to support ethical practice among staff members have been presented. This discussion of external supports and regulations will focus on the following groups: accreditation bodies, the NCBOT, our professional membership organization (the AOTA), and bodies responsible for state regulation of occupational therapists. These bodies assist occupational therapy practitioners in understanding their responsibilities to practice ethically and legally. They also act as resources to the public and provide vehicles for filing complaints when it is believed that rules have been violated.

ACCREDITATION

Accreditation is a process by which an institution or organization seeks to demonstrate to an accrediting agency that it complies with generally accepted standards set forth by appropriate professional organizations. Accreditation is a status awarded to an organization that demonstrates compliance with standards established by the accrediting body. Accreditation may be voluntary (e.g., Commission on Accreditation of Rehabilitation Facilities), mandatory at a state level (e.g., licensure to operate), or required in practicality (e.g., JCAHO accreditation is tied to reimbursement). Accreditation signifies to consumers of services that agencies have met predetermined, generally recognized standards. Accreditation is relevant to initiatives to develop and maintain ethical practices because many accrediting agencies require accredited institutions to have policies (e.g., patient nondiscrimination policy) and processes (e.g., case consultation) that support ethical practice. For example, the JCAHO requires that all health care organizations have a process to address ethical issues related to patient care and organizational ethics. JCAHO rules specifically require that institutions must have a process to examine ethical issues in marketing, admissions, discharges, billing, relationships with third-party payers, and managed care organizations.

A single health care institution may be accredited by more than one accreditation body. It is important for managers to know which accreditation bodies their organization is accredited by (and accreditation goals set by their organization), the expectations guidelines set forth by each accrediting agency, and how their department-specific accreditation activities fit in with their organization's overall accreditation policies and activities. Often hospital-wide accreditation activities compliment, and can build upon, the accreditation activities going on within individual departments.

REGULATION OF OCCUPATIONAL THERAPY PRACTICE

Occupational therapists and occupational therapy assistants are typically regulated by both state regulatory boards (SRBs) and the NBCOT. These regulatory agencies share the function of protecting the public; however, they perform this function in different ways.

State Regulatory Boards. Occupational therapy is regulated in all 50 states and three U.S. territories, but the level of regulation varies significantly. Most states have determined that licensure is the most effective approach to regulating occupational therapy practitioners. Of the 53 jurisdictions in the United States, 46 states, the District of Columbia, Guam, and Puerto Rico *license* occupational therapists; one state (Indiana) has *certification laws* governing

occupational therapists; two states (Hawaii and Michigan) have *registration laws*; and one state (Colorado) has a *trademark law*. Collectively known as SRBs, these regulatory bodies serve, safeguard, and promote the public welfare by ensuring that qualifications and standards for professional practice are properly evaluated, accurately applied, and vigorously enforced. In some states, SRBs protect the public by prohibiting practice by unlicensed occupational therapists or occupational therapy assistants.

It is important to appreciate the distinction between licensure and other forms of regulation. Generally, unlike certification, registration, and trademark laws, a licensure law defines a lawful scope of practice for practitioners. Defining a scope of practice legally articulates the domain of practice and provides guidance to facilities, providers, consumers, and major public and private health and education facilities on the appropriate use of services and practitioners. Defining practice can further ensure important *patient protections* by offering guidance on appropriate care, particularly in the investigation and resolution of consumer complaints involving fraudulent or negligent delivery of services.

SRBs have the authority provided by state law to discipline occupational therapy practitioners who violate regulations. States that include codes of ethics (or statements describing the ethical conduct expected by occupational therapy practitioners) in their laws can discipline practitioners who violate those codes. Drawing on the example of provider competency used earlier in this chapter, working outside a scope of practice often raises serious concerns regarding provider competency, increases risk of harm to the patient, and thus is one example of a violation that represents both legal and ethical misconduct.

Although state procedures for processing complaints are not uniform, the process used in Illinois is provided as an example of how a state might process a complaint. After an initial review within the Illinois Department of Professional Regulation, a complaint is assigned to a department investigator. The investigator is responsible for determining whether or not there has been a potential violation of a licensing law, or department rules and regulations. After developing the facts in cases in which there appears to be a violation, the investigator refers the case to a prosecuting attorney. If the staff attorney concludes that the matter has been sufficiently investigated and there is evidence supporting the complaint, formal charges are filed. Disciplinary actions imposed by states range from censure (a formal expression of disapproval that is publicly announced) to temporary suspension of practice privileges (the loss of certification for a certain duration, after which the individual may be required to apply for reinstatement) or permanent prohibition from practice in the state.

The National Board for Certification in Occupational Therapy. The NBCOT is a national organization that protects the public by legally monitoring entrée to public practice through its certification process, establishing minimum certification standards for entry-level practice, and monitoring those standards via an ongoing disciplinary process. NBCOT's goal is to promote the health, safety, and welfare of the public by establishing, maintaining, and administering standards, policies, and programs for certification and registration of occupational therapy personnel (NBCOT, 2004a). The NBCOT has jurisdiction over all individuals who are certified by it, as well as those individuals who have applied to take the certification examinations. Although the NBCOT is centrally concerned with "safe, proficient and/or competent practice in occupational therapy practice," the NBCOT Candidate/Certificant Code of Conduct contains many principles that reflect expectations of ethical practice.

The NBCOT's disciplinary actions (reprimand, ineligibility for certification, censure, probation, suspension, and revocation of certification) are overseen by the Qualifications and Compliance Review Committee. An explanation of the NBCOT's Disciplinary Action Program is easily accessed via its Web site (*http://www.nbcot.org/*). It is interesting to note that, although the NBCOT's disciplinary actions are independent of those taken by SRBs or the AOTA's Commission on Standards and Ethics, the NBCOT does notify SRBs of any complaints received and disciplinary actions taken. The NBCOT encourages SRBs to share information regarding their disciplinary action with the NBCOT.

If a manager has concerns about unethical conduct by an occupational therapy practitioner, he or she can call the NBCOT and discuss those concerns with staff involved in the Disciplinary Action Program. NBCOT staff would be available to offer direction on filing a complaint with the NBCOT, and where else it may be appropriate to file a complaint (such as with an SRB and/or the AOTA). In addition, NBCOT staff would convey information about the NBCOT's disciplinary action process, direct the manager to the NBCOT Web page for additional information on the disciplinary process, and offer other possible options that an administrator may want to consider given the concerns conveyed.

The AOTA and Ethics. The AOTA advances the quality, availability, use, and support of occupational therapy through standard setting, advocacy, education, and research on behalf of its members and the public. The Commission on Standards and Ethics (SEC) is the body within the AOTA whose function is to "recommend the development of standards and ethics to the Association ... and provide the process whereby the standards and ethics of the Association are enforced." The SEC has produced three key documents that describe, define, and support the values to which those within the profession should aspire. These are the *AOTA Occupational Therapy Code of Ethics* (AOTA, 2004a), the *Guidelines to the Occupational Therapy Code of Ethics* (2000), and the *Core Values and Attitudes of Occupational Therapy Practice* (AOTA, 1993). The Code of Ethics is reviewed by the SEC every 6 years to make sure that the content is current and relevant to member concerns (Deborah Yarett Slater, personal communication, May 26, 2004).

As a voluntary professional organization, the AOTA has no direct authority over occupational therapy personnel who are not members. It does, however, have limited authority over members regardless of what role they are in: practitioner, educator, fieldwork educator, supervisor, administrator, consultant, fieldwork coordinator, faculty program director, researcher/scholar, entrepreneur, student, support staff, or occupational therapy aide. (In contrast, other bodies that regulate occupational therapy are primarily concerned with the actions of practitioners.) The AOTA SEC is responsible for enforcing the Code of Ethics, and has well-documented enforcement procedures that can be reviewed on the AOTA Web site (*http://www. aota.org/*). The AOTA Web site also features links to frequently requested documents that support the professional community, a link to a page featuring frequently asked questions about ethics, and a description of disciplinary actions that can be taken by the AOTA (reprimand, censure, probation, suspension of membership, permanent revocation of membership), and the functions and membership of the SEC. Managers are encouraged to recognize that one of the key functions of the SEC is also to "inform and educate Association members and consumers regarding standards and ethics." It does this by writing and publishing advisory opinions and articles in *OT Practice* (the association's biweekly magazine) on current ethical issues with a focus on interpretation of relevant ethics principles. Advisory opinions are available on the AOTA Web site as well as in the *Reference Guide to the Occupational Therapy Code of Ethics* (AOTA, 2003), which is an important resource for managers and their staff. In addition, managers and their staff may contact the staff liaison to the SEC at the association headquarters or by e-mail for assistance and resources to resolve ethical concerns.

Some Final Thoughts on Occupational Therapy Managers and Ethics

Occupational therapists, occupational therapy assistants, and occupational therapy fieldwork students do not work in a vacuum. We are holistic practitioners who interact with many other disciplines in the ever-changing field of health care. Occupational therapy managers need to be comfortable with ethical reasoning and conflict analysis so they can effectively lead and mentor their staff. Leading staff in activities related to ethical reasoning allows for better clinical care to be delivered. It also helps direct care providers cope with job stress. In a supportive workplace environment that facilitates the exploration of values and resources available to promote best practices, employee "burnout" can be minimized and professionalism can be fostered in a collaborative fashion. In summary, supporting ethical programs and fostering ethical reasoning among practitioners is an inherent part of good occupational therapy practice and administration.

Chapter Summary

This chapter introduced you to common characterizations of a *profession* and what it means to be a *professional*. It was suggested in this chapter that being a member of a profession carries with it associated responsibilities, including joining and sustaining membership in your state occupational therapy association and in the AOTA. The purpose and structure of the AOTA and the purpose of other related organizations and bodies were reviewed.

A primary focus of this chapter was an introduction to ethics as a discipline and branch of philosophy that the occupational therapy manager can use to guide practice and to respond to the common ethical dilemmas that managers and practitioners encounter. Terminology related to ethics principles and concepts was defined and numerous ethics theories were listed. Supports for the manager to guide ethical practice both internal and external to the profession were provided, and case examples illustrated some of the common dilemmas that managers and the staff they supervise face.

Occupational therapists, occupational therapy assistants, occupational therapy fieldwork students, and especially occupational therapy managers must understand the professional systems in which they operate if they hope to have an influence on the contexts in which they practice. There are numerous ways that we can support our profession, ranging from joining and sustaining membership in professional organizations to volunteering for a wide variety of leadership roles available at both the state and national levels. If we choose not to be active participants and responsible professionals, we also abdicate our right to complain about the system in which we practice.

At the start of the chapter, you were introduced to Ellyn, who had become frustrated with some of the staff members with whom she worked because they complained about events occurring within their profession but did not have membership in their state occupational therapy association or the AOTA. Ellyn had decided that an in-service education program on becoming responsible professionals was needed.

Real-Life Solutions

The director of the department in which Ellyn worked agreed that an in-service education presentation on becoming "responsible professionals" was a good idea. To prepare, Ellyn gathered information on the AOTA, her state occupational therapy association, and other related organizations and bodies that influenced the practice of occupational therapy in her state. As she did this, she realized that there was much that she did not know about the structure of these bodies and the many volunteer opportunities that were available. She was particularly interested in the process that the Representative Assembly used to make decisions and to charge various AOTA committees and commissions with doing work on behalf of the association.

Initially, Ellyn had felt quite angry at her coworkers about the attitude they had adopted. To her it seemed that they were blaming others for developments when they had not accepted responsibility for participating in the process. As she began to prepare her presentation, however, it struck her that, without understanding how the various bodies were organized and how they completed their business, that it might be easy to assume that an individual could have little impact on the end results. Ellyn decided to focus her presentation on the organization of the AOTA and related bodies, such as the AOTF, the Fund to Promote Awareness of Occupational Therapy, the AOTPAC, her state association, the NBCOT, and the state regulatory board, and on the many ways that individuals could participate in the process of influencing the service provided to society by the profession of occupational therapy.

Acknowledgments

The authors would like to acknowledge Robin Jones, M.P.A., COTA/L, ROH, Deborah Yarett Slater, M.S., OTR/L, FAOTA, Janie Scott, M.A., OTR/L, FAOTA, and Audrey Rothstein for their respective contributions to content related to the National Board for Certification in Occupational Therapy and the American Occupational Therapy Association.

Resources Related to Participating in a Profession

Useful Resources on Participating in a Profession

THE CENTER FOR HEALTH PROFESSIONS

http://www.futurehealth.ucsf.edu/home.html
The mission of the Center for Health Professions is to assist health care professionals, health professions schools, care delivery organizations, and public policymakers to respond to the challenges of educating and managing a health care workforce capable of improving the health and well-being of people and their communities. The Center for Health Professions is associated with the University of California, San Francisco and focuses its efforts on understanding the challenges faced by the health care workforce and developing programs and resources that assist in making successful transitions to the emergent health care systems

THE ETHICS RESOURCE CENTER

http://www.ethics.org/about.html
The Ethics Resource Center is a nonprofit, nonpartisan educational organization. The center has a stated vision of promoting a world in which individuals and organizations act with integrity. The mission of the Ethics Resource Center is to strengthen ethical leadership worldwide by providing leading-edge expertise and services through research, education, and partnerships.
The Ethics Resource Center strives to

- Inspire individuals to act ethically toward one another
- Inspire institutions to act ethically, recognizing their role as transmitters of values
- Inspire individuals and institutions to join together in fostering ethical communities

Journals That Often Include Articles About Professional Ethics

CAMBRIDGE QUARTERLY OF HEALTH CARE ETHICS

The *Cambridge Quarterly of Health care Ethics* is designed to meet the needs of professionals serving on health care ethics committees in hospitals, nursing homes, hospices, and rehabilitation centers. The aim of the journal is to serve as the international forum for the wide range of serious and urgent issues faced by members of health care ethics committees, physicians, nurses, social workers, clergy, lawyers, and community representatives.

JOURNAL OF MEDICAL ETHICS

The *Journal of Medical Ethics* is a leading international journal that reflects the whole field of medical ethics. The journal seeks to promote ethical reflection and conduct in scientific research and medical practice. It features original articles on ethical aspects of health care, as well as conferences, book reviews, editorials, correspondence, news, and notes. To ensure international relevance, the journal has editorial board members from all around the world.

Professional Organizations Concerned with Participating in the Profession Of Occupational Therapy

THE AMERICAN OCCUPATIONAL THERAPY ASSOCIATION

http://www.aota.org/
    The mission of the AOTA advances the quality, availability, use, and support of occupational therapy through standard setting, advocacy, education, and research on behalf of its members and the public. The AOTA provides its members with a variety of resources and supports to promote responsible participation in the profession of occupational therapy. The AOTA promotes the awareness on the part of the general public of occupational therapy, advocates at the national and state legislative levels, supports state occupational therapy associations, and provides members and managers with resources for dealing with ethical dilemmas.

THE AMERICAN OCCUPATIONAL THERAPY FOUNDATION

http://www.aotf.org/
    Through the use of fiscal and human resources, the AOTF expands and refines the body of knowledge of occupational therapy and promotes understanding of the value of occupation in the interest of the public good. The AOTF promotes a society in which individuals, regardless of age or ability, may participate in occupations of their choice that give meaning to their lives, and foster health and well-being. The goals of the AOTF include securing contributions and managing assets; promoting scientific inquiry; and supporting excellence in education about occupation and occupational therapy.

THE FUND TO PROMOTE OCCUPATIONAL THERAPY

http://www.promoteot.org/
    The Fund to Promote Occupational Therapy is a nonprofit organization established to promote awareness and understanding of occupational therapy by the general public. The Fund promotes occupational therapy through various awareness campaigns and is a resource for occupational therapists who want to promote occupational therapy in their local communities.

THE AMERICAN OCCUPATIONAL THERAPY POLITICAL ACTION COMMITTEE

http://www.aota.org/nonmembers/area5/links/link04.asp
    The AOTPAC is a voluntary, nonprofit, unincorporated committee of members of AOTA. The AOTPAC was authorized by the Representative Assembly in 1976 and has been operational since the spring of 1978. The purpose of the AOTPAC is to further the legislative aims of the AOTA by influencing or attempting to influence the selection, nomination, election, or appointment of any individual to any federal public office, and of any occupational therapist, registered, certified occupational therapy assistant, or occupational therapy student member of the AOTA seeking election to public office at any level.

NATIONAL BOARD FOR CERTIFICATION IN OCCUPATIONAL THERAPY, INC.

http://www.nbcot.org/

The NBCOT is a not-for-profit credentialing agency responsible for certification for the occupational therapy profession. The NBCOT develops, administers and continually reviewing a certification process that reflects current standards of entry-level practice in occupational therapy. The NBCOT also works with state regulatory authorities, providing information on credentials, disciplinary actions, and regulatory and certification renewal issues. The NBCOT is responsible for establishing initial competency through its certification examination and has requirements for maintaining certification related to continuing education to promote continued competency.

Reference List

American Heritage college dictionary (3rd ed.). (1993). Boston, MA: Houghton Mifflin.

American Occupational Therapy Association. (1993). *Core values and attitudes of occupational therapy practice*. Bethesda, MD: American Occupational Therapy Association.

American Occupational Therapy Association. (2000). *Guidelines to the occupational therapy code of ethics*. Bethesda, MD: American Occupational Therapy Association.

American Occupational Therapy Association. (2003). *Reference guide to the occupational therapy code of ethics*. Bethesda, MD: American Occupational Therapy Association.

American Occupational Therapy Association. (2004a). *AOTA occupational therapy code of ethics*. Bethesda, MD: AOTA Press.

American Occupational Therapy Association. (2004b). AOTPAC Fact Sheet. American Occupational Therapy Association Web site. Available at *www.aota.org*

American Occupational Therapy Foundation. (2003). American Occupational Therapy Foundation Mission. American Occupational Therapy Foundation Web site. Available at *http://www.aotf.org/html/mission.html*

Aulisio, M. P., Arnold, R. M., & Younger, S. J. (2000). Health care ethics consultation: Nature, goals and competencies. A position paper from the Society for Health and Human Values–Society for Bioethics Consultation Task Force on Standards for Bioethics Consultation. *Annals of Internal Medicine, 133*, 59–69.

Bailey, D. M., & Schwartzberg, S. L. (2003). *Ethical and legal dilemmas*. Philadelphia, PA: F.A. Davis.

Barnitt, R. (1998). Ethical dilemmas in occupational therapy and physical therapy: A survey of practitioners in the UK National Health Service. *Journal of Medical Ethics, 24*, 193–199.

Barnitt, R., & Partridge, C. (1997). Ethical reasoning in physical therapy and occupational therapy. *Physiotherapy Research International, 2*, 178–194.

Beauchamp, T. L., & Childress, J. F. (2001). *Principles of biomedical ethics* (5th ed.) New York: Oxford University Press.

Benjamin, M., & Curtis, J. (2001). *Ethics in nursing*. New York: Oxford University Press.

Braveman, B., & Fisher, G. S. (1997). Managed care: Survival skills for the future. *Occupational Therapy in Health Care, 10*, 13–31.

Christiansen, C., & Baum, C. (1991). *Overcoming human performance deficits*. Thorofare, NJ: Slack.

Christiansen, C., & Lou, J. Q. (2001). Evidence-based practice forum: Ethical considerations related to evidence-based practice. *The American Journal of Occupational Therapy, 55*, 345–349.

Corbett, K. (1993). Ethics in occupational therapy practice. *Canadian Journal of Occupational Therapy, 60*, 115–119.

Diffendal, J. (2002). The rules: Knowing laws and ethics makes good OT practice. *Advance for Occupational Therapy Practitioners, 18*(4), 9–11.

Fletcher, J. C., Lombardo, P. A., Marshall, M. F., & Miller, F. G. (1997). *Introduction to clinical ethics* (2nd ed.). Hagerstown, MD: University Publishing Group.

Foye, S. J., Kirschner, K. L., Brady-Wagner, L. C., Stocking, C., & Siegler, M. (2002). Ethical issues in rehabilitation: A qualitative analysis of dilemmas identified by occupational therapists. *Topics in Stroke Rehabilitation, 9*, 89–101.

Hansen, R. A. (2003). Ethics in occupational therapy. In E. B. Crepeau, E. S. Cohn, & B. A. B. Schell (Eds.), *Willard & Spackman's occupational therapy* (10th ed., pp. 953–961). Philadelphia: Lippincott, Williams & Wilkins.

Jameton, A. (1990). Culture, morality, and ethics: Twirling the spindle. *Critical Care Nursing Clinics of North America, 2*, 443–451.

Joint Commission on Accreditation of Healthcare Organizations. (2004). Guidelines for document review. Section 1. Patient focused functions: Patient rights and organization ethics (RI). Joint Commission on Accreditation of Healthcare Organizations Web site. Available at *www.jcaho.org*

Jonsen, A. R., Siegler, M., & Winslade, W. J. (1998). *Clinical ethics*. New York: McGraw-Hill.

Kanny, E. M., & Kyler, P. L. (1999). Are faculty prepared to address ethical issues in education? *American Journal of Occupational Therapy, 53*, 72–74.

Kornblau, B. A., & Starling, S. P. (2000). *Ethics in rehabilitation: A clinical perspective*. Thorofare, NJ: Slack.

Kornblau, B. L. (2001). Your personal commitment. *American Journal of Occupational Therapy, 55*, 489–492.

Kyler, P. L. (1999). *Teaching ethics*. Bethesda, MD, American Occupational Therapy Association.

Lohman, H., & Brown, B. (1997). Ethical issues related to managed care: An in-depth discussion of an occupational therapy case study. *Occupational Therapy in Health Care, 10*, 1–12.

National Board for Certification in Occupational Therapy, Inc. (2004a). About Us. National Board for Certification in

Occupational Therapy, Inc. Web site. Available at *http:// www.nbcot.org/webarticles/anmviewer.asp?a=45&z=12*

National Board for Certification in Occupational Therapy, Inc. (2004b). OTR and COTA practitioners needed to serve on the Certification Examination Development Committee. National Board for Certification in Occupational Therapy, Inc. Web site. Available at *http://www.nbcot.org/*

Ontario Institute of Agrologists. (2004). Personal professionalism. Ontario Institute of Agrologists Web site. Available at *http://www.oia.on.ca/professionalism.htm*

Pelligrino, E. D. (1995). Toward a virtue-based normative ethics for the health professions. *Kennedy Institute of Ethics Journal, 5*, 253–277.

Purtilo, R. (1999). *Ethical dimensions in the health professions.* Philadelphia: W. B. Saunders.

Rogers, J. (1983). Clinical reasoning: The ethics, science and art. 1983 Eleanor Clarke Slagel lecture. *American Journal of Occupational Therapy, 37*, 601–616.

Russell, C., Fitzgerald, M. H., Williamson, P., Manor, D., & Whybrow, S. (2002). Independence as a practice issue in occupational therapy: The safety clause. *American Journal of Occupational Therapy, 56*, 369–379.

Scanlon, C., & Glover, J. (1995). Ethical issues. A professional code of ethics: Providing a moral compass for turbulent times. *ONF, 22*, 1515–1521.

Shannon, S. E. (1997). The roots of interdisciplinary conflict around ethical issues. *Critical Care Nursing Clinics of North America, 9*, 13–28.

Sim, J. (1997). *Ethical decision making in practice.* Oxford, UK: Butterworth Heinemann.

Starr, P. (1984). *The social transformation of American medicine.* New York: Basic Books.

Trompetter, L., Hansen, R., & Kyler-Hutchinson, P. (1998). *Reference guide to the occupational therapy code of ethics.* Bethesda, MD: American Occupational Therapy Association.

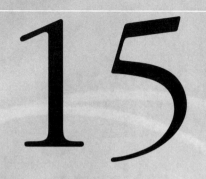

CHAPTER

15

Brent Braveman, Ph.D., OTR/L, FAOTA
Marcia Finlayson, Ph.D., OT(C), OTR/L

Introducing Others to Evidence-Based Practice

Real-Life Management

Angela is an occupational therapist with more than 20 years of experience. She has been a clinical supervisor for 12 years in an occupational therapy department in an acute rehabilitation hospital. She recently completed a postprofessional master's degree and conducted an evidence-based literature review for her master's project. After Angela presented her project to the staff as part of the departmental in-service program, Angela's boss, Lindsay, suggested that they may want to talk about ways to begin to educate and train all the staff in evidence-based practice skills.

Although Angela was excited that her presentation was so well received, and that her boss valued her new skills enough to ask for her assistance, she was also unsure about exactly what she could recommend to Lindsay. Initially, Angela had found the process of finding and evaluating evidence overwhelming. Prior to her return to school, she had not been to a library for many years and only had basic word-processing and Internet skills. Like many persons, Angela had assumed that evidence-based practice was an approach that only persons who had skills in research and advanced statistical knowledge could apply. Through the process of completing her project, she had become more comfortable with conducting and documenting literature searches, reading journal articles, and using books, the Internet, her own clinical judgment, and her professional network

to help her interpret the literature she found. She also now understood that, in addition to research evidence, often therapists have to learn to evaluate and make decisions using other types of evidence when research results are not yet available. However, even with her new skills and comfort level, she did not consider herself an expert. She found the idea of teaching others about evidence-based practice intimidating.

However, Angela was seldom one to back away from a challenge, so she decided to return to the library and to her network of peers to gather some information to prepare herself for her meeting with her boss. She could imagine some of the obstacles they would have to overcome, and she wanted to be able to offer solutions and strategies as well. Some of the obstacles that Angela identified included

- How would they convince staff members that they had the time to participate in evidence-based practice activities?
- Did all staff members have to become equally skilled in finding and evaluating evidence, or could they work as a team?
- What resources existed that she and her boss could use to train and educate staff about evidence-based practice?
- How could Angela and her boss organize tools and aids to help staff members begin to incorporate evidence-based practice into their everyday work?

Key Issues

- Managers must work to make both the time and the tools easily accessible to staff members to facilitate the incorporation of evidence-based practice approaches into their daily routines.
- Clinical experience and judgment, Web sites, case studies, opinion of experts, qualitative reports, and various forms of experimental designs are all valid forms of evidence, and managers must help their staff become comfortable with using all types of evidence to guide practice.
- There are many ways to create a culture in which evidence-based practice is valued, and managers can build structures within their department to support the adoption of an evidence-based approach.

In the spring of 2004, members of the Representative Assembly (RA) of the American Occupational Therapy Association (AOTA) convened. As noted in Chapter 14, the RA is the legislative and policy-making body of the organization, comprised of elected representatives from all 50 states, Puerto Rico, and the primary commissions and committees of the association. A number of initiatives related to evidence-based practice were placed before the RA for consideration. These initiatives ranged from requesting that the AOTA develop and endorse a "white paper" on evidence-based practice, to contracting with an unbiased researcher to conduct a formal evidence-based literature review on the efficacy of sensory integration.

Discussions of the various initiatives took place in smaller task groups. These groups were directed to discuss the initiatives and bring recommendations back to the full assembly for a vote. Through involvement in this process, a number of things became evident. First, there was wide variation in understanding *what* evidence-based practice means across the more than 70 participants (occupational therapists, occupational therapy assistants, and one consumer member). In fact, there even seemed to be varied understandings of how to answer the question, "What is evidence?" Some participants felt that evidence comes in various forms, including clinical experience, whereas other participants held the belief that evidence only meant finding and interpreting complicated empirical studies.

Second, there seemed to be a range of expectations regarding the level of involvement that might reasonably be expected by the "average practitioner." Some participants expressed the conviction that the association's efforts should be placed toward education and training to ensure that all occupational therapy practitioners adopt an evidence-based approach. Other participants had lower expectations, and concerns that many practitioners had limited access to computer technologies, limited skills and knowledge about how to use the Internet, and limited general skills in ways to find and evaluate evidence.

Third, some participants expressed the somewhat paradoxical view that, if we adopt an evidence-based approach, it may negatively impact payment for our services if insufficient evidence exists to justify reimbursement. These participants suggested that we should wait until there were more numerous studies related to the outcomes of occupational therapy intervention before initiating action.

Finally, what was most evident was that, although most participants seemed to think that adopting an evidence-based approach to practice was positive, there seemed to be little agreement on how big of a priority it should be for the profession, the AOTA, and individual occupational therapy practitioners.

Learning the knowledge and skills, and adopting the values and ethical behavior, to make your own practice *evidence-based* is challenging, and can become more challenging when you are not in an environment or working alongside peers who are also seeking to incorporate the use of evidence into their practice. Supervising, teaching, and guiding others to base their practice upon evidence is a responsibility that often falls to occupational therapy managers. Accepting this responsibility can be even more challenging, especially when some of the staff members you are supervising have been practicing for some time without using evidence-based strategies. Throughout this book, you have learned the principles and strategies for finding and evaluating evidence, and you have been introduced to the wide range of occupational therapy and related knowledge that an occupational therapy manager might use in developing, implementing, and improving occupational therapy programming. Chapter 15 will focus on how you can use the information that you have learned and combine it with additional strategies to introduce others to evidence-based practice. We will begin by considering how managers can create an environment that supports evidence-based practice.

Creating an Environment to Support Evidence-Based Practice

The occupational therapy manager can play a pivotal role in helping evidence-based practice to become the accepted approach to practice within the department that he or she manages. The manager can take the lead in creating an environment in which both the process and the outcomes of evidence-based practice are valued. In Chapter 3, you learned that the term *culture* is widely accepted to mean a learned, shared set of basic assumptions or shared way of doing things that is based upon the underlying values and beliefs of the members of a particular society or members of a group. You also learned that shared values serve to influence the actions of the members of an organization in several ways. Specifically, shared values

- Help turn commonplace, routine work into valued activities.
- Create a connection between the mission of the organization and society's values.
- Provide a source of competitive advantage to the organization.

As a manager, if you wish others to come to value evidence-based practice, you must model that value in your own behavior and attitudes. This modeling means accepting the responsibilities that come with evidence-based practice and holding those individuals you supervise responsible as well. In Chapter 1, you were introduced to the responsibilities stemming from evidence-based practice, and they are presented again in Box 15–1.

Box 15–1: Responsibilities Stemming from Evidence–Based Practice

- Staying up to date with the sources of information in your area of practice
- Communicating with others about what you have learned from synthesizing information
- Using good judgment about the information you have gathered by critically evaluating its quality
- Recognizing that translating evidence into everyday practice will not be easy and will require creativity

---

By identifying and articulating the related *values* to adopt, the occupational therapy manager can help make activities related to finding, evaluating, and incorporating evidence into practice both commonplace and valued routines. This is accomplished by connecting those activities to the department's and organization's mission and supporting and rewarding staff for adopting such routines. Most importantly, a manager must find ways to allow staff members the time to learn, practice, and perform evidence-based practice activities. You must take care that you are not sending contradictory messages to staff members by asking them to adopt evidence-based practices but then structuring their jobs so that they do not have the time to perform the tasks related to finding and evaluating evidence or to communicate effectively with their patients and clients to involve them in decisions about how to use evidence in practice.

One of the primary connections between organizational culture (e.g., shared values) and practice (what staff members do) that can facilitate evidence-based practice is the *organizational structure* that you put in place. Classically, organizational structure has been defined as the

> *"centralization of decision-making, formalization of rules, authority, communication, and compensation, standardization of work processes and skills, and/or control of output by acceptance of only adequate outcomes."* (Mintzberg, 1979)

This practice sounds more complicated that it is; in fact, much of Chapter 10 was devoted to describing how managers create organizational structures and turn theory into practice. Such methods and strategies are at the very center of the manager's role. These methods include designing work processes that guide where and when work is performed, articulating the specifications for outputs or the work products that are considered acceptable, making the tools and resources available to support staff in work performance, and assuring that staff have the necessary skills (e.g., competencies) by providing the kinds of training required to perform the work.

The remainder of this chapter will discuss ways that managers can build structures to create bridges from values to practice. We will begin by examining how occupational therapy managers can facilitate the adoption of evidence-based practice strategies within the profession of occupational therapy by actively supporting fieldwork students during their entrée to the profession.

Fieldwork and Entrée into a Profession

Graduates from today's occupational therapy educational programs are entering practice with more sophisticated skills to support evidence-based practice than ever before. This is due in large part to the profession's decision to move requirements for entry-level education to the master's degree level and eliminate baccalaureate education by the year 2007. Accreditation standards for educational programs for occupational therapists (Accreditation Council for Occupational Therapy Education, 1998) require that students be able to

1. Read and understand current research that affects practice and the provision of occupational therapy services.
2. Use professional literature to make informed practice decisions.
3. Know when and how to find and use national and international informational resources, including appropriate literature within and outside of occupational therapy.
4. Understand and interpret basic descriptive, correlational, and inferential statistics.

5. Understand and critique research studies, including various methodologies using both quantitative and qualitative designs.
6. Understand the importance of scholarly activities that will contribute to the development of a body of knowledge relevant to the profession of occupational therapy.

The fact that students are often entering practice settings as fieldwork students better prepared for evidence-based practice than their clinical fieldwork educators and their colleagues can be a challenge for the student, the supervisor, and the fieldwork site. With conscious effort on the part of the occupational therapy manager, however, this challenge can be turned into an opportunity. It is important that managers prepare all current staff, including those who serve as clinical fieldwork educators, to become comfortable with the increasing focus on using evidence in practice. It is also important that managers recognize the potential gap in skills that some practitioners may have and treat it as they would any other skill set that must be learned. By using some creativity and ingenuity, and involving staff members themselves in choosing strategies that best fit your setting, you can use the influx of new skills that fieldwork students may bring as an advantage and an opportunity. A few examples of ways of doing this are included in Box 15–2.

Evidence-Based Practice Competencies

In Chapter 7, you became familiar with the process of identifying and assessing competencies related to various aspects of practice. Including competencies on the knowledge, skills, attitudes, and critical and ethical reasoning necessary for evidence-based practice in your system for the assessment of competencies is a great example of building structures to support evidence-based practice. Furthermore, including competencies in the orientation process and in annual reviews allows you to identify the training needed by staff as they are hired, and to send a clear message to staff about the value of evidence-based practice in your department. Table 15–1 includes sample competencies related to

Box 15–2:	**Strategies for Closing the Gap in Evidence-Based Practice Skills Between Existing Staff and Fieldwork Students and New Graduates**

- Create an evidence-based library for staff members and fieldwork students in your department. Include examples of systematic reviews relevant to your setting, lists of useful Web sites, and examples of evidence-based review forms that they can use in their practice.
- Include an introduction to evidence-based resources, forms, tools, and expectations as part of the orientation process for both new staff members and fieldwork students.
- Encourage fieldwork students to contribute evidence-based resources and tools from their university program to the resources of your department.
- Pair fieldwork students who have more advanced computer skills for conducting formal literature searches with staff who have advanced clinical skills and judgment to find evidence related to a current clinical question.
- Collaborate with nursing, physical therapy, speech-language pathology, and other disciplines to have students work together in evidence-based practice assignments as a way of learning about teamwork and interdisciplinary practice.
- Have a staff member and a fieldwork student collaborate to present an in-service program to other staff and students on types of evidence, resources, and tools or to present a case in which they used evidence to guide decision making.
- Include fieldwork students and staff members on a task force to develop a plan for incorporating evidence-based practice in your setting.

evidence-based practice knowledge, skills, attitudes, and critical and ethical reasoning.

Teaching and Training Basics

Although much of what occupational therapists and occupational therapy assistants do with their patients and clients involves the teaching-learning process, occupational therapy practitioners learn relatively little about formal teaching strategies or how to respond to the learning needs of adult staff members in particular. Luckily, there are many easily accessible resources to guide these activities. Numerous Web pages provide hints and strategies on understanding adult learners, and ways to accommodate the fact that adults are typically motivated to learn for different reasons than children are. In addition, these resources provide suggestions on ways to structure learning experiences for adults more effectively.

Much of today's information on adult learners continues to be based on the work and perspectives of Malcolm Knowles (1913–1997), a central figure in U.S. adult education in the second half of the 20th century. In the 1950s, he was the Executive Director of the Adult Education Association of the United States of America. He wrote the first major accounts of informal adult education and the history of adult education in the United States (Smith, 2004). The available knowledge about adults as learners and the fields of adult learning, training, and training design have grown considerably in the last few decades.

If you are a manager in a hospital or school system, undoubtedly there is someone within your organization or system familiar with the learning needs of adult workers who can assist you in designing effective training materials and approaches for educating your staff. It is likely that that individual has specialized knowledge in training design and delivery. If so, you are encouraged to take advantage of that resource. In addition, an introduction to the basic concepts to consider is provided next.

Knowles (1970) identified the following characteristics of adult learners that must be considered when designing training and learning experiences

Table 15-1	Sample Competencies to Support Evidence-Based Practice			
Knowledge	**Skills**	**Attitudes**	**Critical Reasoning**	**Ethical Reasoning**
Knows occupational therapy conceptual practice models	Demonstrates use of relevant databases to find literature and evidence	Demonstrates appreciation of inclusion of patients in making intervention decisions based on evidence	Describes the process of decision making when there is limited evidence related to an aspect of intervention	Identifies limits to his or her knowledge in relation to various aspects of occupational therapy practice
Identifies evidence-based practice resources	Formulates a clinical question sufficiently narrow to guide a search for evidence	Demonstrates an appreciation for life-long learning and skill development	Describes the process of decision making when there is contradictory evidence related to an aspect of intervention	Identifies steps to take if he or she is feeling unduly pressured into providing intervention that he or she feels is inappropriate or will be ineffective
Is familiar with relevant models in related fields	• Selects and applies appropriate criteria to evaluate the specific form of evidence • Evaluates and summarizes the evidence reviewed to answer the clinical question • Describes summary of evidence using language and concepts appropriate to the audience (e.g., health care team, consumer, payer)		• Is able to give examples of how to combine clinical experience with evidence in order to deduce logical possible intervention options • Demonstrates ability to generalize application of evidence from one clinical case to similar clinical cases	• Demonstrates steps to incorporate evolving evidence into his or her professional development plan to maintain competence • Demonstrates ability to balance clinical expertise, available evidence, and client goals to make a clinical decision

such as those often used to introduce new knowledge in the workplace:

- Adults are autonomous and self-directed. Adults want to become active participants in the learning process and are often effective in guiding their own learning. Adult learners can assist you in identifying their learning needs and will often readily share their interests if asked, and these interests can be used to motivate learning.
- Adults bring their considerable life experiences and knowledge *from the workplace and other environments to the learning situation*. Adults desire to connect new learning to prior experiences. Relating new knowledge, theories, and concepts to existing knowledge will help adults frame the learning experience and make more sense of it.
- Adults are goal-oriented. Adults enter a learning experience with particular goals and learning objectives in mind. Asking adults why they are taking part in learning can help you connect learning activities to these goals and increase learner satisfaction.
- Adults are relevancy-oriented. Adults want to understand *why* they are being taught something and want to see the connection between learning activities and materials, and their goals, daily responsibilities, and future needs.
- Adults are practical. Adults typically prefer to learn what is of most interest and use to them and may not be interested in learning for learning's sake.

In addition, adults typically have motivations for learning that differ from those of children (Cantor, 1992). Understanding these motivations also help in designing effective learning experiences for adult workers. These motivations include

- To make or maintain social relationships
- To meet external expectations such as those mandated in the workplace or by accrediting or licensure bodies
- To learn to better serve others more effectively
- To achieve professional advancement and recognition
- To escape routine responsibilities or for intellectual stimulation
- For pure interest

It is not uncommon for the occupational therapy manager to develop and run educational sessions as part of department staff meetings alone or in conjunction with other managers or supervisors. Whenever possible, you are encouraged to take advantage of local subject matter experts and to be flexible about collaborating with other practitioners and managers in your local area. However, when you do find yourself responsible for leading a discussion or providing staff with instruction, keep in mind that instructors can help to motivate students via several means (Lieb, 2003; Wlodkowski, 2003).

First, you should establish a friendly, open atmosphere that shows the participants that questions and participation are welcome. Setting a tone appropriate to the level of importance of the objective is essential. If the material has a high level of importance, a higher level of tension/stress should be established in the class to indicate the importance of what you are covering. However, people learn best under low to moderate stress; if the stress is too high, it becomes a barrier to learning. You must carefully consider the degree of difficulty of the materials you are covering as well. The degree of difficulty should be set high enough to challenge participants but not so high that they become frustrated by information overload (Lieb, 2003). This balance is especially important when first introducing a topic such as evidence-based practice. It's better not to try to accomplish too much at one time. A good way to start is to identify long-term learning objectives (or the competencies you want staff to develop) and to break those objectives or competencies down into smaller units of learning that can be achieved within the time you have allotted for any given session.

In work settings, adults find themselves participating in learning experiences out of interest and desire to learn, but they are also highly likely to participate because they are instructed to do so by their supervisor. In deciding how to construct the learning experience, you should carefully consider how you present it to staff, as well as the attitude that your staff has toward the training. If staff members are hesitant because of a lack of confidence, because they cannot clearly see the value of training, or because they are pressured for time, you may want to start by providing low-stress and low-demand learning aimed primarily at introducing the value of the topic. Time pressures are among the major barriers reported in the literature to engaging in evidence-based practice. As a manager, you will have to create a structure that will support staff members to learn about evidence-based practice, and then later to apply what they have learned. You play a major role in minimizing these time pressures in the ways that you structure workloads and in-service and continuing education time.

A learner's affect, or emotional experience, while learning can influence the meaning and relevance he or she attaches to the learning. This does not mean that learning must always be "fun," but the introduction to learning about important topics such as evidence-based practice should be consciously and thoughtfully planned. If it is evident that your staff is nervous, distracted by other work responsibilities, or not invested in the learning experience, it will be important for you to resolve these issues before focusing on the specific learning objectives you have identified. Some ideas on different ways to resolve these issues are provided in Table 15–2.

Strategies for Teaching Each Step of the Evidence-Based Practice Process

In Chapter 1, you were introduced to the steps of the evidence-based practice process. These steps are repeated in Box 15–3, and strategies for teaching each step are discussed in this section. Presenting the steps of this process to your staff and using them as a guide for organizing and structuring

Table 15-2	Challenges and Potential Solutions to Introducing Your Staff to Evidence-Based Practice
Challenge	**Potential Solutions**
Staff members are nervous about evidence-based practice (EBP)	1. Start slowly, and use the steps of EBP to guide the development of your educational sessions. Break each step down, and think about how you can grade the skills within each step up and down. 2. Use worksheets, flowcharts, and other visual aids to guide staff along, step by step. 3. Emphasize the importance of clinical expertise in the EBP process, and build on the staff's confidence in this area to build confidence in the other areas of EBP. 4. Use small discussion and problem-solving groups so staff members can build and learn from each other's strengths.
Staff members are distracted by work responsibilities	1. Incorporate the EBP in-services and activities into the normal meetings in your department; ensure that they are not "add-on" activities. 2. Set up the EBP activities so that they are completed by teams of therapists so that the work can be shared. 3. Identify times of the month or year that have lower patient census, and organize EBP activities to correspond to these times. 4. Consider some type of workload incentive for EBP activity involvement.
Staff members are not invested in the learning experience	1. Bring in therapists from other local departments who are using EBP to talk about how and why EBP is useful. 2. Focus each EBP in-service on a specific patient problem that one of the therapists in the department is dealing with, using the in-service to help the therapist solve the problem. 3. Obtain the necessary certification to ensure that the EBP in-services will give the therapists continuing education credits for licensure, if relevant in your jurisdiction. 4. Consider some type of workload incentive for EBP activity involvement.

Box 15–3: **The Evidence–Based Practice Process**

Step 1: Set a question related to a *practice problem.*

Step 2: *Locate resources* that may contain information relevant to the question.

Step 3: Conduct a *critical appraisal* on each resource.

Step 4: *Evaluate and summarize* overall findings.

Step 5: *Answer your practice question,* using your findings, your experience, and the input of your client or clients.

Step 6: *Implement the findings* within your practice.

learning experiences is a helpful way of meeting the need that adult learners have for knowing *why* they are being asked to learn and *how* the new knowledge will be of help and use in their everyday lives.

The first step of the evidence-based practice process is *developing a well-defined and well-built question.* A great first exercise to help teach question development is involving staff in a group examination of their current practice. Reflecting on the current struggles and challenges that staff members are facing will help to make the relevance of the learning clear. Law (2002) noted that well-built clinical questions include three elements: (1) client/population, (2) intervention or exposure (e.g., the use of a specific assessment technique, treatment setting, or model of service delivery), and (3) outcome.

One strategy for helping your staff members develop well-defined and well-built questions is to have them work in groups to begin this process. Perhaps you can start with a large group activity, having staff brainstorm topics for clinical questions. Then the larger group can be broken down into smaller working groups to focus the questions and to prepare a well-built clinical question, using the three previously mentioned points to guide them. You may want to have these small groups share some common experiences—for example, they all work in particular service areas such as pediatrics or mental health, or they are all trying to select a new assessment tool for a particular

client problem. You might also consider pairing within the small groups any occupational therapists and occupational therapy assistants who often collaborate.

Once the small groups have completed their questions, the teaching group can reconvene, share their work, and critique the questions identified by others. The critiques should focus on whether the questions contain the three components of a well-built question. Because the small groups are likely to have identified more than a single question, it may also be necessary for you to lead a discussion about which questions should be a priority to address in your setting. A worksheet for developing clinical questions is presented in Appendix 15–1 at the end of the chapter.

The second step in the evidence-based practice process is *locating resources relevant to the clinical question.* An effective strategy for helping staff become more comfortable with locating resources is to combine didactic instruction with experiential learning. In other words, you should begin by demonstrating and explaining resources to your staff members and then allow them time to experiment and practice on their own. Providing learners with "tip sheets" to guide their practice sessions is recommended. Such sheets may be ones that you develop on your own, or they may come from one of many resources on evidence-based practice that are listed at the end of this chapter. Using the readily available online tutorials from the companies that run the major search databases is also an effective way of providing training in locating evidence; for example, tutorials are available from the OVID Web site (*http://www.ovid.com/*) (OVID, 2004).

Another strategy for helping staff become more comfortable with locating resources is to create a step-by-step example that they can replicate. That is, you can set your own clinical question and conduct a search to address it, keeping careful track of everything that you do and recording it in detail in a handout you can give to your staff to replicate. After they are finished, you can lead a discussion on what ideas they have for improving or refining the search, and then have them make these adaptations. This strategy is particularly useful for staff members who have very limited computer-searching experience, and need to develop their confidence in their ability to think through and conduct searches.

The third step in the evidence-based practice

process is *appraising the resources that have been located during the search*. This is typically the step of the process that staff finds the most difficult, regardless of the type of resource that needs to be evaluated. Having staff members work in small groups is again recommended because it allows them to share their strengths, to see how others process information, to ask questions of others, and to provide and receive support to limit frustration. Providing structured forms to guide documentation of the evaluation of evidence is helpful. These forms should be easily accessible to your staff in hard copy, or they could be loaded on department computers to be filled out over a period of time. Either way, you want to make it easy for staff members to use the forms in a way that fits their work styles and workloads. Samples of questions to guide the development of such forms are provided throughout Chapter 1. In addition, sample appraisal forms that can be used for research articles and program descriptions, as well as a Web site, are presented in Appendices 15–2 through 15–5 at the end of this chapter. As your staff members' skills in evidence-based practice develop, you may want to encourage them to develop their own appraisal forms and customize them to focus on the types of information that are the most salient for their everyday practices.

The fourth step in the evidence-based practice process is *evaluating and summarizing what has been found*. This integration phase can be the most difficult if the information that has been located is contradictory or inconclusive. In order to help staff members think about *how* to evaluate and summarize information, you may want to have them read some existing evidence-based reviews. For example, staff could read the evidence briefs series conducted by the AOTA, or review a couple of relevant Cochrane reviews that are available online. Another resource is the Occupational Therapy Critically Appraised Topics Web site (*http://www.otcats. com/*). By reviewing existing evidence-based practice review summaries, staff members will be able to develop comfort with how such summaries are organized conceptually and how terminology is used. They will then be able to use these examples as a template for thinking about their own summaries for the information they have read.

Another strategy for helping staff members to evaluate and summarize the information they are gathering is to provide them with a glossary of terms that they may be encountering during their reading. An example of such a glossary is provided in Box 15–4. Finally, choosing a standard "levels of evidence" typology for evaluating the literature (see Chapter 1) for use in your department may be helpful. You should use the typology consistently, and consider incorporating it into the forms that staff members will use during the process of appraising the literature they find. This will help staff members start to see the relationship between different types of evidence, and what each of these types can and cannot offer to their clinical decision-making processes.

After evaluating and summarizing the evidence, the next step in the evidence-based practice process is to *answer the initial clinical question*. Helping staff members to become proficient in this step of the evidence-based process involves getting them to connect their findings from the literature, their own clinical experience, and the goals of the client or clients to which the information they have gathered applies. Connecting all of these things can be complicated and may require a range of coordinated strategies that extend over time. No one learns evidence-based practice in an afternoon. Rather, managers help staff learn to apply evidence-based practice by building structures to support its use. Emphasizing the value of evidence-based practice, and building it into the expectations and culture of your organization, will go a long way to incorporating it into the everyday work routines of employees. Using activities similar to those listed earlier in Box 15–2 will help you and your staff develop the *routines* of evidence-based practice. Additional examples of activities to assist with building and supporting evidence-based practice in the everyday routine of work are listed in Box 15–5.

A key part of the final step of evidence-based practice is to communicate the evidence that has been found to others to *integrate and apply it to actual practice*. You and your staff will need to communicate evidence to your clients, your patients, or the consumers of occupational therapy. You will also need to communicate evidence to the other health professionals in your department and organization, as well as those individuals and companies that pay for your services. Communicating

Box 15–4: Glossary of Evidence-Based Practice Terminology

- **Electronic bibliographic database:** Electronic compilations of published research, scholarly articles, books, government reports, newspaper articles, and other recognized sources of information.
- **Critical appraisal:** The process of judging the quality of a piece of information and determining its applicability to practice.
- **Critical appraisal matrix:** A systematic method of summarizing a series of critical appraisals from individual articles to facilitate comparisons and decision making.
- **Electronic table of contents alerts:** A service provided by professional and scientific journals whereby alerts are e-mailed whenever articles that include key words you submit are published.
- **Levels of evidence:** A criterion-referenced typology and classification system that provides guidance for evaluating the quality of a research article; these levels are multilayered, typically including criteria for design, sample size, and internal and external validity.
- **Literature search:** A systematic, explicit, and reproducible method for identifying, evaluating, and interpreting the existing body of recorded work produced by researchers, scholars, and practitioners.
- **Sample size:** The number of participants in a study.
- **Validity:** There are two broad categories of validity: validity of methodology, which includes internal and external validity, and validity of measurement, which includes content, criterion, and construct validity. Ultimately, validity addresses whether or not a research design or a measurement tool was able to capture what it intended to capture (i.e., can the design answer the question posed; does the measurement tool measure what it says it does). Definitions of the different types of validity are as follows:
  - *Internal validity:* Addresses the question of whether or not there are other potential explanations for study findings that are a function of the study design (e.g., biases in sampling or measurement, history or maturation effects, testing effects).
- *External validity:* Addresses the question of generalizability, and to whom the study findings can be applied. External validity is influenced primarily by the sampling method of the study, and whether or not there was differential dropout of participants.
- *Content validity:* A type of validity related to measurement that addresses the question of whether a particular instrument contains all relevant domains of content, given its intent.
- *Construct validity:* Addresses the question of whether or not the instrument produces scores that demonstrate the expected relationships, based on theory, with other concepts and variables. Construct validity is population specific, and built over time through hypothesis testing. There are two types of construct validity: discriminate validity (hypothesize what your tool will *not* correspond with, and test this), and convergent validity (hypothesize what your tool *will* correspond with, and test this).
- *Criterion validity:* Addresses the question of whether the instrument produces scores that approximate or correspond to an existing instrument that measures the same concept or construct, sometimes identified as the "gold standard." There are two types of criterion validity: concurrent validity (when the two instruments are administered at the same time and results compared) and predictive validity (when the current instrument is administered and then another one is used in the future; used when an instrument is being evaluated for its ability to identify characteristics or behaviors sooner than current tests allow).

Box 15–5: Strategies for Building Evidence-Based Practice into the Everyday Routines of Work

- Take advantage of skills and preferences. Not all staff will be skilled at conducting literature reviews or summarizing evidence. Create partnerships in which one staff member covers another's duties so that he or she may spend time in tasks specific to evidence-based practice.
- Train fieldwork students to learn and adopt evidence-based practice by building assignments into fieldwork experiences.
- Use volunteers; put specific requests into your volunteer office for students or others who might have skills in finding or preparing forms of evidence for review.
- Make evidence-based practice activities part of the work routine by scheduling article reviews and case discussions to generate clinical questions.
- Start a journal club to help staff develop skills in critical appraisal.
- Create partnerships with other local occupational therapy departments to share the work and benefits of conducting evidence-based practice reviews.
- Create, load, and maintain a list of evidence-based practice "favorite" Internet links on your department computers so that sites are easily found and accessed.
- Create interdisciplinary evidence-based practice *investigation teams* by having occupational therapists, occupational therapy assistants, physical therapists, nurses, and others work together to research and answer shared clinical questions.
- Encourage, recognize, and reward staff members who become *clinical resource experts* in a topic, in an area of intervention, or with diagnostic groups frequently seen in your practice setting.
- Create and maintain *reference sheets* that spell out the steps to find and evaluate evidence and put them everywhere (i.e., on all computers, on the wall near computers, etc.) so that staff members have easy access.

---

about the evidence is critical so key decision makers (e.g., patients, family members, other care providers, payers) can be involved in deciding whether an intervention is warranted given what you know about the likelihood that it will be effective. More importantly, communicating about the evidence will increase the likelihood that these decisions are well informed, and based on more than just a guess about what might work.

Because you and your staff will be communicating with different sorts of persons with varying interests and investment in the occupational therapy process, you will need to become comfortable with talking about the same evidence in different ways. Organizational leaders and managers from other departments will be concerned about resource utilization, including staff, space, equipment, and supplies. Payers will be concerned about costs to them and will want information such as the frequency and duration of intervention necessary to achieve desired outcomes. Patients will want to know whether the intervention is going to work, and how long it might take to see results. Law (2002) suggested that, regardless of whom you are communicating with, your message is more likely to be understood if it has the following attributes:

1. Nontechnical, simple, and concrete language with simple grammatical structure
2. Terms that cross cultures and perspectives
3. Brevity, with just enough detail for decision making
4. Checks for confusion or lack of comprehension
5. Suggestions for concrete actions related to the information

Most importantly, you must keep in mind your responsibility to involve others in making decisions in a real way. Evidence-based practice *is not* a strategy for justifying to others what you have *already* decided to do, but rather a strategy for involving others in making decisions about what you *should* do in the future given what you know now.

As a second key part of the final step in the evidence-based practice process, it is critically important to ensure ongoing evaluation of the information being applied to practice. It is not enough to teach your staff members to find and evaluate evidence; you must also provide them guidance for evaluating whether the decisions they are making based on what they are learning are really making a difference. Tracking these changes may mean having to go back to the literature and reconsider assessment and outcomes tools, and other systems for monitoring progress and change. Evidence-based practice is a cycle—one does not simply answer a question and move on. One must answer the question, evaluate the response, and perhaps refine the question or develop a new one. Evidence-based practice is an ongoing way of doing and improving practice.

The next section of this chapter will focus on examples of specific structures and tools that managers can create and use to support evidence-based practice and to help it become part of the everyday routines of work.

Creating the Tools to Support Evidence-Based Practice

The following are examples of structures and tools that managers can put in place and use to support evidence-based practice becoming part of the everyday routines of work performed by the staff they supervise:

- *Worksheets for developing clinical questions:* Writing well-built clinical questions can be challenging. A worksheet can break down the components of a question, making it easier for clinicians to develop questions that are targeted and clear to follow.
- *Article review worksheets:* A written worksheet with predetermined questions can be useful to guide readers through the process of reviewing an article and assigning a level of evidence. Worksheets can be developed for different types

of articles (quantitative, qualitative case reports, program descriptions, etc.) and kept in easily accessible files in hard copy or loaded onto computers. Worksheets can also be developed for Web sites, books, or any other type of resource commonly accessed for information in your department.
- *Critical appraisal matrices:* Charts can be constructed to summarize articles that are reviewed (see Appendix 15–6 at the end of the chapter). Matrices can be custom designed to capture the most salient information for your setting and your particular clinical problem. In a department, it would be possible to start a matrix on a computer, and have different therapists add to it as they find new literature.
- *Glossary of evidence-based practice terminology:* A list of definitions of commonly cited concepts, tools, and strategies used in evidence-based practice is also useful. Glossaries are simple ways of reinforcing key concepts as they are learned and help limit confusion among practitioners.
- *Evidence-based practice competencies:* Competencies are explicit statements that define specific areas of expertise and are related to effective or superior performance in a job. Competencies can relate to a point in an employee's employment or routine managerial processes, such as employee orientation or annual performance appraisals, or to the intervention process, such as when learning a new skill.

Chapter Summary

This book overviewed the primary functions of an occupational therapy manager and provided strategies for using theory and evidence related to a wide range of occupational therapy knowledge and knowledge from related fields to guide performance. Although most of the book focused on the use of various forms of data, information, and other evidence used by managers to lead and direct occupational therapy services, this chapter focused on introducing evidence-based practice to others. Specifically, this chapter examined ways that managers can build organizational structures to help integrate evidence-based practice activities into the everyday work routines of occupational therapy staff.

Once a manager and the staff members he or she supervises adopt the values that underlie evidence-based practice and are ready to accept the corresponding responsibilities, they must also adopt new ways of working. Managers can facilitate this process by providing learning opportunities for staff, by making the tools to support evidence-based practice easily accessible, and by integrating the process of finding and evaluating evidence with other systems, such as a system for the assessment of competencies and reward structures.

It was stressed in this chapter that, as adults, staff members have characteristics and needs as learners that must be recognized if a manager is going to develop and deliver an effective educational experience. Fortunately, there are often resources available within larger organizations in which occupational therapy managers work to aid in the development and delivery of staff education and training. For managers who work in settings where this type of assistance is not available on site, or for business owners who often must meet varied staff needs on their own, there are many easily accessible resources available on the Internet. Networking with other managers in your local area or through the use of some of the resources noted throughout this book, such as professional Listservs, are also

strategies that can help managers effectively respond to the educational and training needs of staff.

Learning any complicated skill set can be a challenge, and evidence-based practice indeed requires that practitioners learn a varied set of skills that allow them to find, evaluate, communicate about, and integrate evidence into their service delivery. Managers face the challenge of learning not only to incorporate clinical evidence into their practice but also to recognize that evidence exists on a wide range of topics and issues, including organizational culture, leadership, supervision, program development, and communication, that can guide their practice as a manager. However, with the proliferation of books, articles, and Internet sites, and increased attention paid to evidence-based medicine and practice by accrediting bodies for educational programs and service delivery programs, it seems unlikely that this is a challenge that occupational therapy managers can avoid.

At the start of the chapter, you were introduced to Angela, who had recently learned more about the evidence-based practice process and had begun an endeavor to introduce others in her department to evidence-based practice and to facilitate their skill development.

Real-Life Solutions

As Angela began to search for information on teaching evidence-based practice to others, she noticed that much of what she initially encountered focused on evaluating the most advanced types of evidence, such as quantitative experimental investigations. It struck her that, for a novice, the mistaken idea that other forms of evidence, including qualitative research, program descriptions, case reports, expert opinions, and, most importantly, a therapist's own clinical experience and judgment, were not valid might be reinforced. Angela also felt sure that one of the biggest obstacles to the other staff members in her department investing energy in learning about evidence-based practice would be helping them to find ways that they could find the time to integrate these new strategies into their daily work lives.

Angela decided to pull together some resources that could be used by the staff, including examples of critical appraisal questions and forms for different types of articles, information on free Internet-based tutorials on conducting searches in electronic bibliographic databases, and a list of Internet sites that included summaries of evidence, such as the evidence-based briefs series published by the AOTA or the Cochrane Library. Although it was evident to Angela that making these resources readily available to the staff in paper or electronic formats would help, it also seemed clear that editing some of the forms to minimize the use of scientific language would make it easier for staff members to use the forms and to interpret and discuss with others the results of evidence-based analyses. Angela made a note to herself to start to draft a glossary of terms that staff members would

(continued)

commonly encounter so that they could refer to it and be less likely to feel overwhelmed.

When Angela met with her boss, Lindsay, to discuss what she had pulled together, she found that Lindsay had been busy as well. She had already reviewed some of the resources available on the Internet and had contacted a representative in the human resources and information management department to obtain assistance in designing training sessions on evidence-based practice and designing or purchasing tutorials on searching electronic bibliographic databases that could be accessed through the hospital's Intranet. In addition, Lindsay had started to think about how the adoption of evidence-based practice could be supported and how she could communicate expectations as a manager by building activities related to evidence-based practice into existing departmental structures. For example, she had begun to consider the types of competencies that might be developed and that all staff would expect to be able to demonstrate.

As Angela and Lindsay continued to collaborate, they began to establish a network of other managers and clinicians who were also committed to promoting evidence-based practice. Through this network, they learned about some of the creative ways that other departments were having staff members work in groups to seek evidence to clinical questions they identified. Among other strategies, they found that some clinical departments were partnering with academicians, using volunteers, pairing field-work students with advanced clinicians, having weekly evidence-based practice brown-bag lunch seminars, and creating evidence-based practice teams composed of clinicians from multiple disciplines.

Angela and Lindsay both agreed that they would encounter resistance and roadblocks as they worked to introduce evidence-based practice as an expectation for the department's staff. They knew that some staff members would think that it took too much time, other staff members would lack confidence in their skills to learn to search for evidence and evaluate it when found, and still others would be resistant to adopting the values and responsibilities related to including patients, families, and others in using evidence to make clinical decisions. However, Lindsay recounted the experience she had had just a few years earlier when the hospital introduced its computerized medical record system. She noted that, at first, most of the staff complained about having to spend time in trainings and how one of the staff had simply stated that she was "too old of a dog to learn new tricks!" Yet, in less than a year, all of the staff members were routinely using the computer to document their interventions and she had not heard a complaint in months. Granted, it had taken extra effort by some of the staff members who were less comfortable with newer technology, but even they had eventually recognized the value of the new system. Lindsay was optimistic that it would be the same with evidence-based practice.

Useful Resources for Introducing Others to Evidence-Based Practice

General Information on Finding and Evaluating the Literature

- Cochrane Collaboration and the Cochrane Library (*http://www.cochrane.org/index0.htm*)
- Health Information Research Unit at McMaster University (*http://hiru.mcmaster.ca/*)
- Database of Abstracts of Reviews of Effects (DARE) (*http://nhscrd.york.ac.uk/darehp.htm*)

Occupational Therapy–Specific Resources on Evidence-Based Practice

- OTSeeker (*http://www.otseeker.com/*)
- OT Critically Appraised Topics (*http://www.otcats.com/*)
- AOTA Evidence-Based Practice Project (*http://www.aota.org/*)
- Center for Evidence-Based Rehabilitation at McMaster University (*http://www.fhs.mcmaster.ca/rehab/centre.htm*)

Journals That Are Likely to Include Evidence Relevant to Administration and Management of Health Care Services

THE MILBANK QUARTERLY

The Milbank Quarterly has been published for over seven decades and features peer-reviewed original research and articles that review health care policy and provide analysis of current and evolving policy. Other content includes commentary from a range of professionals representing academicians, practitioners, researchers and policy makers. Articles and commentary found in this journal represent multidisciplinary perspectives on empirical research as well as the application of research and policy in a variety of settings. Social, legal, and ethical issues are addressed.

JOURNAL OF HEALTH SERVICES RESEARCH & POLICY

The *Journal of Health Services Research & Policy* includes articles presenting results of qualitative and quantitative multidisciplinary research from a wide variety of disciplines. In addition to the reporting of empirical results, articles also address current and evolving debates in the scientific, methodological and empirical arenas.

HEALTH SERVICES RESEARCH

The journal, *Health Services Research*, provides researchers, policy makers and analysts, and health care administrators and managers with access to empirical findings as well as articles addressing policy and methodological issues. Readers interested in health care financing, the organization or delivery of health services, or in the evaluation of health delivery outcomes will find *Health Services Research* a useful resource. The journal provides a forum for the exchange of practices related individuals, health systems, and communities.

Professional Organizations Relevant to Administration and Management of Health Care Services

AMERICAN COLLEGE OF HEALTH CARE EXECUTIVES

http://www.ache.org/

The American College of Healthcare Executives (ACHE) is an international professional society of health care executives working in a variety of settings including hospitals, health care systems, and other health care organizations. The ACHE is known for its credentialing and educational programs. The annual Congress on Healthcare Management is a nationally recognized and widely attended event. The ACHE publishes the *Journal of Healthcare Management,* and a magazine titled *Healthcare Executive.*

Government-Related Web sites and Documents

- Centers for Disease Control and Prevention (*http://www.cdc.gov/*)
- National Center for Health Statistics (*http://www.cdc.gov/nchs/*)
- Agency for Health Care Research and Quality (*http://www.ahcpr.gov/*)
- Centers for Medicare and Medicaid Services (*http://cms.hhs.gov/providers/edi/default.asp*)

Resources on Evaluating Information Found on Web Sites

- Beck, S. (1997). Evaluation criteria. In *The Good, The Bad & The Ugly: or, Why It's a Good Idea to Evaluate Web Sources.* Available at *http://lib.nmsu.edu/instruction/evalcrit.html*
- The University of California Berkeley Library *http://www.lib.berkeley.edu/TeachingLib/Guides/Internet/Evaluate.html*

Reference List

Accreditation Council for Occupational Therapy Education. (1998). *Standards for an accredited educational program for the occupational therapist.* Bethesda, MD: American Occupational Therapy Association.

Cantor, J. (1992). *Delivering instruction to adult learners.* Toronto: Wall & Emerson.

Knowles, M. (1970). *The modern practice of adult education: Andragogy vs. pedagogy.* New York: Association Press.

Law, M. (2002). *Evidence-based rehabilitation: A guide to practice.* Thorofare, NJ: Slack.

Lieb, S. (2003). Principles of adult learning. Honolulu Community College Intranet Home Page. Available at *http://honolulu.hawaii.edu/intranet/committees/FacDevCom/guidebk/teachtip/adults-2.htm*

Mintzberg, H. (1979). *The structuring of organizations.* Englewood Cliffs, NJ: Prentice-Hall.

OVID (2004). Online tutorials. OVID Technologies Web site. Available at *http://www.ovid.com/site/help/sp_tutorials. jsp?top=28&mid=29&bottom=31&subsection=58*

Smith, M. K. (2004). Malcolm Knowles, informal adult education, self-direction and andragogy. In *The Encyclopedia of*

Informal Education. infed.org Web site. Available at *www.infed.org/thinkers/et-knowl.htm*

Wlodkowski, R. (2003). Strategies to enhance adult motivation to learn. Nebraska Literacy Home Page. Available at *http://literacy.kent.edu/~nebraska/curric/ttim1/artsum2.html*

Appendix 15–1: Sample Worksheet for Developing Clinical Questions

Identify the client population: _____

Identify the intervention or exposure: _____

Identify the comparison intervention or exposure (if applicable): _____

Identify the outcome of interest: _____

Using the information above, write your clinical question:

_____

_____

_____

Appendix 15–2: Sample Article Review Worksheet 1

Article Describing the Outcomes of an Intervention Using Quantitative Methods

Citation:

Study Purpose/Question/Hypothesis:

- What was the guiding purpose, question, or hypothesis for this study?

Sampling:

- What was the sampling procedure?
  - ☐ Probability based (e.g., simple random sample)
  - ☐ Non–probability based (e.g., convenience sample, consecutive sample)

Sample:

- What is the average age of the sample?
- What is the gender distribution of the sample?
- What is the racial or ethnic distribution of the sample?
- What is the setting in which the sample is based (e.g., community, institution)?
- Based on the above information, is my patient similar to those described in the study?

Intervention:

- What was the experimental intervention used in the study?
- Was there a comparison intervention? If yes, what was it?
- Is there enough detail provided about the intervention that I could replicate it?
- Based on my interactions with my patient, would the experimental intervention be a good match?
- Would the experimental intervention be a good match for my time, resources, and capabilities or those of others in my setting?

Outcomes:

- What outcomes were expected from the experimental intervention?
- Are the outcomes consistent with the goals of my patient?
- Are the outcomes consistent with expectations of outcomes of third-party payers?
- What instruments were used to measure the outcomes?
- Were the reliability and validity of the measurement tools provided?

Results:

- Are the results of the study clearly stated?
- Was a prior hypothesis tested, or were the findings accidental?
- Is it clear how subjects were included in the analyses (i.e., can I account for all subjects in the study)?
- Is there a significant difference before and after the experimental intervention?
- Is there a significant difference between the experimental intervention group and the comparison group (if applicable) at the end of the study?
- If results were not statistically significant (either before/after or between groups), are there other reasons to still consider the intervention?

Overall Appraisal:

- Are there biases that I believe influenced the quality and believability of the study? Consider: sampling method, sample composition, consistency between the intervention and the outcome measures, assignment of subjects to groups, measurement process (i.e., use of blinding, if realistic), quality of analysis, and so forth.
- Based on my clinical experience, do the experimental intervention and the outcomes reported make sense?

Reasons to Adopt This Intervention (Benefits)	Reasons Not to Adopt This Intervention (Risks and Costs)
1.	1.
2.	2.
3.	3.
4.	4.

Decision and Rationale:

Based on the information at this time, I will make the following recommendation to my patient regarding the benefits, risks, costs, and alternatives of this intervention:

Appendix 15–3: Sample Article Review Worksheet 2

Article Describing Experiences of People and/or Phenomena of Interest
Using Qualitative Methods

Citation:

Study Purpose/Question/Hypothesis:

- What was the guiding purpose or question for this study?

Sampling:

- How were people recruited for this study?
- What are the potential limitations or biases inherent in this approach relative to the experiences being studied?

Sample:

- What is the average age of the sample?
- What is the gender distribution of the sample?
- What is the racial or ethnic distribution of the sample?
- What is the setting in which the sample is based (e.g., community, institution)?
- Based on the above information, is my patient similar to those described in the study?

Experiences or Phenomena of Interest:

- What was the experience or phenomenon that the researchers were trying to understand?
- How does understanding this experience or phenomenon relate to my practice?
- How did the researchers go about learning about these experiences/phenomena?
- What did the researchers learn? What were their key findings?
- Are the findings supported through the presentation of raw data (e.g., quotes, etc.)?

Overall Appraisal:

- Are there biases that I believe influenced the quality and believability of the study? Consider: sampling method, sample composition, methods of data collection, characteristics of the data collector, methods of analysis, and so forth.
- Based on my clinical experience, do the findings make sense?

Reasons to Use the Findings	Reasons Not to Use the Findings
1.	1.
2.	2.
3.	3.
4.	4.

Decision and Rationale:

Based on the information at this time, I will make the following recommendation to my patient regarding the benefits, risks, costs, and alternatives of the findings presented in this article:

Appendix 15–4: Sample Worksheet for Evaluating a Web Site

Web Address:

Web Developer:

Areas for Appraisal:

- Is the purpose of the Web site clear?
- Who is the target audience for the Web site?
- Does the Web site present information about a particular intervention or exposure (e.g., an assessment process)? If yes, does the Web site discuss outcomes of the intervention or exposure?
- What are the key points or messages presented on the Web site?
- How reliable are the key points or messages? Consider: number, type, and age of citations; expertise of author(s); where material is published (e.g., peer-reviewed journal, professional magazine); consistency with other materials I have read.
- To what population or populations are the key points and messages relevant? Consider: age; sex; setting, ethnicity/racial mix; diagnosis.
- What types of outcomes are addressed? Are these outcomes supported by data?

Overall Appraisal:

- Are there biases that I believe influenced the quality and believability of the information on the Web site? Consider: age of material, authors of material, support for claims, and so forth.
- Based on my clinical experience, does the information make sense?

Reasons to Use the Information (Benefits)	Reasons Not to Use the Information (Risks and Costs)
1.	1.
2.	2.
3.	3.
4.	4.

Decision and Rationale:

Based on the information at this time, I will make the following recommendation to my patient regarding the benefits, risks, costs, and alternatives of the information presented in this Web site:

Appendix 15–5: Sample Worksheet for Evaluating a Program Description

Source of Program Description (i.e., colleague, book, journal article):

Areas for Appraisal:

- Is the purpose of the program clear?
- Who is the target population for the program?
- Does the target population match the types of patients I see?
- How are program participants identified and selected? Who performs this function?
- What exactly is the "program"? In other words, what are the parameters, interventions, and characteristics of the program?
- What are the intended outcomes of the program? Who evaluates the outcomes?
- What is the setting in which the program is delivered?
- Does this setting match mine?
- What are the staffing needs for the program?
- What are the other costs of the program?
- Are the resources needed by the program available in my setting?
- Is any evidence provided about the efficacy or effectiveness of the program?

Overall Appraisal:

- Based on my clinical experience, does the program make sense?

Reasons to Develop a Program Like This (Benefits)	Reasons Not to Develop a Program Like This (Risks and Costs)
1.	1.
2.	2.
3.	3.
4.	4.

Decision and Rationale:

Based on the information at this time, I will make the following recommendation to my patient regarding the benefits, risks, costs, and alternatives of a program like this:

Appendix 15–6: Sample Critical Appraisal Matrix

Citation	Question or Purpose	Sample	Intervention	Findings	Implications for Practice

Note: A critical appraisal matrix includes only the *key* information from individual critical appraisals of articles. By summarizing articles in a single table, a matrix facilitates comparisons between and across articles, and makes it easier to come to a conclusion about the evidence available.

Index

Note: Page numbers followed by b refer to boxes; page numbers followed by
t refer to tables.